Health Education: Theories, Principles and Applications

Health Education: Theories, Principles and Applications

Edited by Roberta Hansen

hayle
medical

New York

Hayle Medical,
750 Third Avenue, 9ᵗʰ Floor,
New York, NY 10017, USA

Visit us on the World Wide Web at:
www.haylemedical.com

This book contains information obtained from authentic and highly regarded sources. Copyright for all individual chapters remain with the respective authors as indicated. All chapters are published with permission under the Creative Commons Attribution License or equivalent. A wide variety of references are listed. Permission and sources are indicated; for detailed attributions, please refer to the permissions page and list of contributors. Reasonable efforts have been made to publish reliable data and information, but the authors, editors and publisher cannot assume any responsibility for the validity of all materials or the consequences of their use.

ISBN: 978-1-63241-543-1

Trademark Notice: Registered trademark of products or corporate names are used only for explanation and identification without intent to infringe.

Cataloging-in-Publication Data

Health education : theories, principles and applications / edited by Roberta Hansen.
    p. cm.
Includes bibliographical references and index.
ISBN 978-1-63241-543-1
1. Health education. 2. Health literacy. 3. Health promotion. I. Hansen, Roberta.
RA440.5 .H43 2019
613--dc23

Table of Contents

Preface

The profession of educating people about health is referred to as health education. The areas included in this form of profession are reproductive health, spiritual health, emotional health, intellectual health, social health and environmental health. Some of the areas of concern that fall under this discipline are assessing individual and community needs for health education, planning and implementing health education strategies, interventions and programs, conducting evaluation and research related to health education, etc. The topics included in this book on health education are of utmost significance and bound to provide incredible insights to readers. Different approaches, evaluations, methodologies and advanced studies on health education have been included herein. This book, with its detailed analyses and data, will prove immensely beneficial to professionals and students involved in this area at various levels.

All of the data presented henceforth, was collaborated in the wake of recent advancements in the field. The aim of this book is to present the diversified developments from across the globe in a comprehensible manner. The opinions expressed in each chapter belong solely to the contributing authors. Their interpretations of the topics are the integral part of this book, which I have carefully compiled for a better understanding of the readers.

At the end, I would like to thank all those who dedicated their time and efforts for the successful completion of this book. I also wish to convey my gratitude towards my friends and family who supported me at every step.

Editor

An Examination of College Student Health Knowledge

Kathy Sexton-Radek*

A Reporting of College Student Health Knowledge, Elmhurst College, USA

Abstract

College students possess an omnipresence reference that influences their assumptions that their youth is equated to good health. For the most part, this logic prevails, until a closer examination of college life experiences reports high risk behaviours, struggles with health issues and the onset of conditions that were preventable by a healthier lifestyle. Suicide deaths, risky sexual practices, sleep deprivation, substance use represent more of the impactful unhealthy practices and missed meals, non-nutritious food intake and untreated colds/coughs represent the more moderate health concerns of college students. The current investigation explored the health knowledge of college students. Results from a pre-test to post-test case control design indicated a statistically significant difference in health knowledge following a Health Psychology course/educational intervention. The overall number correct on a textbook publisher instrument of Health Knowledge was used as the dependent variable. With no significant differences found for demographic variables of age, gender, number of health related courses taken the data was collapsed into a single group for analysis. The results are presented and discussed in terms of low and high areas of knowledge.

Keywords: Examination; College; Student; Health knowledge

An Examination of College Student Health Knowledge

The emerging adult college student has several challenges to navigate during their college career besides academic performance. The hazards to the health of the college student stem from irregular schedules of late night hours, mental health issues of depression, anxiety, substance experimentation/use to lifestyle factors of low activity level/ exercise, stress triggering unhealthily habits, poor sleep quality [1-4] and nutritional intake. It is estimated that 1100 deaths annually occur due to suicide during the college years [5]. The incidence of suicidal ideation and depression has doubled since the 1990s with the average age of onset of depression now at age 20 years rather than 29 years noted twenty years ago [3]. The incidence for the onset of eating disorders during college year is 0.5-4.2% for anorexia nervosa and bulimia [6]. The use of narcotics has risen to record levels in the last ten years [3]. 1700 college students die from alcohol-related injuries each year [7]. It is estimated that 45% of students are binge drinkers, 19% are frequent binge drinkers and 16% abstain from alcohol use. Added to these figure is a reporting of 4 in 5 fraternity/sorority members as binge drinkers [1]. Estimates of 15% of college students have experimented with Ecstasy, a sevenfold increase since 2001 [8]. Some 100,00 students are victims of alcohol-related sexual assault or date rape (i.e., Rohypnol, gamma hydroxybutyrate admissions to emergency rooms has quadrupled). Thus, serious health issues exist in the College student population.

With an estimate of 9 million 18-24-year-old students enrolled in college nationally, important surveys such as the National College Health Assessment provide descriptive information about this population [3,9]. While some 92% report good to excellent health, estimates of 40% of students currently take prescription medication for depression and stress conditions [8]. 32% of this sampling reported using alcohol frequently as stress management [3,9]. Increased use of risky sexual practices, substance abuse and poor sleep/eating habits occur during college years [10]. Given the association between the development of at risk behaviors during youth and onset of adult illnesses of Cardiovascular disease, Diabetes, Cancer, the engagement in unhealthy behaviors continues [5] used real time diaries of participants to examine health information seeking practices. This is in contrast to the traditional means in the literature of recall techniques on surveys and interviews. The findings indicated that college students, as a population, encounter many health risks and they lack adequate information on health topics [3,8]. For example, instead of health information on activity levels they were commonly presented with websites for fitness and fitness program memberships. Additionally, Baxter et al. reported that college student's health information seeking was influenced by their interest and satisfaction with the search topic -specifically, the college student more commonly searches for fitness information rather than nutrition or mental health information.

Physical activity levels and exercise are a commonly Health intervention. The activity deploys the college student's attention from everyday matters and positive physiological benefits ensue. Zimmerman-Sloutskis, Wanner, Zimmermann and Martin reported the prevalence of inactivity/"no sport" and non-membership in a sport club increased with age. The reported low levels of physical activity trends from their cross-sectional study of a national representative data base points to alarming results. Sedentary activity has been identified as a risk factor associated with mid-life development of cardiovascular and metabolic disorders. Grossman reported the utility of massage relieving not only activity related strain but also as a stress management intervention. Increases in blood flow, lymph flow, white blood cells and T lymphocytes were measured following massage. The associated between causes of preventable death and risk factors has been identified. Tobacco, poor diet and physical inactivity, alcohol consumption, sexual behavior, illicit drug use and other factors account for 48.2% of the variance in predicting mortality [7].

Perhaps a pathway to facilitating the college student to engaging in a greater number of health practices consistently could be found in the adherence literature. Adherence rates typically start low and reduce further with the passage of time [11]. Patients that adhere to

***Corresponding author:** Kathy Sexton-Radek, PhD, C.BSM, A Reporting of College Student Health Knowledge, Elmhurst College, USA,
E-mail: kathysr@elmhurst.edu

treatment reported improved psychological functioning and reduced hospital rates. Medication non-adherence is predictive of relapse and hospitalization. With the deterioration of adherence rates overtime, consideration of influencing factors such as literacy, education level, social support, belief systems and knowledge about their condition have to be examined. The recognition that a condition is or may compromise one's health, the awareness of the impact of a condition on the body and a confident understanding of what to do to ameliorate the situation are fundamental to understanding adherence [11].

With the college student being in an education environment, investigations have examined how college students learn about their health so as to circumvent these serious health risk behaviors largely induced by stress and low regard of Health or Health knowledge [3,5,6,10]. College students seek health information on the internet [6]. The common areas include: relationship issues, financial concerns, sexually transmitted diseases and their treatment, medical concerns related to pain, rashes, cold symptoms. Less common health areas that are searched include: learning difficulties, independent living issues such as budgets/affording an apartment. Mandanello and Clayman reported findings from their secondary analysis of the Health Information National Trends Survey. The findings indicated differing skills and abilities among college students to use and understand health information. Specifically, the numeracy level indicated a statistically significant difference between the groups with those of lower numeracy more commonly reporting negative interactions with health providers including feeling less able to rely on their providers (65% vs. 86%, p<0.0001) and less likely to say to their provider that they understand their provider (70% vs. 88%, p=0.0001). Thus, the impact of numeracy on health information seeking and health provider communication suggests the need to evaluate the college students' numeracy level. Gowen reported that college student health information seeking on the internet was influenced by the way the information was presented and the possible reduced validity of the information. Thus, little screening and still yet, a smaller amount of critical thinking has been reported in the health information internet searches. Gowen reported that college students search for mental health information was more commonly sought in areas of medications, diagnosis, treatment options, access to health care and supports and resources. In further analyses of college student's motivations for seeking online health information, Gowen reports that seeking additional information, reducing isolation by connecting to the online community, lack of other resources and to prepare for an upcoming health visit were most commonly indicated by college students.

Thus, the issues of college students' health knowledge are largely represented by college students Health information internet searches that represent both the quality of the website displaying Health Information and the College student user of internet sites for Health information that display highly verbal and numeric presentations of information that may not be understood by those using the site. With these issues a question emerges as to what college students Health Knowledge is when presented with validated, contemporary resources such as in a college course.

The current investigation examined the premise of college students' health knowledge given the documentation of their reliance on online resources and the health risk behaviors associated with this group. It was hypothesized that college students level of health knowledge is poor and a small, significant increase would occur with educational instruction that has been validated as accurate (i.e., course materials, published peer reviewed textbook used the instruction).

Methods

Participants

Twenty participants from a small Midwestern college agreed to complete a questionnaire asking about several health conditions before and following a Health Psychology course. The students elected to be in the course, it was not required for their major. There were eleven females aged 19-24 years and nine males ages 19-23 years in the study. The students received course credit for an alternative assignment by participating in the study. The study was approved by the IRB and all students completed an informed consent.

Instruments

A 30 item true/false Health Knowledge Questionnaire was used in the study. Each item represented a major health finding. The students responded to each statement by selecting a true or false response. The Health Knowledge Questionnaire is published by Cengage press, correct responses are provided; there is no reporting of psychometric properties (norm group, reliability, validity) (Tables 1 and 2).

Procedure

A Case Control design was used to measure pre and post intervention Health Knowledge using the Health Knowledge questionnaire during the first week of class and during finals week. All twenty participant's names were removed from the materials and a subject number was assigned to provide privacy and confidentiality. The twenty participants were members of a Health Psychology course with a total enrollment of 33 students. The course was taught in a traditional face to face manner meeting twice a week for lecture presentations and discussions. All students were required to complete three exams, a final exam and develop a health promotion project proposal in teams of 3-4 students that culminated into a presentation on the last class meeting day. The course intervention used a typical undergraduate Health psychology textbook (Cengage Publishers, Brannon, Feist and Upgraft authors) and pdf files of contemporary empirical articles that addressed common Health Psychology topics as supplemental reading.

Results

Each item response was treated as a separate variable and coded as correct or not. An overall score of the number correct was computed by a summation of the correct responses. The pre to posttest analysis was

Testing	Mean score correct (30 possible points)
Pre	17 (2.889)
Post	24 (3.427)

Table 1: Health knowledge questionnaire results, t=0.452*.

Pre and Post testing's
United States Life expectancy
Reasons for increases in life expectancy
Smoking related death and cardiovascular disease
High and Low cholesterol age effects on health
At Post testing:
Alcohol and vehicle crashes
Low cholesterol levels and death rates
Most common areas of learning:
Alcohol and poor health risks
Heart disease prevalence in males
Direct and indirect cigarette smoke exposure and health

Table 2: Most frequently incorrect health knowledge questions.

computed using a paired t- test analysis of the overall score at pre and at post testing (t=0.452˙). The mean overall score at pretest was 17 correct (SD=2.889) and 24 (SD=3.427) at posttest. A percent correct overall for the group was calculated at pre and post testing, these values were 57% and 83%, respectively.

The participants were incorrect on the following statements at pre and post testings: United States Life Expectancy, Reasons for increases in Life Expectancy, Smoking related death and Cardiovascular disease, High and Low Cholesterol age effects on health. The most common incorrect responses at post testing were on items about Alcohol and Vehicle crashes and Low Cholesterol and Death rates. The most common areas of learning were in terms of items about Alcohol and poor health risks, Heart disease prevalence in males and Direct/Indirect cigarette smoke exposure and health.

Discussion

College students have an understanding of health information. College students need to have an understanding of Health information to balance their stressful lifestyle and prevent the development of risky behaviors that could lead to poor health. The hypothesis that college student Health Knowledge would increase as a result of a college course in Health Psychology was supported (t=0.452˙). Given the limitations of the design and sampling, this finding is to be held with caution. It is equally plausible that the participants in the study as a result of being in the course, independently sought Health Information and perhaps understood what they were reading more so as the time passed while being in the course. This factor was not measured. The comparisons of each participants scores at pre and post testing, individually did not yield a pattern by demographic level to overall score. However, the case control design limited the framework for comparisons and a between groups analysis with a control group for future studies in this area, which affords more meaningful comparisons should be used in future studies. Additionally, the design of the study using a measure with questions linked to the intervention materials (i.e., Textbook authors Health Knowledge questionnaire contained in the textbook) should be replaced with a psychometric measure with demonstrated reliability, validity, established norms. The instrument used in this study has a strength in terms of its congruence to the intervention materials presented but conclusions should be guarded given the limitation of an absence of psychometric properties of the measure.

The pre to post testing of Health Knowledge following a completion of a Health Psychology undergraduate course findings indicated an overall change of 17 correct responses of 30 possible at pretest, or 57% correct was compared to the average number correct at post testing, 25 correct of 30 possible point (83%). With an estimate that 25% of college students have intermediate literacy and 56% have intermediate numeracy, the findings in the study were higher than was expected [8]. Health Information instruction through a college course would yield elevated results both in terms of comprehension of information as well as retaining the information [12].

Our findings support that college students can broaden their health information knowledge with course work given that a full complement of topics in Health are studied as compared to preferred topics internet searches. The consistency of error on some of the questions from pre to post may reflect this intermediate level of proficiency, on average of college students [13]. The uplifting results that students' performed better at post testing on serious, severe conditions of alcohol risk behaviors and consequences, prevalence of heart disease and risks to heath from cigarette smoking. These larger scale areas reflect morbidity rates and a recognized understanding of these areas is associated with having a health perspective.

An implication of this reporting examination of college student health information suggest a need for an emphasis in teaching information literacy directly as part of formal academic course work. While the college student naturally seeks health information form internet sources, the efficacy of that practice has to be improved. Further, if adherence and types of interchanges with health providers are influenced by the college student's understanding of health information from the internet, modification and means to determine that level will need to be put into place in health care. For example, the common approach of Motivational Interviewing use by healthcare practicitors could be expanded to include an open ended question to the potential college student patient of what health information they know and how they obtain that information. With the myriad of challenges to health that the college student may encounter, adjustments to understanding how they know the information about their health or risk factors will improve their approaching a healthier lifestyle.

References

1. Valerio T, Kim MJ, Sexton-Radek K (2014) Poor sleep quality and academic performance in college students.

2. Sexton-Radek K, Kraprelian J (2013) Emerging adult sleep quality: health and academic performance factors. Journal of Sleep Disorders and Therapy 2: 112.

3. Sexton-Radek K (2012) An epidemiological perspective on college student health and sleep. Journal of Psychology and Psychotherapy 2: 103.

4. Sexton-Radek K (2003) Sleep quality in young adults. New York: Mellon Press.

5. Baxter L, Egbert N, Ho E (2008) Everyday health communication experiences of college students. Journal of American College Health 56: 427-436.

6. Gowen LK (2013) Online mental health information seeking in young adults with mental health challenges. Journal of Technology in Human Services 31: 97-111.

7. Mokdad AH, Marks JS, Stroup DF, Gerberding JL (2004) Actual causes of death in the United States, 2000. Jama 291: 1238-1245.

8. Mannganello JA, Clayman ML (2011) The association of understanding medical statistics with health information seeking and health provider interaction in a national sample of young adults. Journal of Health Communication 16: 163-176.

9. Wallace R (2006) Colleges struggle to meet mental health needs of students. Fox News.

10. Buhi ER, Daley EM, Fuhrmann MA, Smith S (2009) An observational study of how young people search for online sexual health information. Journal of American College Health 58: 101-111.

11. McNicholas F (2012) To adhere or not, and what we can do to help. European child and adolescent psychiatry 21: 657-663.

12. Zeitlin D, Keller SE, Shiflett SC, Schleifer SJ, Bartlett JA (2000) Immunological effects of massage therapy during academic stress. Psychosomatic Medicine 62: 83-84.

13. Zimmermann-Sloutskis D, Wanner M, Zimmermann E, Martin BW (2010) Physical activity levels and determinants of change in young adults: a longitudinal panel study. International Journal of Behavioral Nutrition and Physical Activity 7: 1.

A Study Protocol to Assess the Determinants of Glycaemic Control, Complications and Health Related Quality of Life for People with Type 2 Diabetes in Saudi Arabia

Mohammed J Alramadan[1], Afsana Afroz[1], Mohammed Ali Batais[2], Turky H Almigbal[2], Hassan Ahmad Alhamrani[3], Ahmed Albaloshi[4], Fatimah A Alramadan[3], Dianna J Magliano[5] and Baki Billah[1*]

[1]Department of Epidemiology and Preventive Medicine, Monash University, Melbourne, Australia
[2]College of Medicine, King Saud University, Riyadh, Saudi Arabia
[3]Diabetes Centre, Directorate of Health Affair, Hofuf, Saudi Arabia
[4]Diabetes Centre, Directorate of Health Affair, Jeddah, Saudi Arabia
[5]Baker Heart and Diabetes Institute, Melbourne, Victoria, Australia

Abstract

Background: The prevalence of type 2 diabetes mellitus is high in Saudi Arabia, and a large proportion of those affected by the disease are not controlling their blood sugar, which exposes them to diabetes complications. The aim of this study is to evaluate factors associated with poor glycaemic control, complications and poor quality of life among people with type 2 diabetes in Saudi Arabia.

Methodology: Using a cross-sectional study design, 1082 participants with type 2 diabetes attending diabetes centres in Riyadh, Jeddah and Hofuf will be recruited in the study. They will be interviewed to complete a pre-tested electronic questionnaire. The questionnaire collects information related to socio-demographics, medical history, lifestyle, family support, utilisation of healthcare services, anxiety, depression, quality of life, cognitive function, independence in daily living activity, neuropathy, anthropometric measures, up-to-date documented lab test results and current medication. Data will be summarised and presented as mean ± standard deviation (or median and percentiles) for numerical data and frequency and percentage for categorical data. T-test, ANOVA and chi-square tests will be used to explore associations between risk factors and outcomes. Any association will be evaluated further using regression analysis.

Discussion: Knowledge of the risk factors pertaining to poor glycaemic control, diabetes complications and poor quality of life for people with type 2 diabetes is crucial. This knowledge will assist healthcare providers to identify and provide more intensive care plans to those who need it, as well as guide the development of new strategies to improve management of the disease. This will improve the health of people with type 2 diabetes and lower their risk of complications, and reduce the burden of this highly prevalent disease on families and the community.

Keywords: Type 2 diabetes; Saudi Arabia; Glycaemic control; Complication; Quality of life

Introduction

Diabetes mellitus is one of the most common chronic non-communicable diseases [1,2]. An estimated 415 million adults had diabetes worldwide in 2015 and this number is expected to rise to 642 million by 2040 [3]. In 2015, approximately five million individuals between the age of 20 and 79 years died because of diabetes [3]. Furthermore, roughly 14.5% of global all-cause mortality among adults is attributed to diabetes and half of these deaths occur among those aged below 60 [3].

Similar to other countries in the Middle East, modernisation has taken its toll on the population of Saudi Arabia. The vast lifestyle changes of Saudis over the last few decades, accompanied by rising rates of obesity, have led to a rapid and progressive increase in the prevalence of diabetes. A recent study showed that 13.4% of Saudis aged 15 years and above have diabetes, which is significantly higher than both the global prevalence (8.8%) and the prevalence in the Middle East (10.7%) [3,4].

The control of blood glucose levels is the cornerstone of diabetes management. Studies have shown that there is a strong association between an elevated blood glucose level and the risk of diabetes-related complications and mortality for people with diabetes [5,6]. Of particular concern is that between 50% and 70% of people with type 2 diabetes mellitus (T2DM) in Saudi Arabia have uncontrolled blood glucose

levels [7-9], and the prevalence of diabetes-related complications among them is high [10-13].

A few studies that have examined factors affecting glycaemic control for people with T2DM in Saudi Arabia have indicated poor control to be associated with increasing age, insulin use, smoking, lower levels of physical activity, poor diabetes self-care behaviour, low adherence to medicine, anxiety and depression [7-9]. A number of other factors that may have an impact on glycaemic control, diabetes complications and quality of life-such as the duration of diabetes, family support, cognitive function and lifestyle factors (diet and physical activity)-were not investigated adequately in existing studies from Saudi Arabia [14-16].

Furthermore, it is well-established that haemoglobin A1c (HbA1c) is a more accurate measure of blood sugar control, compared to fasting

*Corresponding author: Baki Billah, Department of Epidemiology and Preventive Medicine, Monash University, Melbourne, Australia, E-mail: baki.billah@monash.edu

and random blood sugar measurements, because HbA1c reflects the level of glycaemic control over several weeks [17]. However, some of the studies from Saudi Arabia used random blood sugar for determining the level of control, which was a limitation to these studies. In addition, the majority of studies from Saudi Arabia involved a single centre, or were hospital-based [8-10,13,18-26] and may not accurately represent the large and diverse population of the country.

To address the above gaps, a multi-centre study is required which will comprehensively investigate the effect of all possible risk factors. Thus, the aim of this proposed study is to conduct a multi-centre study in Saudi Arabia to explore the effect of lifestyle factors, family support and cognitive impairment, as well as other risk factors for glycaemic control, diabetes complications and quality of life for people with T2DM mellitus (T2DM). The knowledge of these risk factors will help healthcare providers, the individuals with the disease, and society as a whole. Understanding the burden of the associated risk factors is also important for public health policymakers who develop healthcare priorities that yield the greatest benefits.

Objectives

This study has three main objectives. Firstly, to evaluate the determinants of poor glycaemic control among people with T2DM in Saudi Arabia. Secondly, to investigate the prevalence of coronary artery disease, neuropathy, nephropathy and cognitive impairment, as well as their associated factors among people with T2DM. Thirdly, to examine factors associated with poor health-related quality of life for people with T2DM. Furthermore, secondary objectives of this study is to examine factors associated with poor control of blood pressure as well dyslipidaemia among people with T2DM.

Methodology

Ethical approval

Both the Monash University Human Research Ethics Committee and the Research Ethics Committee of the Ministry of Health in Saudi Arabia approved this project. The approval of the College of Medicine Institutional Review Board at Kind Saud University was also obtained.

Study design

A cross-sectional study will be conducted to address the research questions. Cross-sectional study design has the advantage of being inexpensive and less time-consuming compared to other epidemiological study designs. Moreover, in using this study design, the prevalence of outcomes such as poor glycaemic control and complications, as well as the prevalence of risk factors, can be measured.

Study population

The study population will consist of people with T2DM in Saudi Arabia attending diabetes centres in the cities of Hofuf, Riyadh and Jeddah (Figure 1). These cities are among the top most populated in the country and their diabetic centres serve a mixture of people who come from urban, as well as rural settings. Inclusion criteria include confirmed diagnosis of T2DM, age 18 years and above and duration of diabetes of one year and more. Participants will be excluded if they have other types of diabetes (type 1 or gestational), or if there is no HbA1c test results in their medical records for the past 6 months. Pregnant women will also be excluded.

Sample size

A total of 1082 subjects with T2DM will be recruited for the study which was calculated based on 90% power, 5% significance level and a margin of error of 2.5% for prevalence of glycaemic control. A back calculation of power shows that a sample size of 1082 participants will maintain a power of 90% or above for all other primary and secondary objectives of this study.

Recruitment

A systematic random-sampling method will be used to recruit participants. The number of participants recruited each day is expected to be 10. Every day during the data-collection period, the data collectors will begin by randomly selecting a participant with T2DM from the first K participants attending the diabetes centre and invite them to participate. The value of K will depend on the number of people attending the centre every day, which varies between centres. Following on, every K-th patient will be approached. If the K-th person declines or does not have T2DM, the next person will be invited. The recruitment will be continued for a period of six months or until data have been collected from 1082 patients, whichever comes first.

Informing participants about the study and obtaining the consent

Data collectors will fully inform each of the participants about the purpose of the study, how the data will be collected and how the collected information will be used while maintaining participants' confidentiality. Then, participants will be given an explanatory statement and allowed some time to read and ask questions. Upon their agreement to participate, they will be required to read and sign a consent form.

Data collection instrument

A pre-tested questionnaire will be used to collect data. The original English version of the questionnaire has been translated into Arabic. The Arabic version was then translated into English to check that the Arabic and the original English versions have exactly the same meanings. Prior to collecting the data, data collectors will be trained by the primary investigator on how to approach participants, inform participants about the study, fill in the electronic questionnaire and take the anthropometric measurements.

Research Electronic Data Capture (REDCap) will be used to collect and manage the data [27]. REDCap is a secure web-based application

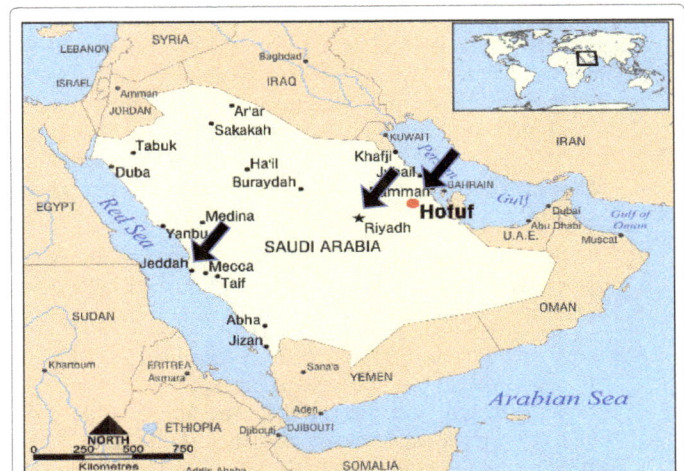

Figure 1: Map of Saudi Arabia showing the main cities and the cities where the research will be conducted (red arrows).

for constructing electronic surveys and collecting data for research studies. It provides a user-friendly interface with validated data entry, audit trails for tracking data manipulation, and an automated export procedure for seamless data downloads to common statistical software packages.

Using a standard questionnaire, the following information will be collected for all participants:

- Diabetes centre and data collector details.

- Participant's socio-demographics data, including name, age, gender, marital status, education, nationality, work status and household income.

- Medical history: duration of diabetes, place of follow-up, frequency of follow-up, diabetes treatment, self-monitoring blood glucose, hypoglycaemic events, medical history of other diseases, diabetes complications and medication adherence (Morisky Medication Adherence questionnaire).

- Family support for diabetes, utilisation of healthcare services, knowledge of HbA1c.

- Lifestyle data including smoking status, dietary habits (UK diabetes and diet questionnaire at: https://sps.onlinesurveys. ac.uk/the-uk-diabetes-and-diet-questionnaire-ukddq) and physical activity (WHO STEPS questionnaire for diet at: http://www.who.int/chp/steps/STEPS_Instrument_v2.1.pdf).

- Psychological aspect data that include depression (the Patient Health Questionnaire-2 (PHQ-2)) [28] and anxiety (Generalized Anxiety Disorder Scale (GAD-2)) [29].

- Patient's quality of life (EQ-5D-5L) [30] and independence regarding activities in daily life (Katz Index) [31].

- Rowland Universal Dementia Assessment Scale (RUDAS) [32].

- Neuropathy screening tool (the Michigan Neuropathy Screening Instrument [33]).

- Anthropometrics: height, weight, blood pressure and waist and hip circumference.

- Materials and equipment: digital scale, measuring tape, and digital automatic blood pressure monitor

- Height: height will be measured for all participants using a portable stadiometer. Standing height is measured with the subject in bare feet, back-square against the wall and eyes looking straight ahead. A set square resting on the scalp and a tape measurement from the wall/bed is used to measure height to the nearest 0.5 cm. This will be done twice and if the measurement varies more than 2 cm, a third measurement will be taken. A stool will be used where necessary.

- Weight: participant will be instructed to remove their shoes and outer layers of clothing (such as jackets or jumpers). Weight will be recorded to the nearest 0.1 kg.

- Waist circumference: will be measured against thin clothing (for cultural reasons), on exhalation, midway between the lower rib margin and the anterior superior iliac spine (hip bone) or narrowest abdominal point. Subject should be relaxed with arms held loosely at sides. The tape measure must be kept horizontal for standing measurement. This will be done twice and if the measurement varies by more than 2 cm, a third

measurement will be taken. The waist circumference will be recorded to the nearest 0.5 cm.

- Hip circumference: measure at the widest circumference around the hip bones, so that the tape passes over the greatest protrusion of the gluteal muscles. The tape measure must be kept horizontal for standing measurement. This will be done twice and if the measurement varies more than 2 cm, a third measurement will be taken. The hip circumference will be recorded to the nearest 0.5 cm.

- Blood pressure: participants should be seated for at least five minutes, legs uncrossed, feet flat on the floor and any excess clothing items that may interfere with measurement must be removed. Three systolic and diastolic blood pressure readings will be taken using an automated blood pressure monitor machine.

- Information from patients' medical records, including the three most recent blood pressure measures, fasting blood sugar measures, HbA1c, serum creatinine, albumin/creatinine ratio, eGFR, lipid profile, current prescribed medications and documented diagnosis of hypertension, coronary artery disease and stroke.

Data management and analysis

During the data-collection period, the data will be saved in the secure REDCap web-based application hosted by Monash University. The application is accessible only by the research team. When the data collection is completed the data will be exported to the IBM SPSS statistical package and will be saved on the secure School of Public Health and Preventive Medicine at Monash University allocated network storage (Monash (S:) drive). Participants' names will be removed from the database and each participant will be identified by a numeric code generated by REDCap. The database containing all information will be saved in a separate secure electronic folder, which will not be used for data analysis. Only the research team will have access to the identified and de-identified electronic databases.

Data will be summarised and presented as either mean ± standard deviation or median and percentiles for numerical data and frequency, and percentage for categorical data. Depending on the type of data, t-test, ANOVA, nonparametric tests or chi-square tests will be used to examine for associations between risk factors and outcomes. Any association will be further evaluated using simple and multiple logistic regression analysis.

Outcomes assessment

Definitions of the main study outcomes that will be considered:

- Glycaemic control: the proportion of the glycosylated haemoglobin (HbA1c) measured as a percentage and categorised as good control (HbA1c<7.0%), reasonable control (HbA1c 7%-8%) and poor control (HbA1c>8.0%).

- Nephropathy: documented eGFR (calculated by the CKD EPI formula) below 90 ml/min (categorised as mild renal impairment (60-89 ml/min), moderate renal impairment (30-59 ml/min), severe renal impairment (15-29 ml/min) and renal failure (<15 ml/min).

- Coronary artery disease: documented diagnosis of coronary artery disease (CAD).

A Study Protocol to Assess the Determinants of Glycaemic Control, Complications and Health Related...

7

- Neuropathy: a score of 7 or more using the Michigan Neuropathy Screening Instrument.

- Quality of life: EQ-5D-5L health states scores will be converted into a single index value between 0 and 1, and the quality of life will be categorised as Good quality of life (0.67-1.00), fair quality of life (0.34-0.66) and poor quality of life (≤ 0.33).

- Hypertension: either a documented diagnosis of hypertension, on antihypertension medications or three previous high blood pressure readings (systolic ≥ 140 and diastolic ≥ 90). Persons with poor blood pressure control are defined as having hypertension and their current systolic blood pressure as ≥ 140 mm Hg or diastolic ≥ 90 mm Hg.

- Dyslipidaemia: Documented total cholesterol>4.0 mmol/L, low density lipoproteins (LDL)>2.0 mmol/L, high density lipoprotein (HDL)<1.0 mmol/L, triglycerides>2.0 mmol/L or taking lipid lowering medication.

- Impaired cognitive function is defined as a score of ≤ 22 in the Rowland Universal Dementia Assessment Scale (RUDAS).

Pilot Study

The questionnaire was piloted on 29 participants attending diabetes centre in Hofuf over a period of two weeks. The sociodemographic characteristics of the participants in the pilot study are presented in Table 1. Mean age was 55.7 (± 11.6) years. Approximately 38% of participants were female and the majority of participants were married (93.1%). Roughly a quarter (24.1%) of participants was illiterate and 41.4% had only achieved primary school. The majority of participants (82.8%) reside in Hofuf city, while the rest lived in remote villages. With regard to work status, 17.2% worked and 34.5% were homemakers (house-wives). The rest of the participants were either retired (27.6%) or not working (20.7%). A large proportion of participants (41.4%) had a total household income between 3000 and 6000 Saudi Riyals.

A summary of some disease characteristics and main study outcomes is presented in Table 2. Participants had a mean duration of diabetes of 17.7 (± 10.5) years. Mean HbA1c was 9.6% (± 2.0%). The majority of participants (69.0%) had poor glycaemic control (HbA1c>8), while 10.3% had good glycaemic control (HbA1c ≤ 7%) and 17.2% had reasonable control (HbA1c 7.1%-8.0%). More than half of the participants (58.6%) had dyslipidaemia and close to half (48.3%)

had hypertension, while the diagnosis of CAD was documented in 31.0% of participants. Using the Michigan Neuropathy Screening Instrument, 31.0% of participants had a score (≥ 7), suggestive of neuropathy. eGFR calculated from most recent serum creatinine showed that 55.2% of participants had some renal impairment. Of those, 27.6% had mild impairment, 24.1% had moderate impairment, and 3.4% had severe impairment. Cognitive function was impaired in about half (51.7%) of participants using the Six-item Cognitive Impairment Test (6CIT) [34]. The quality of life was fair for 34.5% and poor for 3.4% of participants, while the majority (62.1%) had good quality of life. There were some missing values in some important investigations including HbA1c, cholesterol and triglycerides. The range of missing values was between 3.4% for HbA1c and 5.0% for triglycerides.

The questionnaire was found to be acceptable by most of the participants and practical by data collectors. However, the average time required to complete data collection for one participant was more than one hour. In order to ensure the collection of data from the planned number of participants, the length of the questionnaire was reduced after the completion of the pilot study. The STOP-BANG Sleep Apnea and the chest pain (Rose) questionnaires were removed [35,36]. Questions related to the duration of complications reported by participants were also removed.

Based on our findings in the pilot study that a relatively large proportion of people were illiterate, a decision was made to use the Rowland Universal Dementia Assessment Scale (RUDAS) instead of the Six-item Cognitive Impairment Test (6-CIT) to evaluate cognitive function. RUDAS is a multicultural cognitive assessment tool that is not affected by literacy level, and has been validated among Arabic-speaking people [32,37]. Approval to use the amended questionnaire was obtained from all ethical committees that have approved this project.

Discussion

This project is a comprehensive multi-centre study that will improve our understanding of the factors associated with poor control of blood glucose level, the factors that increase risk of diabetes complications and the factors associated with poor quality of life among people with T2DM in Saudi Arabia. The anticipated valuable information that will be obtained from this study will help healthcare providers to identify people with diabetes who are at risk of poor control and complications,

Variable	Descriptive statistics	Variable	Descriptive statistics
Age in years (mean ± SD)	55.7 ± 11.6	**Work status %** Working Not working (able to work) Not working (unable to work) Homemaker (house-wife) Retired	5(17.2%) 2(6.9%) 4(13.8%) 10(34.5%) 8(27.6%)
Gender % Female Male	11(37.9%) 18(62.1%)		
Marital status % Married Divorced (separated) Widowed	27(93.1%) 1(3.4%) 1(3.4%)		
Highest education level achieved % None (illiterate) Primary school Intermediate school Tertiary school University degree	7(24.1%) 12(41.4%) 1(3.4%) 8(27.6%) 1(3.4%)	**Total household monthly income %** ≤ 3000 Saudi Riyals 3000–6000 Saudi Riyals 6001–9000 Saudi Riyals 9001–12000 Saudi Riyals ≥ 12001 Saudi Riyals	3(10.3%) 12(41.4%) 4(13.8%) 7(24.1%) 3(10.3%)
Home location % Inside the city Remote village	24(82.8%) 5(17.2%)		

Table 1: Pilot study participants' sociodemographic characteristics.

Variable	Descriptive statistics	Variable	Descriptive statistics
Diabetes duration in years (mean ± SD)	17.7 ± 10.5	Hypertension % No Yes	15(51.7%) 14(48.3%)
HbA1c % (mean ± SD)	9.6 ± 2.0		
Glycaemic control % Good Reasonable Poor	3(10.3%) 5(17.2%) 20(69.0%)	CAD % No Yes	20(69.0%) 9(31.0%)
Quality of life % Good Fair Poor	18(62.1%) 10(34.5%) 1(3.4%)	Neuropathy % No Yes	20(69.0%) 9(31.0%)
Cognitive impairment % No Yes	14(48.3%) 15(51.7%)	Nephropathy % No Mild Moderate Severe	13(44.8%) 8(27.6%) 7(24.1%) 1(3.4%)
Dyslipidaemia % No Yes	12(41.4%) 17(58.6%)		

Table 2: Characteristics related to diabetes, complications and health related quality of life.

and provide them with more intensive care plans. It will also identify priority issues that will guide the development and implementation of new national strategies to promote the health of people with T2DM in Saudi Arabia.

The strength of this study lies on the relatively large number of participants and the recruitment from three highly populated cities in three different regions of Saudi Arabia. The evaluation of a wide range of risk factors and outcomes using validated tools also provide strength to this study. Since this study is cross-sectional, we will be assessing association; no causal relation can be inferred. Observational study designs are also prone to bias. Nevertheless, this study will not only provide valuable information that will be used by healthcare providers and health policy makers, but will also generate hypotheses that will guide future advance research projects in the field of diabetes in Saudi Arabia, in the Middle East region and globally.

Competing Interests

All authors declare that they have no competing interests.

Author Contributions

All authors were involved in the conception and design of the study. MJA and AA reviewed the literature and MJA drafted the manuscript. All authors critically reviewed the manuscript and approved the final version.

References

1. Shaw JE, Sicree RA, Zimmet PZ (2010) Global estimates of the prevalence of diabetes for 2010 and 2030. Diabetes Research and Clinical Practice 87: 4-14.

2. Whiting DR, Guariguata L, Weil C, Shaw J (2011) IDF diabetes atlas: global estimates of the prevalence of diabetes for 2011 and 2030. Diabetes Research and Clinical Practice 94: 311-321.

3. Cho NH, Whiting D, Forouhi N, Leonor G, Hambleton I, et al. (2015) IDF Diabetes Atlas. 7th edn.

4. El Bcheraoui C, Basulaiman M, Tuffaha M, Daoud F, Robinson M, et al. (2014) Status of the diabetes epidemic in the Kingdom of Saudi Arabia, 2013. International Journal of Public Health 59: 1011-1021.

5. Control D, Group CTR (1993) The effect of intensive treatment of diabetes on the development and progression of long-term complications in insulin-dependent diabetes mellitus. N Engl J Med 329: 977-986.

6. Group UPDS (1998) Intensive blood-glucose control with sulphonylureas or insulin compared with conventional treatment and risk of complications in patients with type 2 diabetes (UKPDS 33). The Lancet 352: 837-853.

7. Al-Nuaim AR, Mirdad S, Al-Rubeaan K, Al-Mazrou Y, Al-Attas O, et al. (1998) Pattern and factors associated with glycemic control of Saudi diabetic patients. Ann Saudi Med 18: 109-112.

8. Al-Hayek AA, Robert AA, Alzaid AA, Nusair HM, Zbaidi NS, et al. (2012) Association between diabetes self-care, medication adherence, anxiety, depression, and glycemic control in type 2 diabetes. Saudi Medical Journal 33: 681-683.

9. Alsulaiman TA, Al-Ajmi HA, Al-Qahtani SM, Fadlallah IM, Nawar NE, et al. (2016) Control of type 2 diabetes in King Abdulaziz Housing City (Iskan) population, Saudi Arabia. Journal of Family and Community Medicine 23: 1.

10. Alwakeel J, Sulimani R, Al-Asaad H, Al-Harbi A, Tarif N, et al. (2008) Diabetes complications in 1952 type 2 diabetes mellitus patients managed in a single institution. Annals of Saudi Medicine 28: 260.

11. Al Ghamdi AH, Rabiu M, Hajar S, Yorston D, Kuper H, et al. (2012) Rapid assessment of avoidable blindness and diabetic retinopathy in Taif, Saudi Arabia. British Journal of Ophthalmology 96: 1168-1172.

12. Halawa MR, Karawagh A, Zeidan A, Mahmoud DH, Sakr M, et al. (2010) Prevalence of painful diabetic peripheral neuropathy among patients suffering from diabetes mellitus in Saudi Arabia. Current Medical Research and Opinion 26: 337-343.

13. Ahmed AA, Algamdi SA, Alzahrani AM (2015) Surveillance of risk factors for diabetic foot ulceration with particular concern to local practice. Diabetes & Metabolic Syndrome: Clinical Research & Reviews 9: 310-315.

14. Sanal T, Nair N, Adhikari P (2011) Factors associated with poor control of type 2 diabetes mellitus: a systematic review and meta-analysis. Journal of Diabetology 3: 1-10.

15. Stopford R, Winkley K, Ismail K (2013) Social support and glycemic control in type 2 diabetes: a systematic review of observational studies. Patient Education and Counseling 93: 549-558.

16. Awad N, Gagnon M, Messier C (2004) The relationship between impaired glucose tolerance, type 2 diabetes, and cognitive function. Journal of Clinical and Experimental Neuropsychology 26: 1044-1080.

17. Association AD (2016) Standards of medical care in diabetes - 2016. Diabetes Care.

18. Al-Rubeaan K, Al-Hussain F, Youssef AM, Subhani SN, Al-Sharqawi AH, et al. (2016) Ischemic stroke and its risk factors in a registry-based large cross-sectional diabetic cohort in a country facing a diabetes epidemic. Journal of Diabetes Research.

19. Al-Rubeaan K, El-Asrar A, Ahmed M, Youssef AM, Subhani SN, et al. (2015) Diabetic retinopathy and its risk factors in a society with a type 2 diabetes epidemic: a Saudi National Diabetes Registry-based study. Acta Ophthalmologica 93: e140-e147.

20. El-Asrar AMA, Al-Rubeaan KA, Al-Amro SA, Kangave D, Moharram OA (1998) Risk factors for diabetic retinopathy among Saudi diabetics. International Ophthalmology 22: 155-161.

21. Wang DD, Bakhotmah BA, Hu FB, Alzahrani HA (2014) Prevalence and correlates of diabetic peripheral neuropathy in a saudi arabic population: a cross-sectional study. PloS ONE 9: e106935.

22. Al-Homrany MA, Abdelmoneim I (2004) Significance of proteinuria in type 2 diabetic patients treated at a primary health care center in Abha City, Saudi Arabia. West African Journal of Medicine 23: 211-214.

23. Al-Rubeaan K, Youssef AM, Subhani SN, Ahmad NA, Al-Sharqawi AH, et al. (2014) Diabetic nephropathy and its risk factors in a society with a type 2 diabetes epidemic: a Saudi National Diabetes Registry-based study. PloS ONE 9: e88956.

24. Al-Shehri A, Taha A, Bahnassy A, Salah M (2008) Health-related quality of life in type 2 diabetic patients. Annals of Saudi Medicine 28: 352.

25. Al Hayek AA, Robert AA, Al Saeed A, Alzaid AA, Al Sabaan FS (2014) Factors associated with health-related quality of life among Saudi patients with type 2 diabetes mellitus: a cross-sectional survey. Diabetes & Metabolism Journal 38: 220-229.

26. AL-Aboudi IS, Hassali MA, Shafie AA, Hassan A, Alrasheedy AA (2015) A cross-sectional assessment of health-related quality of life among type 2 diabetes patients in Riyadh, Saudi Arabia. SAGE Open Medicine.

27. Harris PA, Taylor R, Thielke R, Payne J, Gonzalez N, et al. (2009) Research electronic data capture (REDCap)-a metadata-driven methodology and workflow process for providing translational research informatics support. Journal of Biomedical Informatics 42: 377-381.

28. Kroenke K, Spitzer RL, Williams JB (2003) The Patient Health Questionnaire-2: validity of a two-item depression screener. Medical Care 41: 1284-1292.

29. Skapinakis P (2007) The 2-item Generalized Anxiety Disorder scale had high sensitivity and specificity for detecting GAD in primary care. Evidence Based Medicine 12: 149.

30. Herdman M, Gudex C, Lloyd A, Janssen M, Kind P, et al. (2011) Development and preliminary testing of the new five-level version of EQ-5D (EQ-5D-5L). Quality of Life Research 20: 1727-1736.

31. Shelkey M, Wallace M (1999) Katz index of independence in activities of daily living. Journal of Gerontological Nursing 25: 8-9.

32. Storey JE, Rowland JT, Conforti DA, Dickson HG (2004) The Rowland universal dementia assessment scale (RUDAS): a multicultural cognitive assessment scale. International Psychogeriatrics 16: 13-31.

33. Moghtaderi A, Bakhshipour A, Rashidi H (2006) Validation of Michigan neuropathy screening instrument for diabetic peripheral neuropathy. Clinical Neurology and Neurosurgery 108: 477-481.

34. Abdel-Aziz K, Larner A (2015) Six-item cognitive impairment test (6CIT): pragmatic diagnostic accuracy study for dementia and MCI. International Psychogeriatrics 27: 991-997.

35. Rose G, McCartney P, Reid D (1977) Self-administration of a questionnaire on chest pain and intermittent claudication. British Journal of Preventive & Social Medicine 31: 42-48.

36. Chung F, Subramanyam R, Liao P, Sasaki E, Shapiro C, et al. (2012) High STOP-Bang score indicates a high probability of obstructive sleep apnoea. British Journal of Anaesthesia: aes022.

37. Chaaya M, Phung T, El Asmar K, Atweh S, Ghusn H, et al. Validation of the Arabic Rowland Universal Dementia Assessment Scale (A-RUDAS) in elderly with mild and moderate dementia. Aging & Mental Health 20: 880-887.

3

Awareness, Beliefs and Barriers of Organ Donation among Saudis in Madinah City, Saudi Arabia

Ghaida Jabri*, Alaa Sandokji, Nourah Alzughaibi, Ibrahim Alsehli, Hanan Neyaz, Khadijah Alhusaini, Mohammed Jabri and Mohammed Kareems

Faculty of Medicine, Taibah University, Kingdom of Saudi Arabia

Abstract

Background: Although organ transplantation is considered as the only preferable treatment for end-stage organ disease, there are not many organ donors among Saudis.

Objectives: To assess knowledge and attitude of Saudis in Madinah, Saudi Arabia, towards organ donation and to determine factors intervene with willingness of family to donate a member's organ.

Methods: A cross-sectional study, data were collected through a valid structured interview questionnaire from 290 participants during organ donation campaign in May 2015. The questionnaire included socio-demographic data and data about participants' awareness and knowledge on organ donation. Data were analyzed and compared by participants' sex using appropriate statistical tests.

Results: Of the interviewed 385 Saudis, 290 agreed to participate in the study with a response rate of 76.3%. The mean age of the participants was 27.2 ± 8.8 years. The study revealed 74.1% of the participants were willing to donate their organs with no significant differences between males and females, although only 2.7% of them reported to have a donation card. Religion, money, and age of the recipient appeared to have no role in their willing of organ donation. However, lack of awareness (21.7%), family refusal (20.6%) and fear of unknown (19.7%) were the most important barriers of organ donation.

Conclusions: The study showed a considerable number of participants were willing to donate their organs that religion and financial reasons were not factors. More organ donation campaigns are needed to maximize public positive beliefs.

Keywords: Awareness; Knowledge; Organ donation; Saudi Arabia

Introduction

The development of organ transplantation in the second half of the 20th century has been a remarkable achievement [1]. Recently; organ transplantation is one of the most effective options for those with an end-stage organ failure [2]. Its success has been basically dependent on public awareness, support and active participation. Without these factors, the efficiency of organ transplantation and the consequent saving or extension of lives would have undoubtedly suffered adversely [3].

In Saudi Arabia, the Saudi Center for Organ Transplantation (SCOT), established in 1984, and it was known as National Kidney Foundation with the objective to observe activities of organ donation and transplantation in Saudi Arabia. SCOT has many strategies that included research works, donation cards distribution, health professionals' education and public awareness [4-7]. Despite huge efforts of education and motivation of public about organ donation, the organ donors still not covering the growing waiting list [8-10], and insufficiency of organ donation in Saudi Arabia still a major barrier for transplantation.

Although organ transplantation has brought new horizons of hope to save many patients life, it is accompanied with a variety of cultural, ethical, and religion-related problems [11]. A systematic review of eighteen studies that involved 1019 participants, has detected eight prominent factors that affect the individual's decision about organ donation [12]. These factors include relational ties, religion-related beliefs, cultural influences, family refusal, body probity, health-care system interaction, knowledge about organ donation, and reservations about the process of organ donation [12]. Of these eight factors, the family refusal is found to be the most effective one. Family refusal, however, could be modified with educational and informative incentives where the donation is recognized socially, as a gesture of otherness and solidarity [13].

As the first step in designing and planning interferences in order to increase the acceptance of organ donation, it is necessary to determine the influencing factors on organ donation. By identifying these factors, healthcare team, managers, and planners can help families in their decisions regarding their loved one's organ donation to go through this agonizing decision much easier. Therefore, the goal of this study was to appraise the knowledge and attitude of Saudis in Madinah city, Saudi Arabia, towards organ donation and to determine factors that may facilitate the willingness of family to donate a member's organ.

Methods

During "Organ Donation" campaign on the first tow days of May 2015, a cross sectional study was conducted over a sample Saudi male and female visitors of AL Rashid mall, the largest shopping center

*Corresponding author: Ghaida Jabri, Medical Student, Faculty of Medicine, Taibah University, Kingdom of Saudi Arabia, E-mail: ghaid2@hotmail.com

in Madinah city, Saudi Arabia, and aimed to raise the community awareness about the importance of organ donation. All participants were Saudis and of at least 18 year of age, who visiting the site of the campaign between 6 pm to 10 pm for two days, were interviewed at the entrance before heading to the awareness part of the organ donation campaign. Of the interviewed 380 subjects during the campaign, 290 subjects agreed to participate in this study and filled the study questionnaire, with a relatively high response rate of 76.3%. The information was collected using face to face interview based on a structured pilot tested questionnaire. The used study questionnaire was adopted and modified from previous national and international studies [10-14]. Questionnaire was translated and verified and the instrument was initially tested and any areas of disagreement were resolved with the cooperation of translators and the research team. The validity of the used Arabic questionnaire was obtained with the help of epidemiologist and family and community medicine consultants. The questionnaire included two basic sections; one comprising the socio-demographic data and the other section including data about knowledge, attitude, practice, and factors that affect the decision of organ donation. Socio-demographic data included age, gender, marital status, education level, and economical status.

Knowledge of the responders was assessed by questions regarding the meaning of the term "Brain death", awareness of the concept of organ donation, knowledge of the Islamic fatwa regarding organ donation, sources of information and the best ways to raise knowledge and awareness in their opinion. Attitude of the respondents regarding organ donation was determined through questions regarding opinions on the willingness to donate organs after death, family member's willingness to donate organs, holding an organ donor card, and the factors influencing their decision for donating their own organs or granting a family member well of donating. Enquiring about actual donation of any organ or holding an organ donation card was used to assess participants' practices.

SPSS program (version IBM SPSS statistics 19) was used to analyze the data. Data was presented using frequencies, mean and standard deviation as appropriate. Awareness and attitude of participants towards organ donation were assessed, analyzed and compared by participants' sex and age categories using appropriate statistical tests (chi square or Fischer exact test). P values ≤ 0.05 were used as indicators of statistical significance differences between the groups of the study. Research approval was taken from Taibah University, College Dentistry Research Ethics committee (TUCD-RE). In purpose to avoid physical or emotional harm and to ensure confidentiality and privacy of the collected data ethical consideration was considered.

Results

The socio-demographic characteristic of studied 290 Saudi participants was presented in Table 1. The mean age of the studied participants was 27.2 ± 8.8 years, of them 9.3% were above the age of 40 years. Of the studied cohort, 39.3% were females and 60.7% were males. About two-thirds the studied cohort (64.7%) was of university and higher educational level. Less than one half of them (43.4%) were students, 40.3% were employers and 16.3% were none employers. Three-forth of the participants reported monthly family income of less than 10000 SR. Single participants of the study were representing 63.1%, while 33.2% were married and 3.7% were divorced and widow. Almost all of the studied participants in the sample has heard about organ donation. 4.7% of participants defined organ donation as "taking the tissues of the human body from a cadaver" while 1.1% defined it

as "taking tissues from a living human body donor" and the rest of the participants (94.1%) were defined donation as "taking tissues from human body for transplantation to another person either from living donor and/or" cadaver (Table 2).

Of the studied 290 participants, 215 (74.1%) were willing to donate their organs with significant higher rate was among males (p=0.03). Nearly one half of the studied participants (140 participants (48.3%)) were willing to donate their organs or their family member and the lower percent was among female participants, although not statistically significant. Only 2.7% of the studied participants reported to have had donated an organ (5 males (2.8%) and 3 females (4.3%)). Also, a low percent of the studied sample (4.1%) was reported to have donor card, where only 7 males (3.9%) and 5 females (4.3%) have this card. The majority of the studied participants (82.8%) perceived organ donation as saving lives and which more significantly marked among female participants (p=0.03). The most important factors affecting participant's donation to an organ were the recipient's health condition (50.6%), relation to the recipient (41.1%), religion of the recipient (3.5%) and age of the recipient (4.5%), with no significant differences between males and females, however male participants reported the relation to the recipient was of greater importance.

Table 3 presented the knowledge and belief of the studied participants on organ donation by their sex. Two hundred and eighty-two participants (97.2%) were belief that the most organs can be donated is the kidney with a significant more belief about that organ among males. For donation from living, the respondent's belief the great importance of donor personal consent before donation with a significant difference between males and females (p=0.01), while for donation from cadaver, the need of family consent was an important for 69% of respondents, with statistically significant difference between males and females (p=0.03). More males in comparison to females' participants with a statistically significant differences reported that the donated organs should be promoted and there is need for having effective laws to protect the organ donation process. Two hundred

Characteristics*	N=290
Age in years, mean ± SD (range)	27.2 ± 8.8 (19-60)
Age in years (categories)	
≤ 40	263 (90.7)
>40	27 (9.3)
Participant's sex	
Male	176 (60.7)
Female	114 (39.3)
Educational level	
Illiterate	5 (1.5)
Less than university	98 (33.8)
University and higher	187 (64.7)
Occupation	
Students	125 (43.4)
Employed	116 (40.3)
Unemployed	49 (16.3)
Monthly family income (SR)	
<10000	219 (75.0)
10000-15000	43 (14.9)
>15000	28 (10.1)
Marital status	
Single	182 (63.1)
Married	96 (33.2)
Divorced and widow	12 (3.7)

Table 1: Characteristics of studied Saudi participants (n= 290). *Data are presented by mean ± SD or by n (%).

Attitude and awareness questions	Total n= 290 No. (%)	Male n= 176 No. (%)	Female n= 114 No. (%)	P value
1. Willing to donate your organs				
No	30 (10.3)	14 (7.9)	16 (14.0)	
Yes, under special circumstances	70 (24.1)	40 (22.7)	30 (26.3)	
Yes, irrespective of circumstances	145 (50.0)	100 (56.8)	45 (39.4)	
Not decided	45 (15.6)	22 (12.5)	20 (17.5)	0.02*
2. Donate your organs to				
Family member	140 (48.3)	90 (51.1)	50 (43.8)	
Friend	120 (41.4)	80 (45.5)	40 (35.1)	
Anyone	30 (10.3)	6 (3.4)	24 (21.1)	0.18
3. Have you ever donated an organ?				
Yes	8 (2.7)	5 (2.8)	3 (4.3)	
No	282 (97.3)	171 (98.9)	111 (97.4)	
4. Do you have organ donor card?				
Yes	12 (4.1)	7 (3.9)	5 (4.3)	
No	278 (95.9)	169 (96.1)	109 (95.7)	0.61
5. Your perception of organ donation				
To save someone's life	240(82.8)	142 (80.6)	98 (85.9)	
Out of compassion/sympathy	30 (10.3)	24 (13.6)	6 (8.6)	
For money	15 (5.2)	8 (4.5)	7 (6.2)	
As a responsibility	5 (1.7)	2 (1.1)	3 (4.3)	0.03*
6. Factors holding you to donate your organs				
Age of recipient	13 (4.5)	8 (4.5)	5 (4.3)	
Religion of recipient	10 (3.5)	5 (2.8)	5 (4.3)	
Health status of recipient	147 (50.6)	83 (47.2)	64 (56.2)	
Relation to recipient	120 (41.4)	80 (45.5)	40 (35.2)	0.32

Table 2: Awareness of the studied participants about organ donation by their sex. *Significant.

	Total n= 290 No. (%)	Male n= 176 No. (%)	Female n= 114 No. (%)	P value
1. Organs could be donated				
Kidney	282 (97.2)	171 (98.9)	107 (93.6)	0.01*
Blood	240 (82.8)	142 (80.6)	90 (78.9)	0.60
Heart	145 (50.0)	85(48.2)	60 (52.6)	0.06
Eyes	130 (44.8)	80 (45.4)	55 (48.2)	0.06
Liver	220 (75.9)	130 (73.9)	82 (71.9)	0.75
Skin	135 (29.3)	40 (22.7)	39 (34.2)	0.01*
Bone marrow	265 (57.5)	87 (49.4)	60 (52.6)	0.08
Lungs	224 (48.5)	88 (50.0)	57 (50.0)	1.00
2. Who give consent for living donation				
Donor	270 (93.1)	160 (90.9)	110 (96.5)	
His family	15 (5.2)	12 (6.9)	3 (2.6)	
His spouse	5 (1.7)	4 (2.2)	1 (0.9)	0.01*
3. Who give consent for donation after death				
Family	200 (69.0)	126 (71.5)	74 (64.9)	
Spouse	70 (24.0)	40 (22.8)	30 (26.3)	
Friend	20 (7.0)	10 (5.7)	10 (8.8)	0.03*
4. Should organ donation be promoted?				
Yes	258 (88.9)	150 (85.2)	108 (94.7)	
No	32 (11.1)	26 (14.8)	8 (5.3)	0.01*
5. Effective laws to govern the process of organ donation are necessary				
Yes	273 (94.1)	168 (95.4)	107 (93.8)	
No	17 (5.9)	8 (4.6)	7 (6.2)	0.20
6. Promoting organ donation could be by				
Monetary benefit to donor family	30 (10.3)	10 (5.6)	20 (17.5)	
Giving awards	3 (1.0)	2 (1.1)	1 (1.0)	
Free health treatment for donor family	70 (24.2)	30 (28.3)	40 (35.0)	
All of above	187 (64.5)	134 (63.3)	53 (46.5)	0.23

*Significant
Table 3: Knowledge and belief of the studied participants towards organ donation by their sex.

and seventy-three participants (94.1%) did belief that effective laws are necessary to promote the process of donation, with no significant difference between males and females. Also, to promote donation, the studied participants suggest the monetary benefit to donor family and free health treatment for donor family, with a very few participants suggesting giving money.

Table 4 presented the distribution of the reasons and barriers intervening with organ donation by the studied participants. No reasons were reported by 70 participants (24.1). However, the most important reasons were lack of awareness on organ donation among 63 participants (21.7%), refusal of family members among 60 participants (20.6%), fear of unknown among 57 participants (19.7%), religious

Barriers and reason	Total n= 290 No. (%)	Male n= 176 No. (%)	Female n=114 No. (%)	P value
Lack of awareness	63 (21.7)	40 (22.7)	23 (20.2)	
Fear of unknown	57 (19.7)	34 (19.3)	23 (20.1)	
Religious reasons	20 (6.8)	14 (7.9)	6 (5.2)	
Refusal of family members	60 (20.6)	35 (19.9)	25 (21.9)	0.23
Cultural reasons	20 (6.8)	12 (6.9)	8 (7.1)	
No reasons	70 (24.1)	41 (23.3)	30 (26.3)	

Table 4: Barriers and reasons for not donating organs by donors.

reasons among 20 participants (6.8%), and cultural reasons (6.8%). These percentages were similar between both studies male and female participants with no statistically significant differences.

Discussion

The study findings revealed that 74.1% of the participants were willing to donate their organs with significant higher rate being among the studied males (79.3%). This rate appeared higher than that observed in a recent Saudi study [15] where 66.7% of the study respondents were willing to donate an organ and this rate was decreased to 42.8% among the rural respondents, and similar low willing rate was also reported in the previous Saudi studies [4,15-17]. The detected high rate in this study might be explained by the high literate rate (98.5%), and in particular the university and higher education 64.7% among the study participants. Studies from neighboring countries reported low rate of willingness toward organ donation [18,19] as well as studies of Western countries [20,21]. All the above-mentioned Saudi and non-Saudi studies have revealed education as a main factor in increasing public awareness toward organ donation. Concerning these variations, it was observed that higher awareness and willingness to donate organs were more among people who reported higher educational level. In this study, the rate of university and higher education among the participants was high. Similarly, willing of organ donation was correlated with education and socio-economic status in a similar study from Pakistan [22]. Also, a previous study conducted in Turkey [23] has reported that education and training significantly motivate public for organ donation.

The perception of organ donation as to "save someone life" was reported by the majority of the studied participants and it was marked among females (85.9%). Perception of organ transplantation as "a way for money collection ", however, was very among all studied participants (5.2%), particularly among males (4.5%). This finding has been reported in Scottish study [24], and is thought to be because financial payments appear to undermine the individual and cast doubt over their intentions to donate [25].

The most important factors holding the studied participants to donate were the health status of the recipients (50.6%), and the relation with the recipients (41.4%). The age and religion of the recipient, however, was representing very low motives for participants in this study to donate an organ. Similarly, religion and cultural reasons appeared to have no role in other studies concerned with eye and kidney donation [26,27]. In contrast to these findings, however, the religious beliefs were found to be the most important motivation factor to donate in the previous Pakistan study [22]. Other reported factors were worries about decreasing the level of the received healthcare after donation, lack of family support, and lack of information about organ donation were the primary reasons for lack of willingness to donate [15].

Most of Saudis in the study have appeared to know the different organs which can be donated. The highest level of knowledge about this item was for kidney, liver, blood, bone marrow and heart. The majority of study participants (93.1%) reported the mandatory of donor consent for living donation and 69% reported the necessity of family consent for donation after death. Again, the fact that most of the respondents were literate individuals, a factor made them well educated about organ donation and understood what was displayed in the mass media. Mandatory consent for donation expressed before the death of the donor should ideally form the basis for donation. However, in the case of unavailability of such consent, consent from adult family members of the deceased donor should be obtained for organ donation. In a study done on the responses of relatives of post-mortem cases, it was revealed that out of the potential post-mortem donors, 44.3% of relatives of such cases gave consent for donation after intensive counseling [15].

The study participants have acknowledged some measures to be presented by government to promote organ donation. These measures include; monetary benefit to donor family, giving awards, and free health treatment for donor family. Therefore, it is possible that starting legislations and regulations which will guarantee the donors best health care and easy access to health facilities could encourage people to donate organs in their lifetimes. In a previous study, financial and non-financial support has been reported by their participants to encourage public for organ donation [15].

The study findings have revealed that the most important barriers of not donating organs among the studied participants were lack of awareness (21.7%), and refusal of family members. On the other hand, however, religious (6.8%), and cultural (6.8%) appeared to have a minimal role in this respect. Family members continue to play a prominent role in donation decisions at time of death. In a previous Spanish study, Martinez et al. [28] found that donation was less likely when there is more family conflict. In similar previous studies, adequate knowledge and adequate understanding of the process of organ donation and brain death have been thought to be essential for obtaining donation consent in previous studies [29,30].

The present study appeared to have a number of strengths. The anonymous and comprehensive questionnaire and face-to-face interview that insured correct and complete method for data collection. The study questionnaire has also been tested by a pre-test study and validated by experts. To the best of our knowledge, this study is the first to study the awareness and to explore different barriers intervene with organ donation among Saudis in Madinah city, with a relatively high response rate of 76.3%. Moreover, and unlike other similar studies, this study has analyzed awareness and barriers intervene with organ donation according to participants' sex.

The study questionnaire has also been tested by a pre-test study and validated by experts. To the best of our knowledge, this study is the first to study the awareness and to explore different barriers intervene with organ donation among Saudis in Madinah city, with a relatively high response rate of 76.3%. Moreover, and unlike other similar studies, this study has analyzed awareness and barriers intervene with organ donation according to participants' sex.

As a limitation of this study, as this study was limited by the organ donation day, the study sample was relatively small size that future large and national studies are needed before generalization of these results can be assumed. Furthermore, though this study has probed the awareness and attitudes of general population towards organ donation, studying these issues among terminally ill patients are needed as these sectors of population represent the potential donors in most number of cases. This important point has to be considered in future research to assess awareness and attitudes of palliative care and terminally ill patients towards organ donation.

In conclusion, the study showed a considerable number of participants were willing to donate their organs. Religion and financial factors appeared not to have much effectiveness on organ donation decision among the studied participants. Lack of awareness and family refusal were the most important barriers intervene with organ donation. These findings highlight the need for continued public education through several organ donation campaigns to maximize positive beliefs on organ donation.

Acknowledgments

We would like to express our appreciation to Taibah Medical Club for arrangement of this campaign and we would like to acknowledge all TMC members for their crucial role in helping us in the collection of data.

References

1. Aldawood A, Al Qahtani S, Dabbagh O, Al-Sayyari AA (2007) Organ donation after brain death: experience over five-years in a tertiary hospital. Saudi J Kidney Dis Transpl 18: 60-64.

2. Abouna GM (2001) The humanitarian aspects of organ transplantation. Transplant Int 14: 117-123.

3. Broumand MA, Asgari F (2012) Do Tehranian people agree with organ donation of their relatives after brain death? J Med Ethics Hist Med 5: 51.

4. Alam AA (2007) Public opinion on organ donation in Saudi Arabia. Saudi J Kidney Dis Transpl 18: 54-59.

5. Shaheen FA, Souqiyyeh MZ, Abdullah A (2000) Strategies and obstacles in an organ donation program in developing countries: Saudi Arabian experience. Transplant Proc 32: 1470-1472.

6. Aswad S, Souqiyyeh MZ, Huraib S, el-Shihabi R (1992) Public attitudes toward organ donation in Saudi Arabia. Transplant Proc 24: 2056-2058.

7. El-Shoubaki H, Bener A (2005) Public knowledge and attitudes toward organ donation and transplantation: a cross-cultural study. Transplant Proc 37: 1993-1997.

8. Shaheen F (1994) Organ transplantation in the Kingdom of Saudi Arabia: new strategies. Saudi J Kidney Dis Transpl 5: 3-5.

9. Al Shehri S, Shaheen FA, Al-Khader AA (2005) Organ donations from deceased persons in the Saudi Arabian population. Exp Clin Transplant 3: 301-305.

10. Aldawood A, Al Qahtani S, Dabbagh O, Al-Sayyari AA (2007) Organ donation after brain-death: experience over five-years in a tertiary hospital. Saudi J Kidney Dis Transpl 18: 60-64.

11. Kim JR, Elliott D, Hyde C (2002) Korean nurses' perspectives of organ donation and transplantation: A review. Transpl Nurses J 11: 20-24.

12. Irving MJ, Tong A, Jan S, Cass A, Rose J, et al. (2012) Factors that influence the decision to be an organ donor: a systematic review of the qualitative literature. Nephrol Dial Transpl 27: 2526-2533.

13. Moraes EL, Massarollo MC (2006) Bibliometric study on family refusal of tissue and organ donation for transplants from 1990 to 2004. J Bras Transpl 9: 597-609.

14. Balwani MR, Gumber MR, Shah PR, Kute VB, Patel HV, et al. (2015) Attitude and awareness towards organ donation in western India. Renal failure 37: 582-588.

15. Alghanim SA (2010) Knowledge and attitudes toward organ donation: a community-based study comparing rural and urban populations. Saudi J Kidney Dis Transpl 21: 23-30.

16. Al-Sebayel MI, Al-Enazi AM, Al-Sofayan MS, Al-Saghier MI, Khalaf HA, et al. (2004) Improving organ donation in Central Saudi Arabia. Saudi Med J 25: 1366-1368.

17. Al-Sebayel MI (2002) The status of cadaveric organ donation for liver transplantation in Saudi Arabia. Saudi Med J 23: 509-512.

18. El-Shoubaki H, Bener A, Al-Mosalamani Y (2006) Factors influencing organ donation and transplantation in the state of Qatar. Transplant Med 18: 97-103.

19. Bilgel H, Sadikoglu G, Goktas O, Bilgel N (2004) A survey of the public attitudes towards organ donation in a Turkish community and of the changes that have taken place in the last 12 years. Transplant International 17: 126-130.

20. Schauenburg H, Hildebrandt A (2006) Public knowledge and attitudes on organ donation do not differ in Germany and Spain. Transplant Proc 38: 1218-1220.

21. Sandera S, Miller B (2005) Public knowledge and attitudes regarding organ and tissue donation: an analysis of the northwest Ohio community. Patient Educ Couns 58: 154-163.

22. Saleem T, Ishaque S, Habib N, Hussain SS, Jawed A, et al. (2009) Knowledge, attitudes and practices survey on organ donation among a selected adult population of Pakistan. BMC Med Ethics 10: 5.

23. Tokalak I, Kut A, Moray G, Emiroglu R, Erdal R, et al. (2006) Knowledge and attitudes of high school students related to organ donation and transplantation: A cross sectional survey in turkey. Saudi J Kidney Dis Transplant 17: 491-496.

24. Haddow G (2006) Because you're worth it? The taking and selling of transplantable organs. J Med Ethics 32: 324-328.

25. Bénabou R, Tirole J (2006) Incentives and prosocial behavior. Am Econ Rev 96: 1652-1678.

26. Riyanti S, Hatta M, Norhafizah S, Balkish MN, Siti ZM, et al. (2014) Organ donation by sociodemographic characteristics in Malaysia. Asian Social Science 10: 262-272.

27. Khan N, Masood Z, Tufail N, Shoukat H, Ashraf KTA, et al. (2011) Knowledge and attitude of people towards organ donation. JUMDC 2: 15-21.

28. Martınez JM, Lopez JS, Martin A, Martin MJ, Scandroglio B, et al. (2001) Organ donation and family decision-making within the Spanish donation system. Soc Sci Med 53: 405-421.

29. Sque M, Long T, Payne S (2005) Organ donation: key factors influencing families' decision-making. Transpl Proc 37: 543-546.

30. Rosel J, Frutos MA, Blanca MJ, Ruiz P (1999) Discriminant variables between organ donors and nondonors: A post-hoc investigation. Prog Transpl 9: 50-53.

4

Consumer Acceptance of Genetically Modified Foods in the Greater Accra Region of Ghana

Eric Worlanyo Deffor*

University of Ghana Business School, Department of Organization and Human Resource Management Legon, Accra-Ghana West Africa

Abstract

Genetic Modification (GM) is a rapidly growing technology that can improve productivity and profitability for producers. The study assessed consumer acceptance of GM foods in the Greater Accra Region of Ghana. The study is based on a survey conducted in three districts of the Greater Accra Region namely, Accra Metropolitan Assembly (AMA), Ga East (GE) and Tema Metropolitan Assembly (TMA) using purposive sampling method. A qualitative choice (Logit) model was used to estimate the effect of various factors on consumer acceptance of GM foods. The results obtained showed that, about 90% of the respondents had heard or read something about GM foods indicating a high level awareness among respondents' in the Greater Accra Region. The results also show that 85% of the respondents were willing to accept GM foods. From the logit model, consumers with age groups 31-40 and above 50 years, were more likely to accept GM foods in the study area where as male respondents were less likely to accept GMFs. In addition, respondents with secondary and tertiary levels of education were likely to accept GM foods. Household size 1 to 5, reading product labels as well as understanding of science and technology were also significant variables in explaining consumer acceptance of GM foods in the Greater Accra Region. Obviously awareness and education was shown to be a necessary condition for acceptability of GM foods. The recommendation of this study is to promote effective education about the benefits of GM foods to increase the potential for acceptance.

Keywords: Genetically modified food; Consumer acceptance; Logit; Ghana

Introduction

Genetically Modified Foods (GMFs) are defined as plant and animal products obtained from a collection of scientific techniques that involve taking genes from one plant or animal species and inserting them in another species to transfer a desired trait or characteristic. Most often proponents of agricultural biotechnology view its application as the gate way to the future of food production. In other words, its application holds the potential of making available a wide variety of products with high nutritional, environmental, and economic benefits [1]. In fact the role of biotechnology in the future of agriculture and food production according to Hallman et al. [2] has become increasingly significant as billions of dollars has been and is being spent to develop new and improved foods, fuel, feeds, fibers, pharmaceuticals, and nutraceuticals. The benefits the technology holds for agricultural producers, is the potential of reducing production costs, enhanced yields, and also the potential for increased profits. Additionally, other potential benefits include reductions in pesticide and herbicide use, as well as the potential for enhanced nutritional value, flavor, and shelf life of some foods [3].

Despite these stated advantages, genetically modified foods (GMF) have received mixed regulatory and public acceptance even in the United States and elsewhere [2]. Also as more products developed through biotechnology reach store shelves, consumer reception continue to be mixed. This has been the case especially in Europe where adoption has been met with caution and in some cases rejected altogether as observed by [4,5]. Evidence from Kimenju et al. [6] study indicate that consumer organizations, environmentalists and other non-governmental organizations have expressed concerns about GM foods on the grounds of food safety, ethics, religion and the possible effect on the environment; in addition to the above stated concerns the lack of consumer choice due to inadequate labelling is also expressed. Basically, these concerns are mainly due to consumer perceptions and the fear of the unknown i.e. GMO's may pose some long-term unforeseen health risks, as well as the risk of negative effects on wildlife and the environment. These consumer perceptions are very critical if consumers will accept GM foods [7-9].

However, there is a lack of scientific data concerning environmental and health effects from both industrial and public research sources that consuming GM foods can lead to some unforeseen effect. Indeed, there is little evidence that eating today's GM foods is unhealthy, except in rare cases of allergenicity [10,11]. These assurances notwithstanding, consumer concerns are still high; therefore the application of GM technology to produce food can only be successful if consumers accept the end result. In other words, the future development of gene technology depends heavily on public acceptance. Indeed, public attitude toward genetic engineering and the subsequent acceptance of products derived from the technology is becoming increasingly important in determining the future role of the technology in society. If consumer acceptance issues are not adequately addressed, then the potential economic and social benefits of modern biotechnology may not be realized [12]. Clearly, consumers' acceptance of GM foods form a critical factor that will help determine its future, hence the need to establish the level of consumers' awareness, perceptions and concerns about GM foods and their readiness to accept and subsequently use them. This research therefore possess these questions: Is the policies available in Ghana regarding Biotechnology clearly known? What is the level of awareness of consumers in the Greater Accra Region? What

***Corresponding author:** Eric Worlanyo Deffor, University of Ghana Business School, Department of Organization and Human Resource Management P.O. Box LG 78, Legon, Accra-Ghana West Africa, E-mail: ericdeffor@gmail.com

factors affect consumer acceptance of GM foods? What is the effect of these factors on consumer willingness to accept GM foods? This study attempts to provide answers to the questions raised.

A review by Costa-Font et al. [13] systematically summarized evidence on the acceptance of GM food and its underlying processes. The main issues captured by the study were risks and benefits perceptions, trust, knowledge, and valuation, as well as purchasing decisions. The study also identified three kinds of population that are studied in literature namely, anti-GM food or pessimistic, risk-tolerant or information searchers, and GM-accepters or optimistic and indicated that different compositions of such groups in a specific society determines final acceptance of GM food. The review also pointed out that most studies showed that consumers preferred GM free food until the point to pay premium for them. Preferences were analyzed with varying technics such as stated preferences, real markets, blind taste, etc. It also pointed out that consumer behavior can be related to the associated benefits, information, gender, age, knowledge and so on of GM food. Empirical evidence have also supported and further added different dimensions to the earlier studies. Even though consumers in Venezuela are adequately informed about microbial and pesticides contamination, they are highly misinformed about GM foods [14]. Another study in China revealed that information on GM foods is less available but awareness is high among urban consumers. Information and prices of GM foods were two important factors affecting consumers' attitudes toward GM foods. The study concluded that the commercialization of GM foods is not likely to receive great resistance from the consumers in China [15].

Unlike the two studies discussed in the paragraph above, Krualee and Napasintuwong [16] applied multinomial logit regression to examine the factors that affect the willingness of consumers in Thailand to pay for non-GM food labeling in Thailand. The results suggest that non-GM labeling is an appropriate policy for Thailand when the majority of consumers are averse to GM food and willing to pay less for GM contaminated products or if they consider negative health impacts a serious problem. Using experimental auction methodology, Huffman [17] assessed willingness to pay for food products that might be made from new transgenic and intragenic genetically modified (GM) traits among consumers. The study showed that the consumers respond to both food labels and information treatments, but no single type of information is dominant.

Acceptance of innovations or willingness to accept innovations have also been examined in the field of agriculture. Chebil et al. [18] analyzed the factors that affect farmers' willingness to adopt salt-tolerant forage for livestock, using a Tobit model. The study found positive relationship between willingness to adopt and off-farm income and flock size variable. Another study by Asante et al. [19] employed Probit regression to examine the willingness of farm households to adopt improved yam technologies. In addition to information obtained through extension, media and training, willingness to accept the technology was informed by socioeconomic, technical and individual attributes.

This study also applied a Logit regression procedure to assess consumer willingness to accept genetically modified food in the Greater Accra Region. Specifically, the study determined the level of consumer awareness about GM food in the study area and then modeled the effect of the factors that determines consumer acceptance of GM foods in the region.

Methodology

The Logit framework

This model has been used to estimate the effect of socioeconomic variables, sensory variables, and psychographic variables on consumer preferences for GM foods. The empirical model assumes that the consumer's probability to consume (acceptance) genetically modified food, P_i, depends on a vector of independent variables (X_{ik}) associated with consumer i and variable j, and a vector of unknown parameters β [1]:

$$P_i = F(Z_i) = F(\alpha + \beta X_i) = \frac{1}{[1 + \exp(-Z_i)]} = \frac{1}{[1 + \exp-(\alpha + \beta X_i)]} \quad (1)$$

where denotes $F(Z_i)$ denotes the value of logistic cumulative density function associated with each possible value of the underlying Z_i; P_i denotes the probability that an individual would consume the specific GM food product, given the independent variables X_i.

To estimate the model above, multiply both sides of equation (1) by to get:

$$[1 + \exp(-Z_i)]P_i = 1 \quad (2)$$

By dividing by P_i, and then subtracting 1 leads to

$$\exp(-Z_i) = \frac{1}{P_i} - 1 = \frac{1 - P_i}{P_i} \quad (3)$$

By definition, however,

$$\exp(-Z_i) = \frac{1}{\exp(-Z_i)}$$

So that

$$\exp(-Z_i) = \frac{P_i}{1 - P_i}$$

and by taking the natural logarithm of both sides, we obtain

$$Z_i = \log\frac{1}{1 - P_i} \quad or \quad \log[\frac{P_i}{1 - P_i}] = Z_i = \alpha + \beta X_i \quad (4)$$

The dependent variable in the regression equation above is the logarithm of the odds that a particular choice will be made.

In the above equation, is a linear combination of the independent variables so that

$$Z_i = \log[\frac{P_i}{1 - P_i}] = \beta_0 + \beta_1 x_{i1} + \beta_2 x_{i2} + \beta_3 x_{i3} + \ldots\ldots\beta_k x_{ik} + \varepsilon_i \quad i = 1, 2, 3\ldots, n \quad (5)$$

where Z_i denotes unobserved index level or the log odds of choice for the ith observation; X_{ik} denotes k^{th} attribute of the ith respondent; i denotes observation; β denotes parameters to be estimated; ε denotes random error or disturbance term. The dependent variable Z_i in equation (5) is the logarithm of the probability that a particular choice will be made. The maximum likelihood method of estimation was employed to estimate the logit model, since the individual Pi are not observed; rather the measured dependent variable was $y_i=1$ the choice is made and zero (0) otherwise are. The estimated parameters of equation (5) do not directly represent the marginal effects of the independent variables on P_i. For a continuous variable, the marginal effect of x_k on the probability P_i that the dependent variable (y) takes the value $y_i=1$ is given by:

$$\frac{\partial P_i}{\partial x_{ij}} = \frac{[\beta_j \exp(-\beta X_i)]}{[1 + \exp(-\beta X_i)]^2} \quad (6)$$

However, if the independent variables are also qualitative or discrete in nature, as is the case for the independent variables used in this study, the marginal effect of a discrete independent variable is obtained by evaluating P_i at alternative values of x_{ij}. Marginal effects of such variables are determined as:

Characteristics		
Gender	Frequency	Percent
Male	155	64.6
Female	85	35.4
Total	240	100
Age		
20-30	157	65.4
31-41	46	19.2
41-50	21	8.8
Above 50	16	6.7
Total	240	100
Household size		
41644	80	33.3
41800	123	51.3
41958	37	15.4
Total	240	100

Table 1: Distribution of Respondents According To Socio-Economic Characteristics.

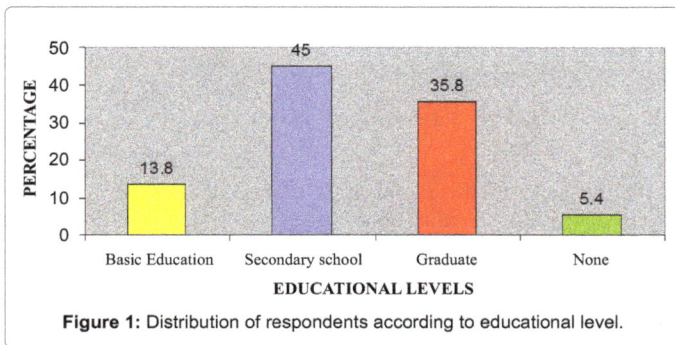

Figure 1: Distribution of respondents according to educational level.

$$\frac{\partial P_i}{\partial X_i} = \beta_i [P_i (1 - P_i)] \tag{7}$$

To obtain the marginal effect or response, we take the means of all the explanatory variables and multiply each mean by its estimated parameter to obtain Pi. The maximum likelihood method of estimation was employed to estimate the logit model.

Empirical Logit Model

In the empirical analysis, the following model is used to predict the probability or the log odds that an individual consumer will consume or accept GM food product:

$$\begin{aligned} WACCEPT = &\beta_0 + \beta_1 PRIC + \beta_2 SEX(MALE) + \beta_3 AGE31\_40 + \beta_4 AGE41\_50 + \beta_5 AGE\_AB50 \\ &+ \beta_6 EDUC2 + \beta_7 EDUC3 + \beta_8 EDUC4 + \beta_9 HHSIZE15 + \beta_{10} HHSIZE\,610 \\ &+ \beta_{11} HEARD + \beta_{12} READL + \beta_{13} RELCON + \beta_{14} SAFCON \\ &+ \beta_{15} ETHICONC + \beta_{16} UNDSC\_TEC + \beta_{17} REGUL + \varepsilon \end{aligned} \tag{8}$$

Statement of hypotheses

The following hypotheses were tested for equation (1) based on apriori expectations:

1. H0: Price has no effect on the willingness to accept GM foods

H1: Price has a negative effect on the willingness to accept GM foods

This hypothesis is also tested for the following variables: Age, and Ethical concerns, safety concerns and religious concerns.

2. H0: Level of education has no effect on the willingness to accept GM foods

H1: Level of education has a positive effect on the willingness to accept GM foods

3. H0: Government control has no effect on the willingness to accept GM foods

H1: Government control has a positive effect on the willingness to accept GM foods

4. H0: Sex has no effect on the willingness to accept GM foods

H1: Sex has a positive or negative effect on the willingness to accept GM foods

This is repeated for the following variables: Reading of labels, Awareness (knowledge about GM), Household size.

Validation of hypothesis

The Z statistic is used to measure the level of significance for each of the estimated coefficients. If Z calculated is greater than the Z critical the null hypothesis is rejected in favors of alternate. Also, the goodness of fit statistic given is the Mc-Fadden R-square. The likelihood ratio (LR) test is computed to determine the joint significance of the independent variables in the model. The LR test statistics follows the chi-square (χ^2) distribution with the degrees of freedom equal to the number of independent variables used in the model. The higher the percentage of prediction the greater the predictive power of the model.

Data collection method

Purposive sampling technique was used to select respondent from three Municipal/District Assemblies in the Greater Accra Region of Ghana, namely the Accra Metropolitan Assembly (A.M.A), the Ga East and Tema Municipal Assembly (T.M.A) with some level of education. The choice was largely influenced by the technical nature of the research topic; hence some level of education on the part of the respondents was needed to facilitate easy explanations and questionnaire administration. However, some data was collected on respondents who had little or no formal education, notwithstanding the difficulty encountered in explaining the terminologies to them.

Results and Discussion

Demographic characteristics of respondents

From Table 1, male respondents formed the largest proportion of respondents having a frequency of 155 representing 65% of the total respondents; with 85 (35%) being females. In the age category 65% of the respondents were within the age group 20-30; followed by 19% within the age group 31-40; with 7% belonging to the age group 50 years and above. The results presented generally indicate that most of the respondents interviewed were relatively young or in their youthful age. The household sizes of the respondents were grouped into 1-5, 6-10 and 11-15. Majority (123) of the respondents had household sizes within 6-10 representing 51%; the least household size group was 11-15 having a percentage of 15. The result is indicative of the fact that most of the respondents have large family sizes. See Table 1 for details. The educational levels of respondents are shown by Figure 1; majority of them had attained some level of formal education ranging from basic to tertiary levels of education. 108 of the respondents had attained secondary (SSS; O/A Level) level of education representing 45%; whereas 36% of them had tertiary level of education. Only a small number (5%) of the respondents indicated they had no form of formal education. Most of the respondents were educated because the respondents were purposively sampled.

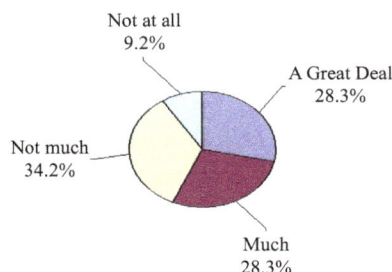

Figure 2: How much have you heard or read about GM foods.

Response	Frequency	Percent
Yes	204	85
No	36	15
Total	240	100

Table 2: Willingness to accept GM foods if their production and importation is regulated by a Government Agency (FDB, SD, AEC).

Variables	Coefficients	Marginal Effect	Probability
MALE	-0.59	-0.143	0.0856*
AGE3140	-1.174	-0.284	0.0039***
AGE4150	0.842	--	0.1813
AGEABV50	-1.828	-0.442	0.0046***
EDUC2	0.866	--	0.2926
EDUC3	1.281	0.31	0.0766***
EDUC4	1.196	0.289	0.1026*
HHSIZE15	0.779	0.188	0.0777*
HHSIZE610	-0.143	--	0.7238
PRICE	0.052	--	0.8687
HEARD	0.026	--	0.9367
UNDSC_TEC	0.725	0.175	0.0496**
READL	0.614	0.148	0.0653**
ETHICGM	0.447	--	0.1991
SAFECON	0.193	--	0.5731
RELCON	-0.62	-0.15	0.1047*
REGUL	0.985	0.238	0.0019***
C	-1.874	-0.453	0.0408
Mean dependent var	0.591667	S.D. dependent var	0.492553
LR statistic (17 df)	58.25616	McFadden R-squared	0.179472
Probability (LR stat)	0.00000203		

Table 3: Logit Results, Dependent Variable: WACCEPT, Method: ML-Binary Logit
* Indicates statistically significant at the 10% level; **Indicates statistically significant at the 5% level; ***Indicates statistically significant at the 1% level

Consumer awareness of genetically modified foods

To find out whether consumers were aware of genetically modified foods, the question how much have you heard or read about Genetically Modified Foods was asked respondents. Out of the total, 240 respondents 34% said they had not heard much about genetically modified foods; 28% a great deal; with less than 10% indicating they had not heard or read anything about genetically modified foods. Generally, most respondents had some basic knowledge (i.e. read or heard) of GM foods, this significant level of awareness is attributable to recent issues on genetically modified foods in the media regarding some alleged contamination of some imported rice with unapproved strain of genetically modified rice in the country (i.e. during the period of data collection) as well as the fact that more educated respondents were sampled hence might have read or heard about genetically modified foods on their own (Figure 2).

Boccaletti and Moro [4] demonstrated that consumer trust in companies and scientists conducting research in the area of gene technologies has a strong effect on perception of risks and benefits associated with those technologies. Therefore if a consumer's level of trust in regulatory bodies is high the likelihood that that consumer will be willing to accept GM foods will be high. The question was asked in the questionnaire; Will you accept GM Foods if their production and Importation is regulated and certified by a Government Agency such as (FDB, SD, AEC). In other words, Do consumers trust (FDB, SD, and AEC) to regulate the importation and productions of GM foods in Ghana? The result as presented in Table 2 show that generally majority of the respondents (85%) indicated they will accept genetically modified foods if their production or importation was regulated by these government agencies such as Ghana Atomic Energy Commission (GAEC), Food and Drugs Board (FDB), and Standard Board (SD). Indicating that most of the respondents have a high level of trust in these government agencies to ensure the safety of the foods and drugs they consume likewise GM foods (Table 2). This result is probably in line with the statement that consumers in developing countries are most likely to have high trust in government agencies to regulate the importation and production of GM foods [20].

Factors affecting consumer's acceptance of genetically modified foods

Most (59%) of the respondents expressed their willingness to accept genetically modified foods if they were introduced into the country. Only 40.2% were not ready to accept genetically modified foods. This result indicates a slightly above average level of consumer acceptance of genetically modified foods in the study area, although they expressed some reservations. The Logit model was employed to investigate the effect of some identified factors on consumer acceptance of GMFs. The results in Table 3 shows that the age variables AGE3140 and AGEABV50, trust in regulatory agencies (REGUL) and secondary level of education (EDUC3) were significant at 1% level of significance, followed by reading of labels (READL) and understanding of science and technology (UNDSC_TEC) been significant at 5% level of significance. Other variables such as Religious Concern (RELCON), Household size of 1-5 (HH15), gender (MALE) and tertiary level of education (EDUC4) was significant at 10% level of significance. The marginal effects, which represent the probability of accepting Genetically Modified foods, were calculated for each significant variable. AGE3140 and AGEABV50 years were significant and meet the apriori expectation. The findings show that the all things being equal, the probability that a consumers or respondents in these age groups accepting GM foods will decrease by -0.284, and -0.442 likelihood respectively in the study area. Secondary school level (EDUC3) of education was also found to be significant with a positive sign meeting the a priori expectation.

The implication is that respondents with at least secondary level of education are likely to accept GM foods in the study area will as well as respondents with tertiary level of education even though their levels of significance vary. The educational variables were also found to have met the apriori expectation of a positive sign. This findings support the assertion that education provides an individual/consumer with the ability to seek, evaluate and understand information about innovation which invariably can influence their likelihood to accept innovations in this context GM foods ceteris paribus. Further analysis of the model results showed that Household size (HHSIZE15) was significant with a positive sign meeting the apriori expectation, indicating the probability or likelihood of a respondent with household size of 1 to 5 accepting GM foods in the study. As households size increases the tendency to be exposed to innovation and information becomes high since members are likely to join the society for their daily activities and are exposed to information about the possible usefulness or benefits of GM foods and can easily fall into the state of acceptability.

The findings also indicate that male respondents had a - 0.14 likelihood of accepting GM foods in the study area. The findings imply that male respondents in households are less likely to take the risk of accepting or by extension purchasing GM foods. It important to indicate that some studies have shown that females are more willing to try innovation nonetheless the decision, of application of innovation has been noted to increases with for males may be due to their access to economic resources [19]. Another key determinant of GM acceptance in the study area is labeling; this was found to be significant in the model with a positive sign; meaning that there is the likelihood of a consumer who reads food labels will accept GM foods; perhaps due to that fact that product labels always portray the benefits of products have the tendency to shape the perception of consumers.

From the model concerns expressed on the grounds of religion was significant with a negative sign. Implying that there is the likelihood for a consumer who express reservations about GM foods based on their religious beliefs not to accept GM foods; this perhaps might be fueled by the perception that GM food production process contradict religious beliefs and teachings. Also, the variable UNDSC_TEC was significant meeting the positive apriori expectation. The result means that ceteris paribus, the likelihood that a consumer with some basic understanding of science and technology accepting GM foods will increase by 0.175 and vice versa. Understanding of science eliminates any fear about the possible hazards of GM foods and this may have contributed to positive relationship. Consumer trust in regulatory bodies was highly significant in the model, meaning that the likelihood of a respondents accepting GM foods if the regulations was certified by these government will increase by 0.24 units confirming reports [6] that higher trust in regulatory mechanisms leads to lower resistance to genetic and biotechnology products.

Conclusion

The conclusion of this study is based on respondents purposively selected from the main districts of in the capital city of Ghana Accra. A Logit model was used to assess the effect of some selected variables on the acceptance of GM foods in the study area. Primarily the issue of acceptance of GM foods and its subsequent use in developing countries such as Ghana is perhaps a critical policy decision to make by government and the relevant regulatory authorities. However, this decision cannot be made without recourse to the end user i.e. consumer. It is important therefore that policy decision in this regard takes into consideration the perceptions and acceptance of consumers based on sound research findings. The study therefore concludes that awareness about benefits or otherwise of GM foods is critical to acceptance of GM foods in the study area especially among individuals with some level of education. Trust and confidence in regulatory institutions on the part of consumers can influence the acceptance of GM foods in the study area; it is important therefore for these organizations to position themselves to allay the fears and concerns of consumers regarding GM foods. Again there would be a need to for proper labeling of GM foods for consumers in the study area to make informed choice during purchase of the groceries etc.

Policy Recommendations

The analysis contributes to a better understanding of the factors influencing consumer acceptance of GM foods in the study area. Therefore before the introduction of GM foods into the country it will be reassuring to consumers if concerns relating to health, safety, and the environment are taken into consideration. It is therefore suggested that policy makers should focus their educational efforts aimed at convincing consumers to accept genetically modified foods through recommended electronic and the print media (i.e. both local and international) should be channels through which to educate consumers to allay them of the concerns and reservations they have towards GM foods. Also policy makers must consider strongly the issues of labeling of GM foods to distinguish it from other food products for consumers to make their choice.

References

1. Hossain F, Adelaja A, Brian H, Onyango B, Schilling W (2002) "Consumer Acceptance of Food Biotechnology: Willingness to Buy Genetically Modified Food Products." New Jersey: Food Policy Institute, Rutgers University.

2. Hallman WK, Adelaja AO, Schilling BJ, Lang J (2002). Public Perceptions of Genetically Modified Foods: Americans Know Not What They Eat. Publication No. RR-0302-001, Food Policy Institute, Rutgers University.

3. Harrison RW, Jae-Hwan Han (2004) The Effects of Risk Perceptions on United States Consumer Preferences for GMO Labelling Paper presented at the 14th International Food and Agribusiness Management Association Annual World Food and Agribusiness Symposium and Forum, June 12-15, 2004.

4. Boccaletti S, Moro D (2000) Consumer Willingness-To-Pay for Gm Food Products in Italy. AgBioForum 3: 259-267.

5. Burton M, Rigby D, Young T, James S (2001) Consumer Attitudes to Genetically Modified Organisms in Food in the UK. European Review of Agricultural Economics 28(2001): 479-493.

6. Kimenju SC, De Groote H, Karugia J, Mbogoh S, Poland D (2004) Consumer Awareness and Attitudes toward GM foods in Kenya. International Maize and Wheat Improvement Centre (CIMMYT) Nairobi, Kenya IRMA Socioeconomics Working Paper 2004-01.

7. Hoban TJ (1998) Trends in Consumer Attitude about Agricultural Biotechnology AgBioForum 1.

8. Caulder J (2001) "Agricultural Biotechnology and Public Perceptions," Agbio Forum.

9. Hallman WK, Metcalfe J (2001). "Public Perceptions of Agricultural Biotechnology: A Survey of New Jersey Residents".

10. Domingo JL (2000) Health risks of GM foods: many opinions but few data. Science 288: 1748-1749.

11. Wolfenbarger LL, Phifer PR (2000) The ecological risks and benefits of genetically engineered plants. Science 290: 2088-2093.

12. Stenholm CW, Waggoner DB (1992) Public policy, in animal biotechnology in the 1990s: challenges and opportunities, in MacDonald JF (Eds), Animal biotechnology: Opportunities and Challenges, National Agricultural Biotechnology Council, Ithaca, New York, NY, 25-35

13. Costa-Font M, Gil JM, Traill WB (2008) Consumer acceptance, valuation of and attitudes towards genetically modified food: Review and implications for food policy. Food Policy 33: 99-111.

14. Pereira de Abreu DA, Rodriguez KV, Schroeder M, de Mosqueda MB, Pérez E (2006) GMO Technology. Venezuelans' Consumers Perceptions: Situation In Caracas. Journal of Technology and Management Innovation 1: 80-86.

15. Huang J, Qiu H, Bai J, Pray C (2006) Awareness, acceptance of and willingness to buy genetically modified foods in Urban China. Appetite 46: 144-151.

16. Krualee S, Napasintuwong O (2012) Consumers' willingness to pay for non-gm food labeling in Thailand. International Food Research Journal 19: 1375-1382.

17. Huffman WE (2010) Consumer Acceptance of Genetically Modified Foods: Traits, Labels and Diverse Information. Working Paper No. 10029. Iowa State University, Department of Economics. August 2010.

18. Chebil A, Nasr H, Zaibet L (2009) Factors affecting farmers' willingness to adopt salt-tolerant forage crops in south-eastern Tunisia. Afjare 3: 19-27.

19. Asante BO, Otoo E, Wiredu AN, Acheampong P, Osei-Adu J, et al. (2011) Willingness to adopt the vine multiplication technique in seed yam production in the forest savanna transition agro-ecological zone, Ghana. Journal of Development and Agricultural Economics 3: 710-719.

20. McFadden D (2001) Economic Choices. American Economic Review 91: 351-378.

5

Environment and Food Poisoning: Food Safety Knowledge and Practice among Food Vendors in Garki, Abuja – Nigeria

Nne Pepple*

Salem University, Lokoja, Kogi State, Nigeria

Abstract

The survey reached fifty food vendors in Garki, Abuja Nigeria to assess their knowledge of food safety, contamination, poisoning and control measures. A simple questionnaire was developed and administered one on one to the target population and data collected on their knowledge food borne disease pathogens, personal hygiene, and food handling practices, safety and risk perception as well as temperature control. 80% reported that they wash and clean their equipment; 52% reported that the exempt a sick staff from work until recovered and certified healthy; 89% reported that they wash their hands regularly with clean water. 42% reported that they use hand sanitizer frequently. 100% (all respondents) said that they washed their hands after handling raw food like fish and meat 53% lacked knowledge of optimum refrigeration temperature while 26% could not adjust refrigerator temperature. 40% had knowledge of Hepatitis A as a food borne pathogen, 20%, had knowledge of Salmonella, and 21%, E. coli, and 12% Listeria and 7% had knowledge of Vibrio as pathogens. Water supply is gotten from local water vendors from private boreholes. Comparison of the knowledge base between the non-educated and educated vendors revealed a great disparity on the level of knowledge between the two. The major source of food supply was from the Open markets while water supplies come from private bore holes. The research also showed a direct relationship between educational level and knowledge of food pathogens as well as hygiene and safety knowledge. Lack of knowledge on safety and hygiene practices among food vendors (owners and staff) indicates the increased risks of food poisoning associated with the food vendors and restaurants.

Keywords: Safety; Contamination; Poisoning; Pathogens; Disease; Risk; Hygiene

Introduction

Food safety has been a growing concern in Nigeria today. The location of some restaurants and food processing industries contributes the transmission of food poisons. According to Professor Alfred Ihenkuronye, more than 200,000 persons die every year in Nigeria of food poison caused by food contamination during processing, preservation and service. Food contaminants are mostly substances from our environments. According to Nigerian health experts, inadequate water supply may affect food safety. Drinking water may also be polluted by human activities therefore, to protect human health is to ensure hygiene, sanitation and adequate drinking are in place. The joint monitoring Program (JMP) for water and Sanitation of the WHO/UNICEF [1], noted that only 58 percent of Nigerians have access to portable drinking water.

Human activities lead to generation of wastes which constitutes a breeding ground for disease vectors and other microorganism that can contaminate food resulting to food poisoning. Pathogens gain access to (contaminate) food through improper handling, during preparation and storage. Food poisoning comes from eating food that have been contaminated with microorganisms like bacteria and viruses; Poisonous metals like cadmium or lead and chemicals. Contaminated food does not always taste bad but mostly smells and tastes very normal. Some food cause poisoning more frequent than others so they need to be properly cooked and/or refrigerated. Examples are dairy foods, sea foods, chicken etc. Universal food safety practices are to be applied to prevent all food poisoning handling practices.

Zainab Akanji, in her study on food safety noted that, 99% of working class Nigerians in urban settings eat outside their homes (mostly from food vendors) and therefore are vulnerable to poisoning if foods are not handled in hygienic conditions. These foods may pose significant public health problems due to poor knowledge of basic food safety measures [2] and inadequate infrastructures. In Abuja, the Federal capital Territory of Nigeria, only the big food companies can afford the exorbitant rent and requirement for setting up a food restaurant with the minimum quality standard. Therefore, food vendors operate in various ways like pushing their food-laden carts, from one location to another; operating under tree shades to which tends to attract more customers than others because they provide a sort of affordable, convenient and often varieties of nutritious food for their customers. Importantly also, this serve as a source of income and an opportunity for self-employment with low capital investment for the vendors [3].

A major barrier to food safety in Nigeria is lack of proper waste disposal and toilet facilities for the customers. Most of the eating stalls in Abuja are marked by unsanitary conditions, like poor drainage systems, overcrowding and poor waste disposal which leads to poor hygiene (personal and environmental) [4]. Of a great concern also is the food ingredients and the source foods. Raw materials and ingredients are usually purchased from the open markets, where the items are displayed openly on tables, ground during rain or shine, in muddy places and around filthy gutters. Buyers are mostly in the habit of touching the food stuffs for with unwashed fingers either to feel the texture or to

*Corresponding author: Nne Pepple, Assistant Lecturer, Salem University, Lokoja, Kogi State, Nigeria, E-mail: nnemikepepple2@gmail.com

ascertain the fineness of the powder in case of grounded stuff. Flies are most often found around the meat and fish areas perching all over the items with absolutely no source of protection. This also present high potential for contamination [5].

What is food poisoning?

Food poisoning (also known as foodborne illness or foodborne disease) is any illness that results from eating contaminated food. Food contamination may be defined as the presence of harmful substance (microorganism or chemical) that can cause illness in food. Food poisoning is an issue of public concern. Over the years, there have been several cases of food borne disease outbreaks and these in turn has kept the public and researchers alert that harmful microbes may be present in food that may cause diseases.

Food poisoning in Nigeria

Although the National Agency for Food and Drugs Administration and Control (NAFDAC) is working hard to monitor the quality of food and drugs sold in Nigeria markets; there is yet no system to survey foodborne diseases in Nigeria. Several cases of food poisoning which led to mortality and morbidity have been reported. According to the World Health Organization (WHO), there are two million reported cases of food poisoning with estimated deaths of two hundred thousand people from food poisoning and twenty thousand deaths from exposure to food pesticides annually – children inclusive. The food borne pathogens (E. coli and Salmonella) were mostly found to be responsible to these deaths. Harmful bacteria, viruses, parasites or chemical substances has also been linked to more than 200 diseases, ranging from diarrhoea to cancers [6]. Meanwhile, Zainab Akanji, in her study on food safety noted that, 99% of working class Nigerians eat outside their homes and therefore are vulnerable to poisoning if foods are not handled in hygienic conditions.. In April 7, 2015, there was a report of food poisoning caused by toxic metals in Zamfara state which resulted to the death of numerous infants and children. There was another outbreak of food poisoning in Ibadan, caused by Salmonella typhimurium, in a sandwich filling that claimed about 20 lives. According to the report, sandwiches were kept at room temperature until consumption following day [5]. Another food poisoning case among three families in Kano State was also reported after yam flour consumption and investigation revealed the use of certain preservatives which had a lethal effect on the consumers [7]. A similar case was also reported among five families in Illorin, Nigeria [6]. There was also a report of 60 cases and 3 deaths due to food borne disease with a symptomatic gastro intestinal disorders among people who ate in a funeral service [8]. The deaths were linked to food contamination during processing, preservation and service [9]. The improper use of agro chemicals and pesticides to control pests on agricultural products and grains were said to be responsible for the rising cases of food poisoning in Nigeria.

Health sector response to food poisoning in Nigeria

The association of food vendors in Nigeria, through various schemes, educates both vendors and consumers on the importance of quality and safe food practices. We create food safety awareness to the public. As such, we promote a clean environment for food preparation, ensuring healthy food handling and processes. The National Agency for Food and Drug Administration and Control, NAFDAC is also concentrating effort to enlighten farmers on the dangers of applying banned agro-chemicals to boost or preserve farm produce. NAFDAC is also intensifying effort in educating food vendors on hygiene and safety practices. Public Nurses under the umbrella of Professional Association of Public Health Nursing Officers of Nigeria (PAPHNON) has concluded plans to sensitise food vendors at the Garki market of the Federal Capital Territory (FCT) on the importance of hygiene practices before selling food to the public.

Research Methods

Subjects

Restaurant/eateries managers in 3 categories of restaurants in Garki were engaged in a face to face interviews using a structured questionnaire to assess their knowledge on food safety and possible causes of food poisoning. The questions were in four categories: Personal Hygiene, food handling/ storage, risk perception and knowledge foodborne disease pathogens. Their sources food and water supply were determined as well. The restaurants were also grouped in to three and their managers were surveyed: Group 1- Major hotels' restaurants; Group 2-regular/fast food type; and Group 3- food hawkers and open space cafeterias.

The survey location

This survey only concentrated in Garki area 3 and Area 10 only. Face-to-face interviews with managers and restaurant heads in the 2 areas were conducted. Data obtained were on Personal Hygiene, food handling/ storage, risk perception and knowledge foodborne disease pathogens [10]. Most of 15 questions were multiple choice questions and the questionnaire was divided into 5 sections: Demographics, Personal Hygiene, food handling/ storage, risk perception and knowledge foodborne disease pathogens. All participants' consents were collected by signing the consent form.

Sixty questionnaires and consent forms were given out, of which 50 (the actual target) consented (83%). In Group 1 (restaurants in major hotels), the managers were 82% Males and 18% Females. Minimum educational level was secondary education and all were certified caterers who had completed course in Food Hygiene. On the average, the managers have at least 8 years working experience in catering and hotel management. In group 2 (regular/fast food type), 62% of the managers were female, 38% were males, all educated with catering and Food Hygiene training experience. Average years of experience were 15 years. Group 3 (food hawkers, gardens and open space cafeterias) were 18% males and 82% females. 45% had at least secondary education. 40% had just basic education and 15% had no education at all. Only 15% in this category had attended catering school and food hygiene course. The rest did not. Participants in this category had an average of 8 years' experience in the business. Restaurants in Group one have an average of 5 staff and said they serve and average of 3000 people, weekly both in indoor and outdoor services, Group two, have average of 7 staff and serves about 8000 people weekly while group three with an average of 4 staff seem to have the largest crowd serving about 12000 people weekly.

Results and Analysis

Risk perception

81% of the respondents agreed that people could easily contract food-borne illnesses if the cooking utensils and equipment are not cleaned regularly; 42% said the illness could be contracted from the restaurant if the attendants do not wash hands after using toilets or handling dirty objects as well as before serving food; 60% said eating raw food or fruits and meat that are not properly cooked. 21% said through eating food that is contaminated by chemicals or petroleum products like kerosene and petrol. Only 52% believed that if a sick staff is allowed to cook food, he/she could lead transmit food-borne illness.

Food handling practices

84% percent of respondents reported that they wash their hands every time with water and soap before preparing foods, 10% said they wash most of the time and 6% said they wash some of the time. Hand washing habit by group of restaurant was 100% in Group 1; 92% in group 2 and 60% in group 3. Regarding the handling of vegetables, various methods were provided by the respondents about how they wash their vegetables before cooking or preparing vegetable salads; such as: Flooding under running water (60%), and soaking in vinegar and salt water (40%).

Refrigerator and temperature control

The recommended temperature for refrigerator is: -18°C/-0.4°F (freezer); 0°C/32°F (meats); 5°C/41°F (refrigerator), 10°C/50°F (vegetables). Given that most of the food items and vegetables must be stored in a cold temperature, it was necessary to assess the managers' knowledge of temperature control. The standard temperature recommended by the National Agency for Food and Drugs Administration and Control (NAFDAC) and the United States Food and Drug Administration is 41°F or 5°C maximum for internal refrigerator temperature. All restaurants in Group 1 and 2 (100%) had at least one refrigerator, gas cooker, micro wave oven, a kerosene or charcoal stove. Some of the restaurants in group 3 (55%) had at least one refrigerator, one of either gas cooker, kerosene or charcoal stove. Only 68% of the restaurant managers knew about the optimal refrigerator temperature while 32% did not know anything about refrigeration temperature. Respondents have various ways of handling left over foods. 72% said left over foods were preserved in the refrigerator and 28% said they were consumed by staff and not served to customers. About how the food is warmed, the respondents said it could be with micro wave, gas cooker, kerosene and charcoal stove depending on the available one at the moment.

Knowledge of foodborne pathogens

The following food borne pathogens were listed by the respondents: Vibrio Cholera (20%); Salmonella (30%), E. coli (25%), Hepatitis A (28%). If a large quantity of food was suspected to be contaminated 35% of the respondents said they could recover it by heating in a higher temperature for some minutes; 15% said onions and palm oil could be added to make it safe again for eating while 25% said such food should be discarded as it is no longer safe for eating.

Personal hygiene and sanitary facilities/equipment

All the respondents agreed that all staff maintain personal hygiene (100%). All restaurants in group 1 and 2 had toilet facilities. Only 12% of the restaurants in group 3 had open latrine system only for liquid wastes, located a few distances from the cooking and eating point. None in group 3 had a convenient toilet.

Pests

The respondents said that the major pests they usually encounter in their business premises, especially the store houses were: Rats (58%) Cockroaches (37%) and flies (53%).

Water supply

All (100%) of restaurants in group 1 and 2 have boreholes located within their facilities. Only 25% of the facilities in group 3 had boreholes and the remaining 75% depend on local water vendors (whose source of water is from private boreholes) for cooking and sometime use water from well for washing dishes and sometimes their vegetables.

Food items supply

55% of the respondents said they buy their food ingredients from the open markets on a daily basis, 28% used regular suppliers, 17% used company registered distributors.

Discussion

In this study, the providers' knowledge base for prevention of food-poisoning at eateries in Garki, Abuja was evaluated. The result of the evaluation indicates that most eatery operators do not have a good knowledge of food-borne pathogens and the practices that affects food safety, or those that facilitates the outbreak of food borne diseases. The knowledge deficiency was greater among street vendors and open canteens operators. This survey also provides an overview of food safety knowledge, Attitude and practices in Nigeria. The result also reveals the gap in knowledge base and the need for educational programs for the food vendors. Although some respondents knew the importance of hygiene and the circumstances that could lead to food poisoning and their preventive strategies, almost half of the respondents didn't find anything wrong with a sick person serving food. It was also discovered that although all the restaurant staff agreed that they practice hand washing, this was only after handling meat or touching what they deem as dirty objects and the proper way of washing hands was not known or followed. 85% of the staff who practiced hand washing only washed hands with water and no soap or detergent was used. But the consequences of not washing hands properly cannot not be under estimated in such a business. One thing also was discovered; most of the restaurants made use of a wooden cutting board for their vegetables and meat cuttings. Sharing this board could easily lead to cross infections. Most of them said they rinse the board with water after cutting a different object but the concern here is that rinsing with water alone could not get rid of pathogens that could hide in the little holes in the board. So, proper sanitation of these tools after each use was necessary to get rid of pathogens. Proper handwashing, hygiene and sanitation may be difficult to adhere to by restaurants in group 3 because these restaurants seldom have a borehole, handwashing or toilet facilities. It is perceived to be very difficult for restaurants in group 3 to achieve sanitation standards.

Education and food safety knowledge

The result of this survey indicates a variation of food safety and hygiene knowledge and practices between the educated and non-educated restaurant staff. Only the educated ones could identify some food pathogens while the non-educated ones named the pests (cockroaches, rats) as pathogens. Beside the formal education, those who attended catering schools had more knowledge on hygiene and safety issues than those that did not attend. Again, these ones were also able to indicate the foods that is prone to poisoning.

Implications to public health

This survey brought to light some issues related to food safety in Abuja. A good number of food vendors lack knowledge about food safety. Most of them lack both formal education and job related training that is needed to ensure safety. Some operate in unhygienic environment without appropriate facilities needed for safety. The study has also provided a guiding light for NAFDAC and other regulatory bodies to tailor their trainings.

Conclusion

Inadequate knowledge of food safety among restaurants staff in Garki is a call to action. An appropriate program to enhance the knowledge base of food vendors on hygiene and safety issues in order to eliminate outbreak of food borne illness is necessary. Individuals (food vendors, restaurant owners), should show the commitment to this course while government and other regulatory bodies should work together to develop a training package in other to avert the potential danger of outbreaks of food borne illness.

References

1. World Health Organization (2009) Global Burden of Disease 2009. Geneva, Switzerland.

2. Osagbemi G, Abdullahi A, Aderibigbe S (2010) Knowledge, attitude and practice concerning food poisoning among residents of Okene Metropolis, Nigeria. Res J Soc Sci 1: 61-64.

3. Sneed J, Strohbehn C, Gilmore SA (2004) Food Safety Practices and readiness to implement HACCP Programs in assisted-living facilities in Iowa. J Am Diet Assoc 104: 1678-1683.

4. Rheinländer T, Olsen M, Bakang JA, Takyi H, Konradsen F, et al. (2015) Keeping up appearances: Perceptions of street food safety in urban Kumasi, Ghana. J Urban Health 85: 952-964.

5. Ehiri JE, Azubuike MC, Ubaonu CN, Anyanwu EC, Ibe KM, et al. (2001) Critical Control Points of complementary food preparation and handling in eastern Nigeria. Bull World Health Organ 75: 423-433.

6. Adeleke SI (2009) Food poisoning due to yam flour consumption in Kano (Northwest) Nigeria. Online J Health Allied Sci 8: 10.

7. Adedoyin OT, Ojuawo A, Adesiyun OO, Mark F, Anigilaje EA (2008) Poisoning due to yam flour consumption in five families in Ilorin, central Nigeria. West Afr Med J 27: 41-43.

8. Fatiregun AA, Oyebade OA, Oladokun L (2010) Investigation of an outbreak of food poisoning in a resource-limited setting. Trop J Health Sci 17: 1117-4153.

9. Raab CA, Woodburn MJ (1997) Changing risk perceptions and food handling practices of Oregon household food preparers. J Consum Stud Home Econ 21: 117-130.

10. WHO/UNICEF (2017) Joint Monitoring Programme (JMP) for Water and Sanitation.

6

Forum on Science and Health Training Program for Neglected and Re-Emerging Diseases

Flávio Rocha da Silva[1,2]*, Marli Brito M. de Albuquerque Navarro[3], Alexandre de Oliveira Saísse[1], Bernardo Elias[2], Correa Soares[3] and Salvatore Giovanni De Simone[4,5]

[1]Instituto Oswaldo Cruz, Fundação Oswaldo Cruz, Rio de Janeiro, RJ, Brazil
[2]Associação Nacional de Biossegurança, Rio de Janeiro, RJ, Brazil
[3]Núcleo de Biossegurança-Escola Nacional de Saúde Pública, Rio de Janeiro, Brazil
[4]Instituto Nacional de Ciência e Tecnologia de Inovação em Doenças Negligenciadas (INCT-IDN)/Centro de Desenvolvimento Tecnológico em Saúde (CDTS), Fundação Oswaldo Cruz, Rio de Janeiro, RJ, Brazil
[5]Departamento de Biologia Celular e Molecular, Instituto de Biologia Universidade Federal Fluminense, Niterói, RJ, Brazil

Abstract

This paper analyzes the impact of initiatives toward raising awareness, refreshing and training by organizing and conducting forums and training courses aimed at health care professionals and community leaders who work in some cities of Rio de Janeiro (extending that initiative to a city in Minas Gerais). It addresses the topic of "neglected and re-emerging diseases", which has been previously deemed of interest to interlocutors involved in that proposal, especially representatives of municipal health secretariats and civil associations of a communal nature.

It should be noted that thematic contents and methodological and pedagogical strategies value objective communication that is easy to understand, without compromising scientific quality. Another aim was to expand scientific information as support to amplify communication with the government in order to help develop public policies, which translate as healthcare actions targeting neglected diseases.

Our conclusion is that it is vital for healthcare professionals, community leaders and government representatives to take part in such events in order to discuss and develop collective proposals based on qualified information about the identified themes as local health priorities to minimize the impact and progress of those diseases.

Keywords: Neglected diseases; Re-emerging diseases; Public health; Professional training

Introduction

The most relevant public health programs in global terms highlight how urgent it is to implement resources, including training healthcare professionals and technological innovation as crucial items to develop controls and/or solutions for neglected diseases and for re-emerging diseases, considering how close the two realities are, since neglected diseases have great potential to resurface. Such concerns are included, for instance, in proposals made by institutions such as the World Health Organization, humanitarian organization Doctors without Borders, among others. For neglected diseases, the conceptual summary is that they are associated with scenarios of poverty, precarious life conditions, as a consequence of profound social and economic inequalities, as a historical condition of poor countries and reflected with significant impact on the health of populations.

The denomination "neglected" is originally linked to the fact that large multinational pharmaceutical companies have no interest in making investments on research targeting those diseases. There is also a lack of financial investment from research supporting agencies to enable technological innovation in a significant scale, represented above all by more effective therapeutic resources. It should be noted that many researchers and managers prefer to use the concept of emerging and re-emerging diseases to refer to this group of diseases. This definition is supported by the concept definition. According to Brazil's epidemiological surveillance, emerging and re-emerging diseases are defined "as clinically distinct infectious diseases which have been recently acknowledged, or an unknown disease whose incidence is increasing in a given place or among a specific population. Specific factors of each disease and the location where they emerge need to be taken into account" [1].

The linearity of those concepts hides the notion that emerging and re-emerging diseases across the world are strongly boosted by the interaction of several phenomena. The context in which infectious diseases emerge and re-emerge is complex in nature and involves multiple unpredictable factors; their incidence depends on complex interaction [2].

Strengthening this complexity, emerging and re-emerging diseases compose an international scenario, mainly regarding the growing globalization which favours the identification of global public health hazards, demanding greater attention from authorities and scientific community to set up a global health program, in order to further understand international health standards related to local contexts that may generate efficient health policies that consider political, economic and social differences between countries. For instance, the tragical Ebola virus epidemic on the African west coast, showed the risk of turning it into a pandemic, having gathered international health authorities to contain spread of the virus worldwide [3].

However, the importance of formulating specific health actions

*Corresponding author: Flávio Rocha da Silva, Instituto Oswaldo Cruz, Fundação Oswaldo Cruz, Rio de Janeiro, RJ, Brazil, Associação Nacional de Biossegurança, Rio de Janeiro, RJ, Brazil, E-mail: flavio.rocha@ioc.fiocruz.br

to contain the disease in African countries must be considered as political singularities, everyone with its own socioeconomic and cultural heritage. Let us also point out that Ebola vírus outbreaks are recurrent, having occurred in 1976, 1994-95 and in 2014. Re-emergence of infectious diseaes, mainly those highly transmisssible, may impact negatively over the affected countries interfering in their comercial relations, sovereignity, safety, security, tourism and environment matters [3].

These contexts point out to the need for educational and health professionals training to make them understand the big effect that infectious diseases may have to the world, choosing among several strategies able to mitigate harm caused by such diseases spread. Ethical issues should also be regarded, specially those related to inequity in distribution of resources as well as the issues requiring decision-making skills within the field of complexity.

Supported by those contexts and conceptual indicators, researchers of InstitutoOswaldo Cruz/FIOCRUZ listed "exploratory" goals as a starting point and conducted a survey from 2010 to 2013 on skills, knowledge and experience necessary to establish a diagnosis and/or suspicion of neglected diseases in some cities of Rio de Janeiro. It was also important to enable those diseases to be recorded as re-emerging or emerging, with the purpose of expanding adequate treatment and relevant communication. The analysis of data obtained during visits, conversations with healthcare professionals and patient care observations resulted in the discovery that there was a lack of techniques, materials, training and continuing professional education toward noticing, suspecting, diagnosis, treatment and communication of neglected and/or emerging and re-emerging diseases.

After the initiative's subject of concern was identified, project "Ciência e SaúdeItinerante" was organized with the support of supervisors from the Teaching Department of InstitutoOswaldo Cruz –FIOCRUZ and participation of professionals from several healthcare institutions. The aim was to spread knowledge about emerging, re-emerging and/or neglected diseases.

The project set the following three goals: developing knowledge about neglected, emerging and re-emerging diseases; training students and healthcare professionals using relevant information about scientific and technological development; improving the scientific knowledge of teachers in public schools by active participation in science and health forums, sharing qualified information about science, health and technology for the population through community associations.

Preparing strategies to refresh knowledge and for training: forum and symposium

Motivated by an assessment of contexts that indicates the need to provide better quality healthcare services in Brazil, especially considering the universal nature of our Unified Health System - SUS, important considerations make it imperative to develop initiatives that translate into programs targeting training public healthcare professionals that work in several healthcare services. L'Abbate believes that any professional who works in a healthcare setting must systematically refresh and improve concepts and practices that reflect innovative knowledge and concepts, especially in the fields of Epidemiology and Social Sciences, in order to understand political-institutional determinants of how the Brazilian healthcare system is organized, in addition to acquiring technical domain over their several areas of work. Based on that affirmation, it is relevant to provide room for reflection that will encourage people to develop critical perceptions of the daily activities experienced by professionals in addition to

absorbing knowledge that represents an expansion of skills that will translate into an increase in the quality of care provided to the population [4].

Guided by this perspective, our account makes an analytical presentation of the proposition that resulted in organizing spaces for reflection that would encourage discussions based on the daily activities of public healthcare professionals in some cities of Rio de Janeiro. With the purpose of achieving the goal of systematic training as a means to improve the quality of services, the following events were organized: Science and Health Forum and Training Course for professionals who work in public health and for community leaders.

Health and Science forums were supported by partnerships with Health Secretariats of the Cities of Paraty/RJ, Angra dos Reis/RJ, and with the involvement of a City in Minas Gerais State, Rio Preto, in addition to other institutions, such as Centro IntegradoEmpresaEscola/RJ(CIEE) and Fiocruz, through the addition of the "Mata Atlântica" campus in Jacarepaguá.

Debated subjects were established with the participation of several local interlocutors in order to address issues that were part of those realities. Valued criteria included the needs and concerns of regions that show the potential or clear conditions or epidemiological conditions and realities that are well defined in terms of neglected and/or emerging and re-emerging diseases, considering as relevant information provided by Municipal Health Secretariats of each city and the institutions involved. It should be noted that the target audience consisted of students, healthcare professionals and community leaders.

Training course

The forums proved to be extremely important in building a proposal for 8-hour Training Courses. They allowed vital assessments used in thematic, methodological and pedagogical proposals, in addition to other strategies that were able to increase participants' interest and encourage new initiatives. Therefore, themes and methodologies for presentation sparked significant interest among healthcare professionals. They also expressed a wish to organize a few initiatives targeting greater epidemiological visibility for the region and expanding knowledge about neglected and/or emerging and re-emerging diseases in order to broaden the view on solutions for problems that are in the realm of public health, of health education and prevention, with the additional aim of raising awareness among the population about the importance of adopting habits that will translate into prevention goals, in addition to establishing a dialog with the government in order to enable public policies, reflected in healthcare action toward neglected diseases.

Strategies organizational procedures

While preparing the contents of presentations, we valued explanatory pedagogical resources whose language was easy to understand, without prejudice to their scientific precision. We should also mention that the thematic universe was established with the contribution of representatives of institutions involved, noting the public health and scientific knowledge needs that were expressed by the Cities and other participating institutions. We also paid special attention to the relevance of information published by highly credible institutions in the field of health, such as the World Health Organization (WHO), the Ministry of Health (MS), the Centers for Disease Control (CDC) and humanitarian organization Doctors without Borders (MSF). Descriptive talks were given, with practical examples of how to apply scientific knowledge.

Course materials were provided to participants with the addressed topics, with the aim to share theoretical and practical reference contents. It should be noted that those materials were tailored to the demands expressed by participants. We should also note that such events, forums and refresher and training courses also targeted the goal of training multipliers, in an attempt to cater to local demand identified among students, healthcare professionals and community leaders.

Results

Three editions of the Science and Health Forum were held between 2010/2012 in partnership with the Paraty City government (RJ), through its Health Secretariat. Forums were aimed at encouraging healthcare professional training in the Costa Verde area on infectious and parasitic diseases and/or neglected, emerging and re-emerging diseases. We intensified collaboration movements with healthcare professionals in those cities, in order to establish intentions toward continuing education and favoring issues regarding emerging, re-emerging and neglected diseases, with special mention to greater demand for knowledge about the following diseases: leishmaniasis, Hansen's disease, viral hepatites, pertussis, in addition to demand for information on vaccines. Information on possible further qualifications on other levels of post-graduate studies with respect to the issues addressed was deemed relevant. In quantitative terms, the first edition of the event in 2010 brought together 150 formally registered participants and a significant number of unregistered participants. Other events unfolding as a result of those partnerships were also organized: refresher courses in epidemiology, diagnosis and treatment of tuberculosis in 2010 and the course on epidemiological aspects, social impact and treatment of Hansen's disease in 2012 [5].

Another important development arose from the need expressed by Municipal Secretariats with respect to improving and training healthcare professionals who work with diagnosis and prevention of Sexually Transmitted Diseases (STDs). This demand is supported by demonstrative data that show a gradual increase of those conditions in the regions of Paraty and Angra dos Reis (Costa Verde in Rio de Janeiro State). Building on this concern and on the continuing partnership with Paraty's Health Secretariat, we held the III Science and Health Forum of Costa Verde in 2012. This expansion of partnerships included other specialists from research, teaching and service provider institutions, such as: EscolaNacional de SaúdePública (ENSP/Fiocruz), Fiocruz Mata Atlântica campus, Hospital Central do Exército (HCE), Universidade Federal do Rio de Janeiro (UFRJ), Universidade Federal Fluminense (UFF). The themes were expanded to include concerns regarding diagnosis, basic family care and neglected diseases training (Table 1) [5].

In the City of Angra dos Reis (RJ) the partnership also relied on contributions from Fundação de Saúde de Angra dos Reis (FUSAR), aiming to organize and stage the I Science and Health Forum in that City, one of the largest in the Costa Verde region. This Forum aimed at expanding the debate on the contexts of some neglected diseases, highlighting the approaches of public policies in the region and their ability to promote discussions about the health problems faced by the city [5,6].

The themes of the talks given at the event were: "Neglected diseases - expression of poverty and inequality"; "Aspects of the ecology of vectors of leishmaniasis in Ilha Grande", "Leishmaniasis in Rio de Janeiro State"; "Tuberculosis in Rio de Janeiro"; "Sexually Transmitted Diseases: HTLV, HPV in women and waiting for SUS vaccination"; "Strategies to control STDs and AIDS in basic care"; "Biosafety for

healthcare professionals". The event had 157 health professionals, with: 24 doctors, 40 nurses, 12 pharmacists, 4 biologists, 2 dentists, 10 nursing technicians and 65 professionals from Fundação de Saúde de Angra dos Reis.

The city of Rio Preto, in Minas Gerais' Mata Mineira zone and outside Rio de Janeiro State, showed great interest in the training program. The Zona da Mata region (MG) gathers over 37 cities. Several of those cities have high incidences of some neglected diseases. Based on this context, in 2011 we held the I Emerging, Re-emerging and Neglected Diseases Symposium. Other themes addressed based on local interests included: "the impact of pertussis in Brazil"; "leishmaniasis epidemiology and vectors in Brazil"; "epidemiology of dengue fever and its vectors"; "clinical and therapeutic care of rational states and collateral effects of polychemotherapy in patients with Hansen's disease"; "rabies and anti-rabies care in humans"; "biosafety in healthcare" [5].

In 2012 there was a Science and Health Forum edition in Rio Preto, which also included healthcare professionals, students and locals. The program established themes about public health issues and diseases such as leishmaniasis, meningitis, spotted fever, parasitoses, accidents with poisonous animals and biotechnological applications in the diagnosis of infectious-parasitic diseases.

The event gathered approximately 120 healthcare professionals, students and locals, in order to share knowledge about epidemiological aspects of infectious and parasitic diseases, in addition to addressing important issues on health and life conditions of the population. According to researcher Alba Valéria Machado, who gave the talk "Epidemiology of Leishmaniasis", the I Forum of Zona da Mata contributed to raising awareness of professionals and the population on aspects related to medically relevant diseases? The researcher thus said: "The Forum helped raise awareness among healthcare professionals and the population with respect to diseases that affect the region" (Table 2) [6].

In the city of Rio de Janeiro there were two events to raise awareness

	I Forum Year: 2010	II Forum Year: 2011	III Forum Year: 2013	Course on tuberculosis	Course on Hansen's disease
Physician	21	26	38	13	5
Nurse	31	45	44	15	14
Pharmacist	5	7	8	4	3
Biologist	2	5	9	1	-
Nursing technician	35	23	33	37	24
Other occupation	62	47	12	3	-
Total	156	153	144	73	46

Table 1: Number of professionals who took part in events in Paraty.

	I Symposium Year: 2011	I Forum Year: 2012
Physician	8	7
Nurse	15	23
Pharmacists	16	12
Biologist	7	5
Veterinarian	13	15
Teachers	10	19
Other health professionals and students	40	24
Total	109	136

Table 2: Number of professionals who took part in events in Rio Preto/MG.

about neglected and re-emerging diseases: the I Symposium on Re-emerging and Neglected Diseases for health professionals and students in Rio de Janeiro State and the I Science and Health Forum of Fiocruz in the Mata Atlântica Campus.

The I Symposium on Re-emerging and Neglected Diseases for health professionals and students in Rio de Janeiro State was held in partnership with Centro de IntegraçãoEmpresa-Escola do Rio de Janeiro (CIEE). The event took place in April 2012 and aimed to expand the public's knowledge on the issue. The meeting was part of Expo CIEE Rio2012's events. Exhibitions and reflections on the proposed thematic framework addressed the following diseases: pertussis, Hansen's disease, tuberculosis and leishmaniasis. Such reflections were summarized in the talk "Neglected Diseases: expression of poverty and of inequality". The eventtookplaceatthe Sul América Convention Center, Cidade Nova - Centro - Rio de Janeiro. Over two hundred students and professionals took part in the event [7].

The I Science and Health Forum, which took place in Fiocruz's Mata Atlântica campus in Jacarepaguá, in the West of Rio de Janeiro, gathered 150 people. The event was organized by Fiocruz in partnership with Rio de Janeiro's City Government and the scientific community of InstitutoOswaldo Cruz (IOC/Fiocruz) also joined in.

The topics were adapted to the region's epidemiological profile. The

Talks were repeated to achieve this goal. Therefore, the topic, neglected diseases in the context of social and economic inequalities and their historical recurrence in Brazil, was accompanied by more detailed technical and scientific approaches, positioning healthcare issues pertaining to, above all, hepatites. This approach was complemented by a talk on biosafety for healthcare professionals, since data show an important incidence of hepatites in infection accidents among healthcare professionals. As reflections and summary talks there were two roundtables delving deeper into the debate over leishmaniasis, re-emerging bacterial diseases, pertussis, tuberculosis and Hansen's disease.

Stemming from the Forum Fiocuz Mata Atlântica campus event, in the second semester of 2012 there were four professional refresher and development courses addressing leishmaniasis, Hansen's disease, medical mycology and biosafety (Table 3).

In all events eighteen topics were addressed (Table 4) across six forums, three symposiums, six professional development courses, with forty speakers from several health and teaching institutions. A total one thousand five hundred professionals were trained in all events.

The impact of those initiatives was that several other cities in Rio de Janeiro State expressed their wish to hold such events (Forum and Training Course). CIEE and Fiocruz Mata Atlântica scheduled the II

	I Forum Year:2012	Course on Leishmaniasis	Course on Hansen's Disease	Course on Biosafety	Course on Medical Mycology
Physician	10	4	6	2	4
Nurse	23	6	4	3	5
Pharmacists	12	2	5	2	4
Biologist	15	3	6	5	4
Veterinarian	5	-	3	1	3
Teachers	10	4	3	6	4
Other professionals and students	77	17	26	35	26
Total	152	36	53	54	50

Table 3: Number of participants at the Forum and refresher courses at Fiocruz Mata Atlântica.

	I Forum Paraty	II Forum Paraty	III Forum Paraty	I Forum Angrados Reis	I Forum Rio Preto	I Forum Fiocruz Mata Atlantica	I Symposium Rio Preto	I Symposium CIEERJ	II Symposium CIEERJ
Leishmaniasis	×	×		×	×	×	×	×	
Dengue		×					×		
Tuberculosis		×		×		×		×	×
Hansens's Disease						×		×	
Spotted fever					×				×
Pertusis	×					×	×	×	
Meningitis	×						×	×	
Neglected diseases				×		×			×
Rabies							×		
STD			×	×					
Hepatitis		×							
Venomous animals	×	×							
Public health policies		×		×					
Verminosis and		×			×				
health promotion						×			
Biotechnological application		×			×				
Graduate education		×					×		
Vaccines		×							
Head lice									×
Biosafety	×			×		×	×		

Table 4: Address topics in forums and symposiums.

Science and Health Forum and the II Symposium on Re-emerging and Neglected diseases for 2013 in Rio de Janeiro.

CIEE chose the Alemão Complex in Rio de Janeiro to host the event in 2013, with the purpose of raising awareness and suggesting pro-active actions in those communities in order to encourage preventive initiatives targeting re-emerging and neglected diseases, especially vector-borne diseases, STDs and tuberculosis. The event took place in April 2013 and featured five speakers form different teaching and research institutions: InstitutoOswaldo Cruz, EscolaNacional de SaúdePública and Hospital Federal dos Servidores do Estado. Topics under discussion included neglected and re-emerging diseases in the city of Rio de Janeiro, the rise in tuberculosis cases in Rio de Janeiro State and the spread of head lice and sexually transmitted diseases.

A scientific exhibition took place alongside the event, with interactive course materials as a way to spark interest and development of science and health in the Alemão Complex region. The following institutions took part in the exhibition: InstitutoOswaldo Cruz, Instituto Vital Brazil and Centro IntegradoEmpresaEscola do Rio de Janeiro.

The exhibition featured information about preventing accidents with venomous animals, dengue control, leishmaniasis control and barnacle activity. Videos were also shown on the topics: "The macro and micro world of *Aedesaegypti* mosquitoes: to fight it we need to know it"; "*Aedesaegypti* and *Aedesalbopictus*: a threat in the tropics" and "Triatominae: the link to a disease".

As pro-active action targeting the community who lives in the Alemão Complex, CIEE made a list of all participants so they could be included in all its different professional training and internship programs.

This proposal to raise awareness reached a total of 70 participants, most of which live in the Alemão Complex region, community leaders and university students from different regions, in addition to a significant number of children who interacted motivated by the activities suggested by the scientific exhibition [8].

The main legacy left by scientific events held in cities and at the institutions involved was affirming the need to continue initiatives to train healthcare professionals, especially with respect to neglected and re-emerging diseases.

It should be conclusively noted that a few topics were re-edited and adapted to the needs of events as they unfolded, such as exhibitions on leishmaniasis and biosafety. Other subjects such as STDs were specified as demands from the cities of Paraty and Angra dos Reis. According to the criterion of thematic adaptation to local demands, the Rio Preto-MG city government expressed interest on the following subjects: spotted fever and meningitis (Table 4).

The analysis of this process highlights the need to develop policies to train new healthcare professionals, emphasizing the importance of neglected and re-emerging diseases and the fact that many healthcare professionals who took part in the events expressed their difficulty recognizing those diseases during routine activities in healthcare units where they worked.

In professional refresher courses held after the forums, the need for continuing professional development became clear, especially about diseases such as tuberculosis, for instance, for which it was thought there was enough training for healthcare professionals. In fact, there are significant vulnerabilities, especially with respect to shortcomings regarding biosafety guidelines, in addition to knowledge on the new treatment program adopted by the Ministry of Health. Such vulnerability factors were highlighted by participants, such as outdated knowledge that interferes with professional performance and quality of care.

In summary, training programs targeting neglected and re-emerging diseases made a real contribution to local public policies. Therefore, the Training Program supported by the events described above should be extended to include other cities, and through the proposed topics meeting possible needs identified in academic education and in the process of developing scientific skills and practical actions required by healthcare professionals in their daily activities.

We emphasize that healthcare professionals must have constant access to room for reflection that will also encourage critical expression of daily experiences, revealing their views, concerns, suggestions, expressing creative proposals of people who build quality and ethics.

Our conclusion is that it is vital for healthcare professionals, community leaders and representatives of resident associations to take part in such events in order to discuss and develop collective proposals based on qualified information about the presented themes aiming to spread that information and promote preventive actions targeting neglected and re-emerging diseases in their communities, thus minimizing the impact and progress of those diseases.

References

1. Ministry of Health (2014) Brasil.

2. Souzaw, Doenças negligenciadas (2010) Neglected Diseases:Science and technology for national development strategic studies. Rio de Janeiro: Academia Brasileira de Ciências, pp. 56.

3. Emerging and Re-emerging Infectious Diseases (1999) BSCS, Mark Dabling Blvd, Colorado Springs.

4. Solange abbate L(1999) Education and Health Services: assaying capacity-building of health professionals. Cad. Saúde Pública, Rio de Janeiro 15:15-27.

5. Fundação (2013) Oswaldo Cruz Foundation & Institute.

6. Prefeitura (2013) Angra dos Reis City mayorship (Municipality).

7. Integrated Enterprise and School Centre (2013).

8. Folha (2013) Education NEWS LETTER.

Human Health Caring as General Education for Engineers: Introduction to a New Theory with Practice of Nursing

Naoko Takayama[1]* and Hiromi Ariyoshi[2]

[1]Department of Education, Asahi University, Japan
[2]Department of Medicine, Saga University, Japan

Abstract

Nursing has been given to nurse students as a professional education. But in today's aging society, not only nurses but also general public need to have the basic knowledge and skills of nursing. People with basic knowledge and technique of nursing will be willing to help people with disability.

Then Takayamahas come to realize that the knowledge and skills of nursing will help engineers develop aiding instruments for physically and mentally challenged people. This made the author start a new subject of Human Health Caring for Engineers in the regular curriculum at a college of technology, which is the first regular course not only in Japan but in the world. For the last thirteen years 1,112 students finished the course 'Human Health Caring'. The introduction and evaluation of this nursing education for engineers are reported in this paper.

Keywords: Nursing education; Engineering; Subject in regular curriculum; Nursing education; Important roles in hospitals; Social changes

Introduction

Since Meiji Era nursing education in Japan has been performed as a vocational education for producing professional nurses, who have been doing their important roles in hospitals and clinics. But with social changes like aging society in Japan, the work of nurses has not been limited in medical facilities but has been extended to social communities. The authors have come to realize that under the present day social changes, it is necessary to give nursing education not only to nurses and nurses-will-be but to the general public. The society needs health promotion, industry nursing, help for recovery from diseases and the skills to take care of the disabled and the aged at home. It is obvious that machines and instruments are one of the effective ways to solve these problems. In order to make engineers to be interested in the solution of these social problems, we started 'Human Health Caring for Engineers' in the regular curriculum at a national college of technology in 1999. The practice of nursing education for engineers is reported [1-3].

The aim and the start of 'human health caring'

The aim of teaching nursing in the regular curriculum is humanity education for engineers. In 1997 the Reformed Gender Equal Employment Opportunity Law was promulgated and the Gender Equal Society Law was enforced in 1999.With these circumstances, gender equality and empowerment have been encouraged at home and in the society, including work places. Changes, though small, have been seen in the male dominant society. This is one of the factors that enabled us to open a nursing course in the college of technology. In Japan, nursing education is categorized into seven fields: Introduction to Nursing, Adult Nursing, Gerontological Nursing, Home Care Nursing, Maternal Nursing, Child Nursing and Mental Nursing [4].

The course was named Human Health Caring and it was a full-year two-credit elective course, the introduction to nursing and nursing art in fundamental nursing being emphasized with gerontological nursing.

Outline of Human Health Caring

Definition of human health caring

The Human Health Caring is an activity to help people to maintain and promote health, understanding them as comprehensive beings, that is, as physical, social and mental beings. It is a pragmatic course of study that through the activities not only to help others at every level of health

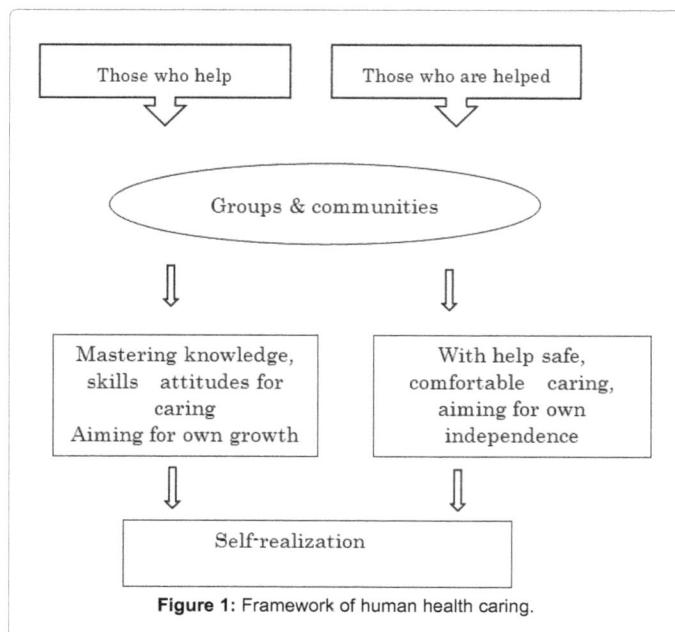

Figure 1: Framework of human health caring.

*Corresponding author: Naoko Takayama, Department of Education, Asahi University, Japan, E-mail: takayama@y-nm.ac.jp

and on the process of self-realization but also to aim at the own self-realization of helping people [2].

Components and framework of human health caring

Three components are set in the course. The first is humanity which means every phase of life, including study and practical training of gerontology and of physical disability. The second is health which does not only mean the state without sickness but to help people to live independent life with their own quality of life. The third is caring

	Reaction of learners	study fields	goals
A	understanding	Knowledge	cognitive domain
B	realizing &feeling	Attitudes	affective domain
C	helping	motor skills	psychomotor domain

Table 1: Study fields, goals& reaction of learners cf. R.S. Bloom (1966).

1st step
Basic knowledge of Human Health Caring
(Understanding of humanity, health and society)
2nd step
Basic skills of Human Health Caring
(Skills for communication and for supporting life)
3rd step
Exercises: Exercises in campus
Practice: Practice at institutions for old age people

Table 2: Three steps of human health caring.

Order	Contents
1.	Introduction to Human Health Caring Definition, framework, caring, humanism, nursing, life and living skills.
2.	Humanity and development task Human development stages, developmental task, life ethics, study of humanity for the equal cooperative society with disabled people.
3.	Helping skills
3-1	Skills of helping human activities 1 Observation with basic knowledge of vital signs Communication skills, role plays and process record Basic knowledge of nutrition and practice of meal
3-2	Skills of helping human activities 2 Basic knowledge of excretion Activities, recreation and body mechanics Practice of moving patients Basic knowledge of wheelchairs, practice with the elderly & with wheelchairs Living environment, sleep, rest, skin care & clothing
4.	Practice at nursing facilities for the aged Communication with elderly people Assistance with wheelchairs Special bathing machines & infectious diseases
5.	Welfare machines & universal design
6.	Social welfare service Social welfare, Normalization& barrier free Nursing care insurance system

Table 3: Contents of the course study.

Year	Nr. of students	Year	Nr. of students
1999	30	2006	69
2000	103	2007	81
2001	88	2008	94
2002	106	2009	86
2003	81	2010	91
2004	86	2011	104
2005	93	total	1112

Table 4: The number of course students.

which means the practical caring skills that enable learners to help the aged and people with disability, establishing good human relationship. Needless to say, both verbal and non-verbal communications are indispensable for good caring [5].

The framework of Human Health Caring is shown by Figure 1. It shows that people who help as well as those who are helped in groups and communities seem to be aiming at their own independence and self-realization.

Characteristics of human health caring and study fields

Study fields and attainable goals are shown in Table 1. The aim of this course is to give engineers the opportunities to learn to understand human beings through theory, practice and experience. In the rapidly aging society, not only caring mind and technology but the helping devices are indispensable. We built up the curriculum intending to put these necessities together in our society [6]. The Theory of Curriculum of Nursing Education by Olivia and Watson [7] and the Theory of Communication by Wiedenbach [8] were adopted for building the syllabus.

The outline and steps of learning of the course

The course was named 'Human Health Caring' in which the course attendants were all engineering major (Table 2).

Syllabus and Teaching Methods in 2012

Credit number and participants

2 credit full-year course: elective for 4th year students.

Aims

One of the most important aims of this course was to make engineer students concerned about the old and the disabled by learning and experiences. And realize the problems of the society.

Goals

A. Students are supposed to have knowledge and skills [9] to help the old aged and the disabled by learning and experiences.

B. Students study and understand barrier free and universal design by learning normalization.

C. From the engineering point of view, students are expected to find social problems and the solution.

Contents of the course

In 2013, 24.1% of the population of Japan is old age people [10]. The life expectancy of male is 79.6 and that of female is 86.4 years old. The objects of caring in this course were elderly and/or disabled people. The students studied about the human development and life cycle and learned the basic knowledge and skills of caring, which is indispensable for developing welfare devices (Table 3).

The number of course students

The majors of these elective course attendants were mechanical engineering, electric and electro engineering, civil engineering and computer science and engineering (Table 4).

Teaching methods and evaluation

In order to get the students well-motivated, as the technical terms in nursing being unfamiliar to them, we used audiovisual aids, giving the opportunities for practices and experiences (Tables 5 and 6).

Methods	Frequency	Contents
Lecture	13	Introduction, human development
Workshop	1	A good life
Exercise	10	Personal history
		Communication analysis by process record
		Self-care and room setting
		Planning daily schedule and events at an elderly home
		Role playing
		Vital sign measuring
		Meal assistance
		Practice of moving patients
		Experience on wheelchairs &, experience with the elderly people
Practice (off campus)	1	Practice at a nursing welfare elderly home
Audiovisual aids	5	Assistance of disabled people
		Meal assistance
		Excretion assistance
		Changes of position

Table 5: Teaching methods.

Evaluator	Content of Evaluation
Students	Excellent- 4.6/5 Eye opener about humanity (Attentive, positive, few failed)
Facility director	Greatly expect on engineers' concern about the needs of the old and the disabled
Facility nurse	Real practical education needed by society
Society	Awarded by the Japan National Higher Education Council(2006)

Table 6: The evaluation of the course.

Results of practice at a nursing welfare elderly home

The institution for student practice was a large nursing welfare elderly home in G city. Thanks to thoughtfulness of the institution, students were given rich practice, which was the afternoon periods in the second semester, after studying about elderly people, infection of diseases and experiencing elderly life and wheel chairs [11].

Aims of practice

1. To cultivate attitude to respect elderly people by learning and experiencing with them.
2. To learn about welfare machines and barrier free
3. To learn about welfare social resources and welfare services at welfare facilities.

After the orientation by the head of a welfare institution, students start practice beginning with wheelchairs to various welfare machines and devices. They learn and experience much of hardware and software of the institution. At the end of practice they establish good communication and relationship with elderly people. They experience pleasure of being thanked.

Conclusion

Significance of human health caring at a college of technology

There has been a great expectation that engineers are able to contribute not only to the development of welfare machines and devices but to the improvement of houses and buildings of these facilities.

Teaching method

Engineering students, unfortunately, have not many opportunities to learn about humanity. The practice at nursing institutions for elderly people has become an eye opener with humanity. Learning by experience has been effective

Nursing education

In today's aging society, non-professional nursing education is indispensable in order to live together, helping one another. Needless to say, a great many people are to be helped with new inventions and innovation by engineers.

Inner changes of students

After the practice at the nursing welfare facilities, the students have come to show deep understanding with elderly people. They also have realized the important social role of engineering by the experience of being thanked by elderly people in the facility.

References

1. Erikson EH (2001) Identity and the Life Cycle. Kanazawa Press 113-417.
2. Hatano K (1998) Basic Nursing 1, Introduction to Nursing. Medical Press 2-158.
3. Takayama N (2008) Human health caring as general science of engineering: introduction to a new theory and practice of nursing. Japan Society for Welfare Engineering 10: 2-7.
4. Takayama N (2004) Human Health Caring. Educational Press Center 1-121.
5. Takayama N (2007) Introduction to Caring Skills Educational Press Center 1-66.
6. Takayama N (2000) A Study on Nursing Education to the Students of a College of Technology. Journal of Japanese Society of Nursing 23: 279.
7. Olivia EB, Watson J (1989) Toward a Caring Curriculum: A New Pedagogy for Nursing. Medical Press 1-396.
8. Wiedenbach E (1964) Clinical Nursing-A Helping Art, pp.13-136 Gendai Press.
9. Takayama N (2001) Human Health Caring as General Science with New Theory and Practice of Nursing. Research Report of Anan National College of Technology. 37: 47-55.
10. Takayama N (2002) A Study of Understanding of the Old-Age People by Engineering Students and the Influence Factors. Research Report of Anan National College of Technology. 38: 43-51.
11. Journal of Health and Welfare Statistics (2011) Health, Labor and Statistics Association 58.

8

Hypertension Prevention and Control: Effects of a Community Health Nurse-led Intervention

Osuala Eunice O*

Department of Nursing Science, Nnamdi Azikiwe University, Nnewi Campus, South East, Nigeria

Abstract

Hypertension is a major risk factor for Cardiovascular Disease (CVD) with complications such as stroke and heart failure. Knowledge and attitude about hypertension have been indicated to influence practice of healthy lifestyle which has implications for hypertension prevention and control. There are anecdotal reports of sudden death and stroke in Isunjaba. However, there is no documentation about their lifestyle practices relating to hypertension. Health information given by nurses may positively influence healthy behaviours such as exercise, weight control, appropriate nutrition and regular Blood Pressure (BP) checks. This study was designed to assess the effects of a Community Health Nursing Intervention (CHNI) on knowledge, attitude and lifestyles relating to hypertension among residents of Isunjaba, Imo State, having the economic advantage of population-focus study in mind. There was significant difference in knowledge, attitude, and lifestyle of the two groups after intervention, P value<0.05. Health Education about hypertension to improve knowledge, attitude as well as positive lifestyles among populations should be supported by nurses, agencies and the Government.

Keywords: Blood pressure-check; Health behaviours; Population-focus; Nurse-led intervention; Lifestyle-modification

Introduction

The concern over cardiovascular disease is especially relevant in the healthcare of a developing nation like Nigeria. In Nigeria, 57 million people are estimated to be hypertensive with many still undiagnosed. Hypertension is a disease that is both common in urban and rural populace [1,2]. It has been linked to unhealthy lifestyles habits (lack of exercise and rest, consumption of alcohol, tobacco products, excess fatty foods and dietary sodium) which are common in our society today [3]. According to Das either due to poverty or affluence our lifestyle (nutrition pattern, social habits and working culture) has changed and thus increased the predisposition to hypertension [4]. Hypertension is identified as the leading cause of Target Organ Damage (TOD) like blindness, kidney failure and coronary artery diseases. Emerging data from hospital studies show that hypertension or its complication is the most common non-communicable disease in Nigeria [5].

By casual observation cases of stroke and sudden deaths have been noted in Isunjaba in Isu Local Government Area of Imo State by the researcher. These cases may be linked to cardiovascular diseases (CVD). The world being a global village, Isunjaba need to be protected from cardiovascular diseases (CVD). Hypertension if left unchecked especially in the rural area where the population is predominantly that of old people, would increase its incidence, cases of stroke, heart failure, glaucoma and renal failure. Even though many studies had been conducted on hypertension in various continents as Asia, America, and Africa by researchers [6-8]; only a few had been done in the rural area of Nigeria [9-13]. Isunjaba of Isu Local Government Area in Imo State being a rural community is not excluded.

Knowledge of risk factors, symptoms, prevention, management, and complications of hypertension may be lacking in rural dwellers in this community. The community blood pressure and attitude to hypertension prevention as well as lifestyle habits of the people is not known as few studies have been done on hypertension among rural dwellers in Nigeria. Since lifestyle influences High Blood Pressure (HBP), if nothing is done, problem of stroke and sudden deaths would continue. There is need for early diagnosis, prevention and control. Hypertension can be prevented as well as controlled through awareness, modification or elimination of unhealthy lifestyle habits. This informed the decision of the researcher to investigate the knowledge, attitude, lifestyle habits and blood pressure of rural dwellers in Isunjaba of Imo State, through a community intervention programme. Findings would be useful to Community Health Nurses in planning health promotion strategies and policy makers in planning health care programmes in relation to hypertension prevention and control.

Ethical Considerations

Approval to conduct the study was obtained from the ethical committee, Nnamdi Azikiwe University Teaching Hospital Nnewi (NAUTH/CS/66/VOL.3/009), Anambra State in line with its ethical protocol. Approval to conduct the study was also obtained from the Kings (Ezes') of respective communities and the Chairman of the Local Government Area. Participants were given essential information about the study procedure, duration, its purpose and benefits. Confidentiality of the respondents was assured by not writing names or addresses on the questionnaire and record cards. The right and integrity of the study participants was fully protected and written consent also obtained from each and every one of them. Only those who were willing to participate were included in the study.

Methods and Materials

The study adopted a quasi-experimental design. Multistage cluster sampling technique was used to select two communities in Isunjaba, assigned into Experimental (EG) and Control groups (CG) by balloting.

---

*Corresponding author: Osuala Eunice O, Department of Nursing Science, Nnamdi Azikiwe University, Nnewi Campus, South East, Nigeria, E-mail: euniceosuala@yahoo.com

A total of 442 rural dwellers (199 from EG and 243 from CG), between ages 20 and 75 years that consented, were selected.

Sample size determination

This was based on the formula for two proportions [14].

$$n = \frac{\left[Z\alpha \sqrt{2\, pc\, (1-pc)} - Z\beta \sqrt{pt(1-pt) + pc(1-pc)} \right]^2}{(pt - pc)^2}$$

Sampling procedure

Multistage cluster sampling: Multistage sampling technique was adopted: Through purposive sampling, out of the 21 Local Government Areas (LGA) in Imo State, Isu LGA and Isunjaba, one of the five towns in Isu LGA were selected. Using simple random sampling method the required number of communities, clusters of villages, households and participants were selected.

Selection of town: Isu LGA comprises of five towns, Isunjaba (a rural community) one of the towns was chosen purposively for the study based on researcher's observation and familiarity with health issues in the community.

Selection of communities: From the four autonomous communities, using simple random (balloting) technique, two communities were selected. One of the communities was assigned head and the other tail by balloting. With tossing of the coin, the first appearance which was the coat of arms (head) was assigned the experimental group, and Isuobishi (subjects) from this process was assigned the Experimental group (Group A) while Isuokporo (control) was assigned the Control group (Group B). The subjects in Isuobishi were therefore assigned into Group A, and those in Isuokporo into Group B, as experimental and control respectively.

Selection of villages: The eight villages in groups A - Isuobishi were categorised chronologically into two clusters, senior and junior groups. Similarly, same was done for the eleven villages in Group B - Isuokporo. Two villages were then randomly selected from each cluster.

Household selection: In each of the two selected villages in the clusters for the study, households were selected, using odd numbers which was determined by tossing the coin. Head (side with coat of arms) was for even while tail (side with unit of amount) was for odd. Households identified as odd from this exercise were selected until required number was got.

Selection of participants: A total of 442 subjects were selected for the study as this figure is the highest calculated sample size figure and as such accommodates the other two values. Experimental group constituted a sample of 199 subjects (45%) while control constituted 243 (55%), respectively. This was based on proportion of 968:1,184 which makes a total for a study population of 2,152. In each village, the centre was identified. Tossing the coin, based on the side of the coin, (the head is right and the tail is left) the first house on the street was identified, followed by selection of men and women alternatively from the selected households until required number was got.

A validated structured questionnaire with Correlation coefficient value of 0.76 was used to assess level of knowledge of risk factors of hypertension, attitude to its avoidance and lifestyle in relation to regular BP check, exercise and healthy diet. Maximum scores obtainable for knowledge, attitude and lifestyle were 25, 80 and 50 while minimum scores were 0, 20 and 0 respectively. Data were collected at baseline, Post Intervention 1 (P1) and post intervention 2 (P2) at three monthly intervals. The Community Health Nursing Intervention (CHNI)

consisted of instruction on risk factors for BP, consumption of healthy diet, regular Blood Pressure check and exercise. The CHNI was administered to Experimental Group (EG) for two weeks and none for the Control Group (CG). Descriptive statistics, student t test and paired t test were used for data analysis with significant level set at p=0.05.

Results

Socio-demographic characteristics

Demographic variable showed that ages of respondents ranged from 20-75 with mean 49.49+14.45. The age of participants in EG was 49.3+14.5 years while CG was 50.5+14.4 years. Ages 50-59 were greatest in number 100 (22.6%) followed by ages 60-69 [94 (21.3%)] while<30 were the least with 42 (9.5%) in number. Participants with primary school education had the highest percentage of 38.5. Participants of low income class were 243 (57.6%) while upper class was 28 (6.6%). This is based on house hold income/ day of Lower class<N 500 (<$3), Middle class N 500-2500 ($3-15), and Upper class>N 2500 (>$15) (United States Census Bureau household income [15] (Table 1). There were more women in the study than men which show cased a typical rural community in Nigeria.

Objective 1

To assess participants' knowledge of risk factors, symptoms, management, prevention and complications of hypertension.

Participants' knowledge of risk factors, symptoms, management, prevention and complications of hypertension: Table 2 shows knowledge scores of respondents. At baseline in the experimental group, 74 (73.3%) knew that blood pressure of 140/90 mm Hg is termed Hypertension, while it was 144 (87.8%) at midterm and 137 (78.7%) at the end-line. For Control group it was 96 (64.4%), 25 (20.3%) and 24 (14.1%) respectively. Response on knowledge of alcohol as a risk factor was 80 (65.0%) and 199 (100%) at end-line in experimental while it was 107 (64.8%) and 85 (48.3%) in the control respectively. In the experimental group 108 (77.1%) responded that heat sensation in the head and severe headache is a symptom of hypertension and this improved to 199 (100%) at end-line. Response by experimental group that regular exercise will help to prevent hypertension was 146 (86.9%) and 199 (100.0%) at baseline and end-line respectively while in the control it was 154 (74.4%) and 159 (78.7%). More participants acknowledged stroke as a complication at end-line. Knowledge of stroke as a complication of hypertension rose from 149 (92.5%) at baseline to 196 (98.5%) at end-line in the experimental and from 154 (88.0%) to 124 (85.5%) in control group.

Respondents' level of knowledge in experimental and Control groups, pre-and post-intervention: In the experimental group 55 (27.6%) and 94 (47.2%) had high and low knowledge at baseline respectively, while it was 131 (65.8%) and none at end-line. In control 61 (25.1%) and 125 (51.4%) had high and low knowledge at baseline respectively while it was 215 (88.8%) at end-line (Table 3). There was increase in level of knowledge in the experimental group at midterm and end-line. High knowledge rose from 55 (27.6%) to 169 (84.9%) and dropped to 131 (65.8%) respectively. In the control, high knowledge decreased from 61 (25.1%) to 1 (0.4%) and zero respectively (Figure 1). There was significant difference in knowledge of the two groups after intervention, P value 0.000 but not at baseline P value 0.68.

Objective 2

To assess the attitude of the participants to hypertension and its preventive measures.

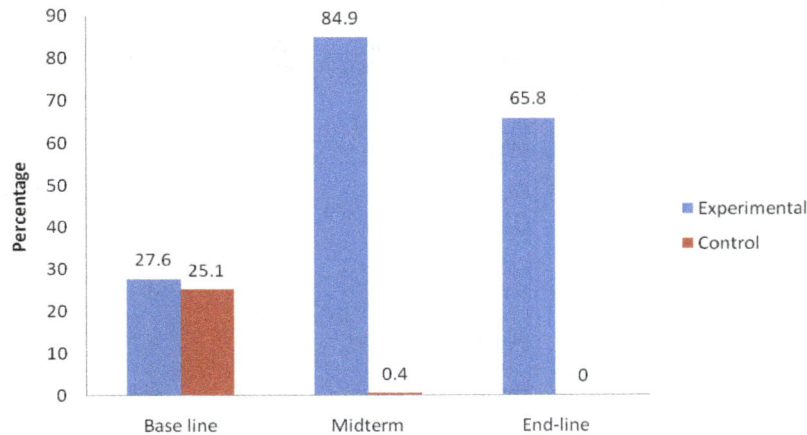

Figure 1: Respondents level of high knowledge, pre and post intervention.

Variables	Experimental N=199	Control N=243	Total N=442	X²	P value
Sex					
Male	74 (37.2)	108(44.4)	182 (41.2)	0.123	2.380
Female	125 (62.8)	135 (55.6)	260 (58.8)		
Marital Status				0.365	0.947
Married	166 (83.4)	198 (81.5)	364 (82.4)		
Single	22 (11.1)	31 (12.8)	53 (12.0)		
Separated	2 (1.0)	3 (1.2)	5 (1.1)		
Widowed	9 (4.5)	11 (4.5)	20 (4.5)		
Age (Yrs)				1.280	0.937
<30	21 (10.6)	21 (8.6)	42 (9.5)		
30-39	30 (15.1)	37 (15.2)	67 (15.2)		
40-49	43 (21.6)	47 (19.3)	90 (20.4)		
50-59	45 (22.6)	55 (22.6)	100 (22.6)		
60-69	40 (20.1)	54 (22.2)	94 (21.3)		
>70	20 (10.1)	29 (11.9)	49 (11.1)		
Occupation				9.197	0.056
Jobless	21 (10.6)	28 (11.5)	49 (11.1)		
Civil Servant	45 (22.6)	39 (16.0)	84 (19.0)		
Farming	68 (34.2)	114 (46.9)	182 (41.2)		
Petty trading	37 (18.6)	32 (13.2)	69 (15.6)		
Artisan	28 (14.1)	30 (12.3)	58 (13.1)		
Income				13.988	0.003
Upper class	14 (7.0)	14 (6.3)	28 (6.6)		
Middle class	31 (15.6)	11 (26.2)	42 (10.0)		
Lower middle class	50 (25.1)	59 (26.5)	109 (25.8)		
Lower class	104 (52.3)	139 (62.3)	243 (57.6)		
Religion				7.077	0.132
Anglican	11 (5.5)	9 (3.7)	20 (4.5)		
Catholic	147 (73.9)	200 (82.6)	347 (78.7)		
Pentecostal	33 (16.6)	26 (10.7)	59 (13.4)		
Moslem	2 (1.0)	0 (0.0)	2 (0.5)		
African Traditional	6 (3.0)	7(2.9)	13 (2.9)		
Level of education				1.655	0.647
Non formal	29 (14.6)	42 (17.3)	71(16.1)		
Primary	73 (36.7)	97 (39.9)	170 (38.5)		
Secondary	47 (23.6)	51 (21.0)	98 (22.2)		
Tertiary	50 (25.1)	53 (21.8)	103(23.3)		

Table 1: Socio demographic characteristics of respondents in Experimental and Control at baseline.

Statement	Baseline			Midterm			End-line		
	Exp Freq (%)	Control Freq (%)	Total	Exp Freq (%)	Control Freq (%)	Total	Exp Freq (%)	Control Freq (%)	Total
Definition Blood pressure of 140/90mmHg is termed hypertension	74 (73.3)	96 (64.4)	170 (68.0)	144 (87.8)	25 (20.3)	169 (58.9)	137 (78.7)	24 (14.1)	161 (46.8)
Risk factors Obesity can bring about hypertension	91 (70.0)	106 (70.0)	197 (70.4)	196 (98.5)	112 (67.1)	308 (84.2)	199 (100.0)	103 (53.6)	302 (77.2)
Tobacco products/snuff can bring about hypertension	72 (62.1)	75 (51.4)	147 (56.1)	197 (99.0)	29 (22.1)	226 (68.5)	199 (100.0)	16 (7.2)	215 (50.9)
Alcohol can bring about hypertension	80 (65.0)	107 (64.8)	187 (64.9)	199 (100.0)	87 (59.6)	286 (82.9)	199 (100.0)	85 (48.3)	284 (75.7)
Use of table salt can bring about hypertension	87 (65.9)	89 (57.1)	176 (61.1)	195 (98.0)	45 (22.8)	240 (60.6)	199 (100.0)	38 (16.1)	237 (54.5)
Hypertension is hereditary	64 (50.0)	85 (55.2)	149 (52.8)	165 (87.3)	50 (32.9)	215 (63.0)	196 (99.5)	43 (27.4)	239 (67.5)
Signs and symptoms Heat sensation in the head with severe headache is a symptom of hypertension	108 (77.1)	156 (85.7)	264 (82.0)	198 (64.1)	111 (72.5)	309 (88.0)	199 (100.0)	107 (54.6)	306 (77.5)
Hypertension may come with pain side of neck	73 (64.0)	102 (70.8)	175 (67.8)	192 (98.0)	28 (23.3)	220 (69.6)	199 (100.0)	21 (10.5)	220 (55.1)
Prevention Regular exercise prevents Hypertension	146 (86.9)	154 (74.4)	300 (80.0)	196 (98.5)	168 (82.4)	364 (90.3)	199 (100.0)	159 (78.7)	358 (89.3)
Management Hypertension is best managed in hospital	168 (88.9)	207 (89.2)	375 (89.1)	194 (97.5)	214 (91.1)	408 (94.0)	197 (99.5)	209 (88.9)	406 (93.8)
Complications Hypertension can cause eye damage	121 (81.2)	146 (80.2)	267 (80.7)	197 (72.4)	75 (51.7)	272 (79.1)	198 (99.5)	51 (23.5)	249 (59.9)
Stroke is complication of hypertension	149 (92.5)	154 (88.0)	303 (90.2)	197 (99.5)	124 (85.5)	321 (93.6)	196 (98.5)	126 (74.1)	322 (87.3)

Table 2: Participants' knowledge of risk factors, symptoms, management, prevention and complications of hypertension.

Statement		Experimental					Control				
		SA	A	D	SD	Total	SA	A	D	SD	Total
HBP is a serious ailment	1st	144 72.4%	45 22.6%	9 4.5%	1 0.5%	199 100.0	172 70.8%	55 22.6%	12 4.9%	4 1.6%	243 100.0
	2nd	195 98.0	4 2.0	0 0.0	0.0 0.0	199 100.0	196 81.0	38 15.7	2 0.8	6 2.5	242 100.0
	3rd	196 99.0	2 1.0	0 0.0	0.0 0.0	198 100.0	195 80.6	39 16.1	2 0.8	6 2.5	242 100.0
You will readily give up a habit that can lead to HBP	1st	99 49.7	78 39.2	13 6.5	9 4.5	199 100.0	104 42.8	110 45.3	19 7.8	10 4.1	243 100.0
	2nd	131 65.8	65 32.7	1 0.5	2 1.0	199 100.0	135 55.8	77 31.8	16 6.6	14 5.8	242
	3rd	179 89.9	18 9.0	0 0.0	2 1.0	199 100.0	137 56.8	75 31.1	15 6.2	14 5.8	241
Regular BP check, even when well if tool is available	1st	91 45.7	73 36.7	15 7.5	20 10.1	199 100.0	91 37.4	89 36.6	15 6.2	48 19.8	243 100.0
	2nd	89 44.7	104 52.3	3 1.5	3 1.5	199 100.0	49 20.2	29 12.0	91 37.6	73 30.2	242 100.0
	3rd	176 88.4	15 7.5	2 1.0	6 3.0	199 100.0	20 8.3	50 20.7	87 36.0	85 35.1	242 100.0
Use of table salt is good if food is tasteless	1st	41 20.6	57 28.6	75 37.7	26 13.1	199 100.0	87 35.8	77 31.7	53 21.8	26 10.7	243 100.0
	2nd	22 11.1	32 16.2	93 47.0	51 25.8	198 100.0	175 72.3	38 15.7	10 4.1	19 7.9	242 100.0
	3rd	36 18.2	14 7.1	12 6.1	136 68.7	198 100.0	193 79.8	19 7.9	22 9.1	8 3.3	242 100.0

Statement	Phase	SA	A	D	SD	Total	SA	A	D	SD	Total
HBP affects women most	1st	33 / 16.6	45 / 22.6	93 / 46.7	28 / 14.1	199 / 100.0	71 / 29.3	42 / 17.4	86 / 35.5	43 / 17.8	242 / 100.0
	2nd	63 / 31.7	23 / 11.6	66 / 33.2	47 / 23.6	199 / 100.0	130 / 53.7	20 / 8.3	32 / 13.2	60 / 24.8	242 / 100.0
	3rd	83 / 41.9	6 / 3.020	18 / 9.1	91 / 46.0	198 / 100.0	146 / 60.3	8 / 3.3	63 / 26.0	25 / 10.3	242 / 100.0
HBP does not affect youth	1st	32 / 16.1	56 / 28.1	87 / 43.7	24 / 12.1	199 / 100.0	58 / 24.0	52 / 21.5	96 / 39.7	36 / 14.9	242 / 100.0
	2nd	42 / 21.2	12 / 6.1	85 / 42.9	59 / 29.8	198 / 100.0	160 / 66.1	31 / 12.8	14 / 5.8	37 / 15.3	242 / 100.0
	3rd	56 / 28.3	5 / 2.5	13 / 6.6	124 / 62.6	198 / 100.0	183 / 75.6	17 / 7.0	35 / 14.5	7 / 2.9	242 / 100.0
HBP will develop whether one adopts a positive health action or not	1st	40 / 20.1	59 / 29.6	67 / 33.7	33 / 16.6	199 / 100.0	91 / 37.4	64 / 26.3	47 / 19.3	41 / 16.9	243 / 100.0
	2nd	31 / 15.6	9 / 4.5	92 / 46.2	67 / 33.7	199 / 100.0	168 / 69.4	43 / 17.8	9 / 3.7	22 / 9.1	242 / 100.0
	3rd	42 / 21.3	3 / 1.5	10 / 5.1	142 / 72.1	197 / 100.0	209 / 86.4	11 / 4.5	16 / 6.6	6 / 2.5	242 / 100.0

Key: 1st, 2nd and 3rd=baseline, midterm and end-term respectively. HBP=Hypertension, SA=strongly agreed, A=agreed, D=disagree and SD= strongly disagree

Table 3: Attitude of the participants to hypertension and its preventive measures.

Statement	Phase	Experimental				Control			
		Always	Occasionally	Never	Total	Always	Occasionally	Never	Total
You do regular exercise	1st	89 / 44.7	90 / 45.2	20 / 10.1	199 / 100.0	106 / 43.6	80 / 32.9	57 / 23.5	243 / 100.0
	2nd	185 / 93.0	12 / 29.3	2 / 1.0	199 / 100.0	4 / 1.7	29 / 12.0	209 / 86.4	242
	3rd	193 / 99.0	2 / 1.0	0 / 0.0	195 / 100.0	0 / 0.0	19 / 90.5	223 / 92.1	242 / 100.0
In the last 3 months you have checked your BP	1st	27 / 13.6	67 / 33.7	105 / 52.8	199 / 100.0	37 / 15.2	62 / 25.5	144 / 59.3	243 / 100.0
	2nd	192 / 96.5	6 / 3.0	1 / 0.5	199 / 100.0	72 / 29.8	4 / 1.7	166 / 68.6	242 / 100.0
	3rd	115 / 59.0	78 / 40.0	2 / 1.0	195 / 100.0	1 / 0.4	17 / 7.0	224 / 92.6	242 / 100.0
You have time for rest during the day	1st	23 / 11.6	126 / 63.3	50 / 25.1	199 / 100.0	31 / 12.8	148 / 60.9	64 / 26.3	243 / 100.0
	2nd	39 / 19.6	150 / 75.4	10 / 5.0	199 / 100.0	7 / 2.9	81 / 33.5	154 / 63.6	242 / 100.0
	3rd	115 / 59.0	78 / 40.0	2 / 1.0	195 / 100.0	1 / 0.4	17 / 7.0	224 / 92.6	242 / 100.0
You take fruits every day	1st	65 / 32.7	130 / 65.3	4 / 2.0	199 / 100.0	63 / 25.9	175 / 72.0	5 / 2.1	243 / 100.0
	2nd	184 / 92.5	13 / 6.5	2 / 1.0	199 / 100.0	2 / 0.8	234 / 96.7	6 / 2.5	8 / 1.8
	3rd	193 / 99.0	0 / 0.0	2 / 1.0	195 / 100.0	0 / 0.0	232 / 95.9	10 / 4.1	242 / 100.0
You add salt at table	1st	24 / 12.1	74 / 37.2	101 / 50.0	199 / 100.0	33 / 13.6	118 / 48.6	92 / 37.9	243 / 100.0
	2nd	2 / 1.0	7 / 3.5	190 / 95.5	199 / 100.0	32 / 13.3	154 / 63.9	55 / 22.8	241 / 100.0
	3rd	2 / 1.0	0 / 0.0	192 / 99.0	194 / 100.0	32 / 13.2	171 / 70.7	39 / 16.1	242 / 100.0
You consider your work stressful	1st	24 / 12.1	84 / 42.2	91 / 45.7	199 / 100.0	63 / 25.9	101 / 41.6	79 / 32.5	243 / 100.0
	2nd	6 / 3.0	93 / 46.7	100 / 50.3	199 / 100.0	51 / 21.1	106 / 43.8	85 / 35.1	242 / 100.0
	3rd	73 / 37.4	61 / 31.3	61 / 31.3	195 / 100.0	87 / 36.0	92 / 38.0	63 / 26.0	242 / 100.0

Table 4: Participants' lifestyle habits in relation to hypertension.

Attitude of the participants to hypertension and its preventive measures: At baseline 206 (46.6%) of the respondents had positive attitude score while 236 (53.4%) had negative. Out of the 442 participants, 316 (71.5%) agreed that hypertension is a serious ailment. Two hundred and three (45.9%) will give up habit if related to hypertension. 182 (41.2%) will have regular blood pressure checks even when well if measuring tool is available while for 90 (20.4%) stated that hypertension is not for young people. One hundred and twenty-eight (29.0%) stated that table salt should be used if food is tasteless. 131 (29.6%) also strongly believed that one will develop hypertension, adoption of healthy lifestyle or not. Attitude improved in the experimental group as positive attitude score rose from 119

(59.8%) at baseline to 185 (90.3%) and 173 (86.9%) at midterm and end-line respectively while in the control the score decreased from 117 (48.1%) at baseline to 40 (16.5%) and 49 (20.2%) at midterm and end-line respectively (Table 3).

Respondents' attitude scores to hypertension in experimental and control, pre and post intervention: In the experimental group, 119 (59.8%), 185 (93.0%) and 173 (86.9%) and of the respondents had positive attitude score while in the control it was 117 (48.1%), 40 (16.5%) and 49 (20.2%) at baseline, midterm and end-line respectively (Table 4) 80 (40.2%), 14 (7.0%) and 26 (13.1%) of the respondents had negative attitude score in experimental group while in the control it was 126 (51.9%), 202 (83.5%) and 193 (79.8%) at baseline, midterm and end-line respectively.

Objective 3

To identify participants' lifestyles habits in relation to hypertension.

Participants' lifestyles habits in relation to hypertension: Identified lifestyle habits among respondents include use of table salt, alcohol, kola, and cigarette and snuff consumption. Among the experimental group, regular exercise was done by 89 (44.7%) at baseline and 193 (99.0%) at end-line while in control it was 106 (43.6%) and 0 (0%) at baseline and end-line respectively. Within three months' participants in the experimental group that checked their blood pressure were 27 (13.6%) and 195 (100.0%) at baseline and end-line respectively while among control it was 37 (15.2%) and 23 (9.5%) respectively. At baseline fruit was never taken by 4 (2.0%) and 5 (2.1%) in the experimental and control respectively and even after the intervention. Few of the respondents in both experimental 24 (12.1%) and control 33 (13.6%) groups use salt at table. The number dropped in the experimental to 2 (1.0%) at end-line of intervention (Table 4).

Respondents' lifestyle scores to hypertension in experimental and control, pre and post intervention: Respondents with positive lifestyle habits score, rose from 119 (59.8%) at baseline 195 (98.0%) to 195 (100%) at end-line in the experimental group. It was 112 (50.2%), 30 (12.4%) and 35 (14.5%) in the control group respectively. There was steady improvement in lifestyle score in the experimental group after intervention.

Ho: There is no significant difference between pre, post-test 1 and post-test 2 in the two groups.

Comparison of mean score of knowledge, attitude and lifestyle variables in groups: This table shows the mean scores of knowledge, attitude and lifestyle variables in experimental and control groups pre and post intervention. At baseline, mean scores of respondents on knowledge in Experimental and Control were 8.7 and 8.3 respectively (SD 8.49 ± 4.03). For attitude it was 46.3 and 51.3 respectively, (SD 45.10 ± 6.51) while for lifestyles it was 21.9 and 20.7 respectively, (SD 21.21 ± 4.92). At end-line, mean scores of respondents on knowledge in Experimental and Control were 15.6 and 5.7 respectively, (SD 5.22 ± 5.22). For attitude it was 44.2 and 41.2 respectively, (SD 45.75 ± 7.35), while for lifestyles it was 21.9 and 20.7 respectively (SD 20.63 ± 5.60). The mean scores of respondents on knowledge, attitude and lifestyle of Experimental and Control groups at the three phases with P value <0.05 in Experimental group and >0.05 in the Control. There was significant difference between the knowledge, attitude and lifestyle scores of experimental and control, P value 0.000 (Table 5).

Discussion

Comparison of findings at the three phases showed significant

difference between the scores of participants in the Experimental and Control group after intervention on knowledge, attitude, lifestyle (p<0.05). Improvement was also noted in the attitude and lifestyle of the control though not significant (P>0.05). This may be attributed to the method of data collection which in its self is a form of intervention or hawthorn effect as observed in studies of this nature. It could also be due to other sources of information which is beyond the control of the researcher. Non responses, even though it did not affect the findings was observed more in the control which may be as a result of apathy observed among members. It was perceived that their expectation was that drugs would be dispensed even though they were informed there will be no payment. Prevalence of hypertension was on the increase. Only very few were obese. This may be because majority are farmers thus physically active. Fifty percent (50.0%) of all the respondents had correct knowledge of hypertension at baseline. This was lower than the findings by Familoni and Olunuga in Benin City where 59.3% of the non-clinical workers and 63.2% of the factory workers in the study had correct knowledge of hypertension [16]. This difference may be attributed to the rural setting in this study. However there was improved knowledge in the experimental group in subsequent assessments. This change may be the influence of the health education received by the Experimental group. Respondents with tertiary education had the highest score in knowledge of hypertension (44%). This is in line with the study by Samal et al. in which knowledge of risk factors was related to level of knowledge. Ninety percent knew that stroke is a complication of hypertension, 61.1% knew of negative impact of table salt on blood pressure as against 77% and 54% respectively [17]. Unlike the study by Familoni and Olunuga in which 50% knew treatment is for life, in this study it was lower [16]. There is need for dissemination of accurate information to the controls that hypertension can only be controlled and not cured.

Variable	Group	Period	Mean ± SD	P-Value
Knowledge	**Experimental**			
		Baseline	8.67 ± 3.92	
		Midterm	15.30 ± 0.99	0.000
		End-line	15.64 ± 0.52	
	Control			
		Baseline	8.35 ± 4.13	
		Midterm	6.09 ± 2.62	0.421
		End-line	5.69 ± 2.15	
Attitude	Experimental			
		Baseline	46.25 ± 4.75	
		Midterm	62.67 ± 5.88	0.000
		End-line	51.28 ± 6.22	
	Control			
		Baseline	44.40 ± 7.55	
		Midterm	43.36 ± 9.32	0.826
		End-line	41.21 ± 4.57	
Lifestyle	Experimental			
		Baseline	21.89 ± 4.53	
		Midterm	17.00 ± 2.19	0.000
		End-line	26.17 ± 1.89	
	Control			
		Baseline	20.65 ± 5.17	
		Midterm	8.85 ± 2.40	0.666
		End-line	16.17 ± 3.02	

Table 5: Mean scores of respondents on knowledge, attitude and lifestyle within groups.

Majority of the respondents with negative attitude to hypertension were of middle age. This age group should be targeted in programmes for behavior change. Many respondents strongly disagreed to having hypertension in their lifetime, whereas only 30% considered themselves at increased risk of stroke [17]. In this study fifty percent believed that the ailment is not for young people despite the fact that hypertension in younger people, especially before the age of 30 is usually more fatal than in the late fifties [18]. Same belief was similar to the participants in the Ibadan study in which 93% had difficulties to accept having new/additional Non Communicable Disease (among which hypertension is one) [19]. Apparently these participants may not go for routine blood pressure check based on their belief. However the negative attitude in this study was lower than that of the Ibadan study.

Twenty four percent strongly agreed that hypertension affects women more. Thirty percent of the participants believe that irrespective of adoption of a healthy lifestyle hypertension will still occur. This implies that some participants will readily adopt prescribed healthy lifestyle while some would not. The percentage of respondents' with positive attitude improved from 60% to 88% after intervention in the experimental group. The positive change in attitude may be attributed to the perception of hypertension as a serious ailment or peer influence during 'walking exercise' as observed by researcher. In this study, 55% have similar believe as participants in the study by Busari et al., in which 53.8% believed that the goal of treatment was to cure the disease [20]. The fact that hypertension can only be controlled need to be emphasized by Community Health practitioners to limit incidence of stroke. Even though statistically there was no association between age, sex and level of knowledge, it was observed from the findings that positive attitude was more marked in female (58%) than in males (42%). This may be due to a culture where men have all the authority as head of the family. Women are house bound in the evenings, with men gathering in their social circles, encouraging unhealthy lifestyle habits as goat head, and cow tail and alcohol consumption amongst cohorts. Negative attitude was also least marked among the respondents with no formal education, which may be due to lack of influence of Western culture which makes one more assertive. Women must be empowered so that they can influence their men's attitude. The unhealthy lifestyles in relation to nutrition include chewing of kolanut, use of table salt, alcohol and cigarette. These risk factors were also identified by Aghaji and Omorogiwa, et al., in their studies [21,22]. Consumption of snuff by some respondents was identified in this study. This may be because rural dwellers are mainly old people who prefer snuff to cigarette. A minor percentage of participants were obese. This may be because majority are peasant farmers. Majority of the respondents in this study have witnessed stroke victims in their community and therefore perceived hypertension as a serious ailment. This experience may have also contributed to eagerness in the experimental group to know remedies for prevention and control of ailment which led to compliance to prescribed regimes that resulted in the improvement in lifestyle habits after intervention. Sixty (60%) include vegetable in their meal always in experimental group and 54.1% in control. The liberal use of vegetable may be rooted in the Ibo culture of adding vegetable to all soup. This may have also contributed to the non significant difference in nutrition score of experimental and control after intervention. Food choices did not constitute a problem to the participants as was the study in China, in which lack of healthy food choices were their major barriers to lifestyle modification [23]. Lifestyle habits improved positively from 60% at baseline to 98% midterm and 100% at end-line in the Experimental group. The relapse which occurs at the maintenance stage of the trans-theoretical model of behavior change was slightly noted. This may likely be due to the flier on healthy lifestyles, the role play which must

have served as 'reminders' and support from significant others since the ailment was perceived as serious. This emphasizes on the importance of follow up and reinforcement in behavior modification or change. Regular follow up, even after this study should be maintained in the experimental community for the behavior change to be sustained and same intervention should also be replicated in the control community.

Conclusion

There was marked improvement in knowledge, attitude and lifestyle relating to hypertension control after community health nursing intervention in Isunjaba. This led to improved regular blood pressure checks by community members, donation of blood pressure measuring tools by philanthropists for distribution in all wards. Regular health promotion information by nurses is recommended for sustainability of knowledge, attitude, health promoting activities and lifestyle. Study need to be replicated in other rural communities in Nigeria to arrest the upward trend in hypertension prevalence in the country and Africa sub-region.

Greater percentage of the respondents had low knowledge at baseline but knowledge improved greatly in the experimental group after intervention. More than half of the participants with high blood pressure were only revealed during screening. Knowledge and awareness of risk factors is a component of behavior change as shown by finding in this study, Self-measurement blood pressure devices should be possessed by each household. Mobile clinics involving collaborative approach should be adopted. Policy on attitudinal and lifestyle changes in relation to hypertension prevention and control amongst the youth and middle aged should be put in place. Even though 70% agreed that hypertension is a serious ailment, only half of the participants have positive attitude and were willing to take up recommended lifestyle habits. Programme for attitudinal change need to be intensified for the youth and middle aged amongst whom the negative attitude and poor lifestyle were most marked. Continuity of the programme is important for sustainability. The intervention programme should also be carried out in the Control community as well.

Acknowledgements

Dr O Abimbola Oluwatosin and Prof S Kadiri of the Faculty of Clinical Sciences, University of Ibadan, Oyo State, Nigeria are being acknowledged for their supervision of this study.

References

1. Jolly S, Vittinghoff E, Chattopadhyay A, Bibbins-Domingo K (2010) Higher cardiovascular disease prevalence and mortality among younger blacks compared to whites. The American Journal of Medicine 123: 811-818.

2. Okpechi IG, Chukwuonye II, Tiffin N, Madukwe OO, Onyeonoro UU, et al. (2013) Blood pressure gradients and cardiovascular risk factors in urban and rural populations in Abia State South Eastern Nigeria using the WHO STEP wise approach. PLoS ONE 8: e73403.

3. World Health Organization (2002) The world health report 2002: reducing risks, promoting healthy life. World Health Organization.

4. Das SK, Sanyal K, Basu A (2005) Study of urban community survey in India: growing trend of high prevalence of hypertension in a developing country. Int J Med Sci 2: 70-78.

5. Abonnema Foundation (2013) Hypertension in Nigeria: Rising to the challenge.

6. Metintas S, Arikan I, Kalyoncu C (2009) Awareness of hypertension and other cardiovascular risk factors in rural and urban areas in Turkey. Transactions of the Royal Society of Tropical Medicine and Hygiene 103: 812-818.

7. Egan BM, Zhao Y, Axon RN (2010) US trends in prevalence, awareness, treatment, and control of hypertension, 1988-2008. JAMA 303: 2043-2050.

8. Iyalomhe GB, Iyalomhe SI (2010) Hypertension-related knowledge, attitudes and life-style practices among hypertensive patients in a sub-urban Nigerian community. Journal of Public Health and Epidemiology 2: 71-77.

9. Ekwunife OI, Udeogaranya PO, Nwatu IL (2010) Prevalence, awareness, treatment and control of hypertension in a Nigerian population. Health 2: 731-735.

10. Osuala EO, Abimbola OO, Kadiri S (2014) Knowledge, attitude to hypertension and lifestyle habits of rural dwellers in Owerre-Nkwoji, Imo State Nigeria. Journal of Public Health and Epidemiology 6: 48-51.

11. Demaio AR, Otgontuya D, de Courten M, Bygbjerg IC, Enkhtuya P, et al. (2013) Hypertension and hypertension-related disease in mongolia; findings of a national knowledge, attitudes and practices study. BMC Public Health 13: 194.

12. Oladapo OO, Salako L, Sadiq L, Soyinka K, Falase AO (2013) Knowledge of hypertension and other risk factors for heart disease among Yoruba rural South Western Nigeria. BJMMR 4: 993-1003.

13. Balogun MO, Olugbenga O (2013) Prevalence of hypertension in three rural communities of Ife north local Government Area of Osun state, south West Nigeria. International Journal of General Medicine 6: 863-868.

14. Maxwell FP (1998) A-Z of Medical statistics. A comparison for critical appraisal. Oxford University Press Inc., New York, USA.

15. US Bureau (2006) United States Census Bureau. Household Income.

16. Familoni OB, Olunuga TO (2005) Comparison in the knowledge and awareness of hypertension among hospital and factory workers in Sagamu, Nigeria. Nigerian Medical Practitioner 47: 43-45.

17. Samal D, Greisenegger S, Auff E, Lang W, Lalouschek W (2007) The relation between knowledge about hypertension and education in hospitalized patients with stroke in Vienna. Stroke 38: 1304-1308.

18. Ige OK, Owoaje ET, Adebiyi OA (2013) Non communicable disease and risky behavior in an urban University Community in Nigeria. Afr Hlth Sci 13: 62-67.

19. Busari OA, Olusegun T, Olufemi O, Desalu O, Opadijo OG, et al. (2010) Impact of Patients' Knowledge, Attitude and Practices on hypertension on compliance with antihypertensive drugs in a resource-poor setting. TAF Prev Med Bull 9: 87-92.

20. Aghaji MN (2008) Hypertension and risk factors among traders in Enugu, Nigeria. Journal of College of Medicine 13: 114-115.

21. Omorogiwa A, Ezenwa EB, Osifo C, Ozor MOE, Khator CN (2009) Comparative study on risk factors for hypertension in University setting in Southern Nigeria. International Journal of Biomedical and Health Sciences 5: 103-107.

22. Chan RSM, Lok KYW, Sea MM, Woo J (2009) Clients' experiences of a commodity based lifestyle modification programme: A qualitative study. Int J Environ Res Public Health 6: 2608-2622.

23. Prochaska JO, Redding CA, Evers KE (2002) The Transtheoretical Model and Stages of Change in Health Behaviours and Health Education: Theory, Research and Practice. New Jersey, USA, pp: 280-282.

9

Impact of Interprofessional Education for Medical and Nursing Students using Simulation Training and a Training Ward

Adina Dreier-Wolfgramm[1], Sabine Homeyer[1], Angelika Beyer[1], Stefanie Kirschner[1], Roman F. Oppermann[2], and Wolfgang Hoffmann[1]

[1]*Department of Epidemiology of Healthcare and Community Health, University Medicine Greifswald, Greifswald, Germany*
[2]*Department of Health, Nursing and Management, University of Applied Science Neubrandenburg, Germany*

Abstract

Background: Interprofessional teamwork has become increasingly important to provide patient centered care. Physicians and nurses as two major professions are needed to be adequately qualified. Interprofessional Education (IPE) is an eligible approach. Nevertheless, there is a lack of the impact for both professions. Therefore, we implemented and evaluated simulation training and a collaborative working sequence on a training ward. The aim was to analyze the course structure and assess learning effects to evaluate the suitability for IPE.

Methods: A mixed methods study with a sequential explanatory design was conducted. A total of five medical and five nursing students were involved. Students completed questionnaire based interviews after IPE lectures. Two group discussions were conducted to specify and expand quantitative evaluation results. For descriptive statistics, we used the software package SPSS. Both group discussions were analyzed by a qualitative content analysis using the software MAXQDA.

Results: Students rated IPE predominantly positive. The learning contents broadness and the links between theory and practice. Students identified six core learning effects: (1) Realization of the importance for collaborative working; (2) Gaining knowledge about the roles of both professions; (3) Realization, that interprofessional care facilitates work; (4) Practicing communication between physicians and nurses; (5) Improving collaborative communication with the patient; and (6) Understanding chances and challenges of joint decision making. Nevertheless, students suggested improvements, e.g., the scenarios of the simulation training should be expanded.

Conclusion: The results provide clear evidence that IPE by simulation training and a training ward is feasible and well accepted by students in a German medical school. Results can be used to adapt IPE lectures and to implement them for a larger number of students. The next step is to generalize findings and to sustainably implement IPE in both curricula.

Keywords: Interprofessional education; Education research; Education medical; Graduate education; Nursing; Baccalaureate; Health education; Empirical research

Introduction

Interprofessional teamwork among health care professionals has become increasingly important. A changing health care system caused by an aging population with increasing demands of health care services in both, primary care and hospitals, are the main challenges. This leads to a growing complexity of health care and the World Health Organization (WHO) already considered in 2006 that interprofessional teamwork is required to ensure appropriate patient centered health care [1]. Therefore, health care professionals must be qualified for an effective collaboration with other health care professions in a multidisciplinary team. Physicians and nurses as the two major professions in the health care system are affected in particular. Current health care education concepts do not adequately prepare medical and nursing students for interprofessional team work [2]. Hence, innovative educational approaches are required [3]. Interprofessional Education (IPE) is an effective tool for teaching team-based care [4,5]. Previous studies have proven that IPE supports a safe and high quality provision of patient care [6-8]. IPE can be divided into three primary areas: (1) Didactic learning; (2) Simulation training; and (3) Authentic clinical experiences [9]. The primary goal is to teach students in teamwork skills and to gain understanding of health care professionals roles [10].

In particular, learning in practice based settings by simulation trainings and clinical exercises on training wards are two important teaching methods for IPE [6,11,12]. Simulation trainings comprise a range of learning opportunities including communication, role identification, team working and conflict resolution [7,13,14] and has been comprehensively explored for the medical and nursing profession [10]. Evaluations have shown their effectiveness for improving medical and nursing student's communication skills [15-17]. A training ward enables an exercise of care for patients in a learning environment under supervision [18]. Over the last 20 years, IPE implemented as clinical training wards has increased [19]. Morphet et al. stated that training ward enhance medical and nursing students' understanding of the importance of team-based care as well as their understanding of their roles and the roles of other health care professionals [18]. The implementation and evaluation of IPE by simulation trainings and training wards are still rare in Germany. Therefore, we implemented and evaluated an interprofessional simulation training and a collaborative working sequence at the palliative care training ward for medical and nursing students.

*Corresponding author: Adina Dreier-Wolfgramm, Department of Epidemiology of Healthcare and Community Health, Institute for Community Medicine, University Medicine Greifswald, Ellernholzstr. 1-2, 17487, Greifswald, Germany, E-mail: adina.dreier@uni-greifswald.de

Materials and Methods

Design and implementation of the IPE

The simulation training took place at the skills lab of the University Medicine Greifswald. Although this facility provides an ideal setting for IPE, this was the first time to use it for this learning approach. The simulation training case was on caring for a patient with a bronchial carcinoma in an advanced stage. The current state of patients' health required a hospital treatment.

In the first scenario, the nurse worked in a hospital setting at the department of internal medicine. It is weekend and the state of patient's health impaired (e.g., difficulty in breathing, strong sweating, fear of death). Now, the nurse is responsible to inform the physician about the patient's history and his current state of health. The challenge is the patient has not been treated by the physician until now. In the second scenario, the physician and nurse conducted an assessment regarding the current patient's health care needs (e.g., patient's posture, monitoring color, respiratory sounds, vital parameters, breathable quality). Subsequently, interventions were developed in collaboration. The patient was then informed about the next medical treatment steps and the nursing interventions. Both scenarios were monitored by the lecturer. Overall, the simulation training took 90 minutes including a (1) theoretical introduction to bronchial carcinoma, the (2) review of the two scenarios, the (3) exercise in the two simulation scenarios and a (4) feedback round among the students, the lecturer and the simulation patient. All students participated in the two simulation scenarios. During the simulation training, interprofessional teams, consisting of one medical and one nursing student were formed. The medical student was asked to act as the physician and the nursing student took the role of a nurse.

The IPE working sequence on the palliative care training ward went for four hours per team (one medical and one nursing student). This lecture took place on the palliative care training ward of the University Medicine Greifswald, which was previously available only for nursing students in their 3-year vocational nursing training.

The working sequence was conducted with a 'real patient' (one patient per team) including an (1) introduction of the training ward, (2) enabling patient file viewing (identification of primary health care needs), (3) first patient contact (collect general data about the disease and patient history), (4) conducting an assessment regarding the current patient's health status (e.g. activities of daily living, pain, mobility, nutrition), (5) reflection of the assessment data and information exchange between the medical and nursing student, (6) collecting vital parameters, (7) identification of treatment goals and development of interventions in collaboration between the medical and nursing student, (8) reflection round between the students and the lecturer. During the patient contact (see 3,4,6), students were entirely interactive with each other, learning from each other's perspective and helping each other (e.g., handling blood pressure monitor) when needed. The lecturer was present the entire time to aid or support in case of questions.

Research questions and study aim

We examine following research questions: (1) How assess students the course structure? (2) What are the learning effects of IPE? and (3) How evaluate students both lectures suitable for IPE? The aim is to prove feasibility of IPE and to prepare a sustainable implementation of IPE by simulation trainings and training wards in Germany.

Research design

We conduct a mixed methods study with a sequential explanatory design to evaluate the course structure, learning effects and the suitability of simulation training and working sequences on a training ward for IPE.

Medical and nursing students

A total of ten students (n=5 medical students of the University Medicine Greifswald, n=5 nursing students of the University of Applied Science Neubrandenburg) participated in the study. Both student groups were in the first year of their academic programs and had no previous experiences in IPE. We verbally invited students in their introduction lectures of the academic programs to participate in the study and they received written project information's and a written informed consent. Upon written informed consent of the first five medical and five nursing students, ten students were enrolled in the study.

Four medical students are male and the average age is 26 (SD: 4.0). Two of them had completed a 3-year vocational training in nursing before their medical academic training. Four nursing students are female and the average age is 25 (SD: 3.0). Four nursing students already had completed a 3-year vocational training in nursing.

Lecturers

We recruited faculty members of the University Medicine Greifswald, who had clinical experiences of both student's groups and had taught in simulation training as well as on a training ward. The lecturer of simulation training was a general practitioner and an expert in palliative care. He had extended experiences in teaching clinical skills by simulation trainings and was one of the lecturers, who implemented and Objective Structured Clinical Examinations (OSCE) for medical students at the University Medicine Greifswald. A practice supervisor of the 3-year vocational nursing training was the lecturer for the collaborative working on the palliative care training ward. She had comprehensive experience on the training ward and with supervision of nursing students. One study team member briefed both lecturers prior to IPE regarding the learning contents, tasks and learning objectives.

Data collection

The Bildungscluster study is one of the first studies in Germany exploring IPE by simulation training and collaborative working on a training ward. No valid and reliable instrument for the quantitative quantitative interprofessional course evaluation was available. Consequently, we developed a questionnaire which consists of 13 Items in three sections: (a) content-related design of the lecture and evaluation of the lecturer (three items), (b) learning effects (seven items) and (c) suggestions for improvement (three items). Eight items were scored on a 4-point Likert scale with anchors 1 (completely agree) to 4 (completely disagree) or 1 (very well) to 4 (bad) or 1 (substantially higher) to 4 (unchanged). The group size assessment for a learning success were evaluated by 1 (spot on), 2 (too small) and 3 (too big). Four items (description of learning effects by IPE [1 item] and suggestions for improvement [3 items]) were captured as free text.

We pre-tested the survey instrument in small groups with representatives of both student groups and then digitized it using TeleForm® (Electric Paper Information Systems GmbH Lüneburg Germany, version 10.2). The students completed the questionnaire after the two IPE lectures. We scanned all questionnaires and verified them in TeleForm®. For analysis, we documented the data in an MS-access data base and transferred them to the software package IBM® SPSS® Statistics (Version 22, Ehningen). To specify aspects, which could not be adequately addressed in the quantitative evaluation, we conducted two group discussions (one with the medical students and one with the nursing students). Semi-structured questions were developed based on the results of the quantitative evaluation and addressed (a) the learning effects of IPE in general, (b) the learning effects by the simulation training and on the training ward as well as (c) the suggestion for improvement. We audio recorded and transcribed both group discussions.

Data analysis

For descriptive statistics, we used the software package SPSS. To analyze both group discussions, we conduct a qualitative content analysis using the software MAXQDA (Version 12, VERBI GmbH, Berlin) [20]. Two study team members conducted the coding of the group discussions according to the consensual coding approach [20]. In a first step, both team members coded the discussions separately. In a second step, both coders compared their category system with respect to similarities and differences. Differences were discussed and the category system was modified if both coders agreed. In the majority of cases, this caused an extension of the category system. Subsequently, we developed a system with categories, sub-categories and codes based on the code systems of both coders. The qualitative results were then integrated to the quantitative results for data interpretation.

Results

IPE lectures-course structure and lecturer

Both student groups rated the course structure and the lecturers predominantly positive. Especially the learning content broadness and the linkage of theory and practice were assessed as 'very well' and 'well' for both, the simulation training and the training ward (Table 1).

In addition, the majority of students reported, that the group size for effective learning was 'spot on' for both IPE lectures (n=10 simulation training, n=9 training ward). Only one medical student stated the theoretical introduction of the simulation training with all students as 'too big'.

Comments for the lecturers were positive by a considerable number of both student groups. All students stated that both lecturers were well prepared, very involved and able to explain complex contents. Differences between medical and nursing students concerned the assessment of lecturer's promotion of student's active involvement in IPE and giving feedback: while all medical students 'completely agree' or 'agree' with the respective statements, three nursing students only 'less agree' and one nursing student completely disagreed with the lecturers' feedback giving. These results are summarized in Table 2.

Learning effects

All participating medical and nursing students reported learning effects and both IPE lectures were rated as interesting as well as the IPE approach promotes the interest for these lectures. Therefore, the majority of students would participate in these two IPE lectures again. Only one nursing student mentioned that it is rather unlikely to participate in IPE by collaborative working on the training ward again (Table 3).

A detailed description of the learning effects by IPE in general and for the two lectures is reported in Table 4. Students identified six core learning effects: (1) Realization of the importance for collaborative working; (2) Gaining knowledge about roles of both professions; (3) Realization, that interprofessional care facilitates work; (4) Exercise communication between physicians and nurses; (5) Exercise collaborative communication with the patient; and (6) Making joint decisions (Table 4).

These learning effects were specified in the qualitative group discussions. For example, the realization of the importance for collaborative working is to student's opinion connected with the recognition that physicians and nurses complement each other in patient care and can work as equal collaboration partners.

Therefore, IPE can promote the openness of medical and nursing students for interprofessional care practice. In addition, both student groups reported special learning effects for both IPE lectures. The simulation training allows students to exercise collaboration by a feeling of a 'real patient' situation.

Five students pointed out (n=2 medical, n=3 nursing) that the learning effect could be enhanced by a real patient instead of a professional actor. The collaborative working on the training ward supports students to realize the importance of patient collaborative assessment (e.g., mutual support in patients' assessment, information exchange) and allows to exercise practical skills (e.g., assessment of vital parameters, correct measurement of blood pressure).

In summary, IPE lectures had a positive effect on the medical and nursing students' level of knowledge. The majority reported, that their level of knowledge is 'substantially higher' or 'higher' (n=9 simulation training, n=7 training ward) after both IPE lectures. One nursing student stated hardly any change in her state of knowledge by the simulation training and the collaborative working on the training ward. Two other nursing students agree with this assessment with respect to the training ward. In consequence, all medical students and eight nursing students rated the simulation training and the collaborative working on the palliative care training ward as suitable for IPE. Only two of the nursing students mentioned, that the collaborative working on the training ward is to their opinion less eligible for IPE (Table 3).

Suggestions for improvement

To further enhance learning effects both student groups suggested improvements. The Table 5 shows that five students (n=2 medical, n=3 nursing) would appreciate when IPE lectures would be taught by lecturers of both professions.

The simulation training would be more effective with a preparatory seminar for theoretical knowledge about the disease of the simulation patient would be preceded before. Three students expressed their wish to expand the number of exercises for the two scenarios which includes a changing role between medical and nursing students. For further development of the simulation training, the expansion of scenarios to other diseases and a more detailed feedback to students' performance in the scenarios would be desirable.

An adaption of the schedule to one day for the collaborative working on the palliative care training ward would enhance the learning effects to one medical student's point of view.

Discussion

The results provide clear evidence that IPE by simulation training and collaborative working on a training ward is feasible and suitable for medical and nursing students in a German medical school. In particular, the study demonstrated that IPE can help to adequately

	Simulation Training								Training ward							
	Medical students (n)				Nursing students (n)				Medical students (n)				Nursing students (n)			
	very well	well	less well	poor	very well	well	less well	poor	very well	well	less well	poor	very well	well	less well	poor
Course structure	3	2			2	3			5				3	2		
Learning content broadness	4	1			4	1			3	2			1	3	1	
Linkage theory and practice	3	2			2	3			3	2			3	1	1	
Learnability in predefined time	1	3	1			5			2	3				5		

Table 1: Quantitative evaluation results of the students regarding the course structure (N=10).

	Simulation Training								Training ward							
	Medical students (n)				Nursing students (n)				Medical students (n)				Nursing students (n)			
	completely agree	agree	less agree	completely disagree	completely agree	agree	less agree	completely disagree	completely agree	agree	less agree	completely disagree	completely agree	agree	less agree	completely disagree
Lecturer … … was well prepared	5				3	2			5				5			
… was very involved	5				3	2			5				5			
… making complicated understandable	5				1	4			3	2			4	1		
… promoting active involvement	3	2			1	2	2		5				5			
… gave feedback to active involvement	5				1	2	1	1	4	1			4	1		

Table 2: Quantitative evaluation results of the students regarding the lecturer assessment (N=10).

	Simulation Training								Training ward							
	Medical students (n=5)				Nursing students (n=5)				Medical students (n=5)				Nursing students (n=5)			
	completely agree	agree	less agree	completely disagree	completely agree	agree	less agree	completely disagree	completely agree	agree	less agree	completely disagree	completely agree	agree	less agree	completely disagree
The lecture was interesting	5				4	1			4	1			3	2		
IPL promoting my interest for the lecture	2	3			1	3	1		2	3			2	3		
I would participate in this IPL lecture again	3	2			2	3			2	3			2	2	1	
There is a learning effect by IPL	4	1				3	2		2	2	1		1	2	1	1
The lecture is eligible for IPL	3	2			3	2			3	2			3		2	

Table 3: Students learning effects (N=10), quantitative results.

prepare medical and nursing students to work in a collaborative team approach. The students of both professions rated the lectures predominantly positive.

One important finding was that a course structure including a linkage of theory and practice is important and the chosen group sizes for the IPE lectures could be implemented well. A second major finding was the identification of the six core learning effects of IPE including the realization of the importance of collaborative working, gaining knowledge about other health care professional's roles and practicing collaborative communication. These findings are comparable to recent studies. Ker et al. mentioned that structured IPE in a realistic clinical environment can support the development of competences in interprofessional working. This approach allows medical and nursing students to exercise skills by a multidisciplinary exchange and getting feedback from different perspectives in order to maximize learning effects [21]. To enhance students' understanding of their own professional roles and the roles of the other profession is one of the most commonly mentioned benefit of IPE. It includes the willingness to learn more about each other's philosophy and to share knowledge within an interprofessional team [22-25]. This supports correct decision making in the treatment of patients [26].

Based on IPE lectures in the Bildungscluster study, both student groups learn more about health care professional roles and conclude that physicians and nurses complement each other. Furthermore, a patient centered care requires a collaborative communication between both professions including making joint decisions. This underlines the urgency to improve teaching interprofessional communication skills by IPE [27,28].

To further develop IPE in Germany, participating medical and nursing students made suggestions for improvement, e.g. that IPE should be taught by lecturers of both professions and the scenarios of the simulation training should be expanded. This result agrees with some prior research. For example, Bastami et al. reported of an IPE lecture for medical and nursing students to exercise communication

Learning effects
Both IPL lectures
Realization of the importance for collaborative working
working as equal collaboration partners
physicians and nurses complement each other
greater openness for interprofessional collaboration
Gaining knowledge about the roles of both professions
capable to understand specific roles of both professions
Interprofessional care facilitate the work
hierarchical structures are counterproductive
Exercise communication between physicians and nurses
active listening
negotiate agreements
respond to each other
have the guts to ask questions
accepting feedback to patient care from the nursing profession
Exercise collaborative communication with the patient
empathic patient care
Make joint decisions
Simulation Training
Feeling of real patient situation
real patients as simulation patient increase the learning effect
Training ward
Realization of importance of collaborative patient assessment and patient admission
collaborative patient file viewing
mutual support by patients assessment
information exchange between both professions
requirement of adaption of assessment documentation as one for both professions
Exercising practical skills
assessment of vital parameters
correct measurement of blood pressure

Table 4: Detailed description of students learning effects (N=10), qualitative data.

Suggestion for improvement
Both IPL lectures
IPL lectures should be taught by lecturers of both professions
Simulation Training
A seminar for theoretical knowledge about the disease of simulation patient should be preceded before
expand the number of the exercises of the two scenarios for increasing the learning effect
changing role of medical and nursing student's development of scenarios for other diseases
expansion of the feedback round for student
expansion of feedback to nursing student performance.
Training ward
Time scale should be expanding to one full day

Table 5: Students suggestions for improvement (N=10), qualitative results.

in breaking bad news. Lecturers of both professions were included to ensure a specific feedback for both students groups as well as to reflect the lecture from different perspectives [29]. The German Medical Association underlines in their position paper 'Interprofessional Education for Health Care Professionals, 2015, that IPE lectures should always involve lecturers from all professions included in IPE. Thereby, a specific qualification for instructors is required and suitable concepts for advanced trainings are needed to develop [30].

The number of scenarios in IPE simulation trainings varies in different studies from one to four or more depending on the schedule and the focus of the IPE lectures [14,26]. The Bildungscluster Study used two scenarios based on the two primary learning aims of collaborative communication (scenario one) and exercising practical skills (scenario two).

The study has several limitations. First, the small number of ten participating students and the selection process maybe, was biased. The Bildungscluster Study addresses the feasibility of IPE for medical

and nursing students in Germany. Based on that, we chosen a small group size of ten. Internationally, IPE in small groups with ten to 15 students is widely used [29,31,32]. A first implementation with a small group size allows to test IPE courses and subsequently to adapt the lectures for a larger number of students [33]. Four nursing students and two medical students completed a 3-year vocational nursing training. Consequently, the chosen recruiting procedure suggests that we enrolled students, who are more interested in IPE in contrast to other medical and nursing students. Therefore, the generalization of the results is limited.

Secondly, no valid and reliable instrument for the quantitative evaluation was available. Internationally, a range of instruments has been proposed to evaluate different aspects of IPE [34]. In Germany, there is only the German version of the "Readiness for Interprofessional Learning Scale" (RIPLS) available. Mahler et al. conducted a validation study and concluded that a further development of the instrument is needed [35]. In addition RIPLS evaluates attitudes to IPE in contrast to the main focus the Bildungscluster Study, which includes the evaluation of the course structure, learning effects and eligibility to IPE. Therefore, we developed and pre-tested a questionnaire with ten representatives of both student's groups. No adaptions were required and subsequently we used the instrument for the Bildungscluster study with no changes.

In summary, we implemented and evaluated as one of the first studies in Germany the feasibility of IPE by using simulation training and a collaborative working on a training ward. We used places of learning, which had been not available for medical or nursing students before. The results are the basis to improve both IPE lectures (e.g., lecturers from both professionals should be involved, expansion of simulation scenarios) and to implemented and to evaluated them with a larger number of medical and nursing students. Further studies are needed to address changes in learning effects by the expansion of simulation scenarios and the involvement of lecturers of both professions. This is required to be able to generalize findings and to sustainably implement IPE in both curricula in Germany.

Acknowledgement

The first implementation and evaluation of IPE between medical and nursing students at the University Medicine Greifswald and the University of Applied Science Neubrandenburg was accompanied and supported by the participating students and lecturers. The authors wish to thank following person listed in alphabetical order: Nanja van den Berg, Ines Buchholz, Andreas Flick, Andreas Jülich, Jens Thonack, Sandra Huber, Nikolas Zimowski. A scientific advisory board with several experts from different fields supported the study by the development of a strategy paper to sustainably implement IPE between medical and nursing students in the curricula of both professions. Therefore, the authors wish to thank: Reiner Biffar, Jean-François Chenot, Wolfgang Gagzow, Peter Hingst, Anja Kistler, Arthur König, Christine Lorenz, Steffen Piechullek, Rainer Rettig, Hagen Rogalski, Helmut Schapper, Dirk Scheer, Sibylle Scriba, Elfi Thomas, Sven Wolfgram, Marek Tadeusz Zygmunt.

Ethical Considerations

Drugs and medical devices were not applied in the study. No interventions were conducted. Only questionnaire based interviews were conducted with students. Side effects of interviews have not been identified yet. Consequently, statement by the ethics committee of the University of Greifswald was not necessary.

Funding

This work was supported by the Association for the Promotion of Humanities and Sciences in Germany (Stifterverband für die Deutsche Wissenschaft) [grant numbers H190 5907 9999 24586].

Authors' Contributions

ADW and WH are the principal investigators of the Bildungscluster study. Both develop the study design and were responsible for the IPE lecturers, data collection, data management and data analysis. ADW was the major contributor in writing the manuscript. SH supervise IPE lecturers and collect data together with AB and SK. SH verify and analyze data. SH, AB, SK, RFO interpreted the results. RFO recruits the nursing students for the Bildungscluster study. All authors read and approved the final manuscript.

References

1. WHO (2006) The World Health Report 2006: Working Together for Health. World Health Organization, Switzerland p: 237.

2. Blomberg K, Bisholt B, Kullén Engström A, Ohlsson U, Sundler Johansson A, et al. (2014) Swedish nursing students' experience of stress during clinical practice in relation to clinical setting characteristics and the organisation of the clinical education. J Clin Nurs 23: 2264-2271.

3. Margalit R, Thompson S, Visovsky C, Geske J, Collier D, et al. (2009) From professional silos to interprofessional education: campuswide focus on quality of care. Quality Management in Healthcare 18: 165-173.

4. Kitto S, Nordquist J, Peller J, Grant R, Reeves S (2013) The disconnections between space, place and learning in interprofessional education: an overview of key issues. J Interprof Care 27: 5-8.

5. Reeves S, Goldman J, Oandasan I (2007) Key factors in planning and implementing interprofessional education in health care settings. J Allied Health 36: 231-235.

6. Kent F, Francis-Cracknell A, McDonald R, Newton JM, Keating JL, et al. (2016) How do interprofessional student teams interact in a primary care clinic? A qualitative analysis using activity theory. Adv Health Sci Educ 21: 749-760.

7. Bolesta S, Chmil JV (2014) Interprofessional education among student health professionals using human patient simulation. Am J Pharm Educ 78: 94.

8. Abu-Rish E, Kim S, Choe L, Varpio L, Malik E, et al. (2012) Current trends in interprofessional education of health sciences students: A literature review. J Interprof Care 26: 444-451.

9. Reese CE, Jeffries PR, Engum SA (2010) Learning together: Using simulations to develop nursing and medical student collaboration. Nursing Education Perspectives 31: 33-37.

10. Miles A, Friary P, Jackson B, Sekula J, Braakhuis A (2016) Simulation-Based Dysphagia Training: Teaching Interprofessional Clinical Reasoning in a Hospital Environment. Dysphagia 31: 407-415.

11. Lapkin S, Levett-Jones T, Gilligan C (2012) A cross-sectional survey examining the extent to which interprofessional education is used to teach nursing, pharmacy and medical students in Australian and New Zealand universities. J Interprof Care 26: 390-396.

12. Cook DA, Hatala R, Brydges R, Zendejas B, Szostek JH, et al. (2011) Technology-enhanced simulation for health professions education: a systematic review and meta-analysis. JAMA 306: 978-988.

13. Poore JA, Cullen DL, Schaar GL (2014) Simulation-based interprofessional education guided by Kolb's Experiential Learning Theory. Clinical Simulation in Nursing 10: e241-e247.

14. Tofil NM, Morris JL, Peterson DT, Watts P, Epps C, et al. (2014) Interprofessional simulation training improves knowledge and teamwork in nursing and medical students during internal medicine clerkship. J Hosp Med 9: 189-192.

15. McGregor CA, Paton C, Thomson C, Chandratilake M, Scott H (2012) Preparing medical students for clinical decision making: a pilot study exploring how students make decisions and the perceived impact of a clinical decision making teaching intervention. Medical Teacher 34: e508-e517.

16. Chakravarthy B, ter Haar E, Bhat SS, McCoy CE, Denmark TK, et al. (2011) Simulation in medical school education: review for emergency medicine. West J Emerg Med 12: 461-466.

17. Alinier G, Hunt B, Gordon R, Harwood C (2006) Effectiveness of intermediate-fidelity simulation training technology in undergraduate nursing education. J Adv Nurs 54: 359-369.

18. Morphet J, Hood K, Cant R, Baulch J, Gilbee A, et al. (2014) Teaching teamwork: an evaluation of an interprofessional training ward placement for health care students. Adv Med Educ Practice 5: 197-204.

19. Elisabeth C, Ewa P, Christine WH (2011) The team builder: The role of nurses facilitating interprofessional student teams at a Swedish clinical training ward. Nurse Educ Practice 11: 309-313.

20. Kuckartz U (2014) Qualitative Content Analysis. Methods, Practice and Computer Support. Volume 2. Weinheim, Basel: Beltz Juventa.

21. Ker J, Mole L, Bradley P (2003) Early introduction to interprofessional learning: a simulated ward environment. Med Educ 37: 248-255.

22. McGettigan P, McKendree J (2015) Interprofessional training for final year healthcare students: a mixed methods evaluation of the impact on ward staff and students of a two-week placement and of factors affecting sustainability. BMC Med Educ 15: 185.

23. Hylin U (2010) Interprofessional education: Aspects on learning together on an interprofessional training ward. Institutionen för klinisk forskning och utbildning, Södersjukhuset/Department of Clinical Science and Education, Södersjukhuset.

24. Wakefield A, Cocksedge S, Boggis C (2006) Breaking bad news: qualitative evaluation of an interprofessional learning opportunity. Med Teacher 28: 53-58.

25. Ponzer S, Hylin U, Kusoffsky A, Lauffs M, Lonka K, et al. (2004) Interprofessional training in the context of clinical practice: goals and students' perceptions on clinical education wards. Med Educ 38: 727-736.

26. Liaw SY, Zhou WT, Lau TC, Siau C, Chan SWC (2014) An interprofessional communication training using simulation to enhance safe care for a deteriorating patient. Nurse Educ Today 34: 259-264.

27. Wang R, Shi N, Bai J, Zheng Y, Zhao Y (2015) Implementation and evaluation of an interprofessional simulation-based education program for undergraduate nursing students in operating room nursing education: a randomized controlled trial. BMC Med Educ 15: 115.

28. Balogun SA, Rose K, Thomas S, Owen JA, Brashers V (2014) Innovative interprofessional geriatric education for medical and nursing students: focus on transitions in care. QJM.

29. Bastami S, Krones T, Schroeder G, Schirlo C, Schaefer M, et al. (2012) Inter-professional Communication processes-difficult Conversations with Patients.

30. Walkenhorst U, Mahler C, Aistleithner R, Hahn EG, Kaap-Fröhlich S, et al. (2015) Position statement GMA Comittee–"Interprofessional Education for the Health Care Professions". GMS Zeitschrift für medizinische Ausbildung.

31. Wagner J, Liston B, Miller J (2011) Developing interprofessional communication skills. Teaching and Learning in Nursing 6: 97-101.

32. Freeth D, Nicol M (1998) Learning clinical skills: an interprofessional approach. Nurse Educ Today 18: 455-461.

33. Kyrkjebø JM, Brattebø G, Smith-Strøm H (2006) Improving patient safety by using interprofessional simulation training in health professional education. J Interprof Care 20: 507-516.

34. Cox M, Cuff P, Brandt B, Reeves S, Zierler B (2016) Measuring the impact of interprofessional education on collaborative practice and patient outcomes. J Interprof Care 30: 1-3.

35. Mahler C, Rochon J, Karstens S, Szecsenyi J, Hermann K (2014) Internal consistency of the readiness for interprofessional learning scale in German health care students and professionals. BMC Med Educ 14: 145.

10

Importance of Supporting School Education on Radiation After the Fukushima Daiichi Nuclear Power Plant Accident

Shimizu Y*, Iida H, Nenoi M and Akashi M

National Institute of Radiological Sciences, National Institutes for Quantum and Radiological Science and Technology, 4-9-1 Anagawa, Inage-ku, Chiba 263-8555, Japan

Abstract

The National Institute of Radiological Sciences (NIRS) in Japan has conducted training courses for professionals to obtain correct knowledge on radiation and its use in various fields. After the Fukushima accident, the demands for education on radiation not only by professionals but also by students increased. NIRS started school visits to conduct classes on radiation basics to ninth-grade (14/15-year-old) students in public junior high schools in cooperation with the Chiba city education board. After the classes, a questionnaire survey was conducted to evaluate the school visits and to improve the contents of the education. Almost half of the students thought that the contents of the lecture were slightly difficult or difficult to understand. Use of devices or instruments such as a cloud chamber, TV phone, or survey meter was helpful to arouse the students' interest. The school visits significantly changed the students' feelings toward radiation from "fear" to "interest". Our preliminary trial to conduct a class on radiation basics in junior high school suggests that detection of radiation by students and its visualization are very helpful in educating school children on radiation.

Keywords: Radiation education; School visits; Students; Japan

Introduction

Radiation exposure is a unique event because it cannot be detected by the human senses. Nevertheless, we are of course always being exposed to natural radiation. Today, moreover, radiation is used not only in medicine but also in science, industry, and for the generation of electricity. Ionizing radiation is useful for mankind and, in fact, is now essential for human life: for example, for roentgenographic examinations, nondestructive inspections, sterilization of medical instruments, and so on. However, radiation had not been taught in schools for 30 years until the Japanese school curriculum guidelines were revised in 2008 [1].

A huge earthquake struck the Pacific coast of eastern Japan at 14:46 on March 11, 2011 and triggered a tremendous tsunami. This earthquake and tsunami caused serious damage to the Fukushima Daiichi Nuclear Power Plant (NPP) operated by Tokyo Electric Power Co. (TEPCO). This damage resulted in large amounts of radioactive material being released into the environment. After this accident, many misunderstandings concerning radiation and its effects were spread in the general public, and even 6 years after the accident, there are still reports by mass media of misunderstandings about radiation that have led to discrimination in schools [2,3]. Thus, education on radiation and its effects is necessary in today's society.

Since its establishment in 1959, the Human Resources Development Center (HRDC) of the National Institute of Radiological Sciences (NIRS) under the National Institutes for Quantum and Radiological Science and Technology has conducted various training courses on the basics of radiation, radiation protection, radiation emergency medicine, and other topics mainly for professionals. In Japan, however, no systematic education on radiation basics was conducted in elementary or junior high schools. Although local governments with nuclear facilities such as NPPs ran a training/education system on radiation and its effects before the accident, this system was limited to 19 prefectures and focused on first responders and health care providers. In this article, we clarify and discuss problems raised in society after the accident and introduce our trial and efforts to educate students on the basics of radiation.

Materials and Methods

A questionnaire was prepared for the students (n=258) who took the class on radiation basics that NIRS conducted at school visits. The students were ninth-graders (14/15 years old) from 8 classes in Chiba city junior high schools.

The questionnaire consisted of the following closed questions: What is your most favorite subject?; What is your least favorite subject?; How was the special lesson?; Which subject was most interesting? (Multiple answers were allowed for this question.); Before you took the special lesson, how had you felt about radiation?; After you took the special lesson, how do you feel about radiation?; and Is the knowledge on radiation useful for your life?

Results

Training courses at NIRS

We have conducted both regularly scheduled and on-demand courses even before 2011. After the Fukushima accident, the number of training courses held at NIRS increased dramatically; the number of regularly scheduled or Fukushima-related courses increased to more than 30 in 2014 [4,5] (Figure 1A). These courses included those for first responders or communicators in local governments. Meanwhile, it is noteworthy that on-demand training courses have also increased: almost 20 courses were conducted in 2016. Figure 1B shows the on-demand courses according to the target population. Half of these courses were for students from elementary school to university level, and they were held at the request of the schools or local education boards.

*Corresponding authors: Yuko Shimizu, National Institute of Radiological Sciences, National Institutes for Quantum and Radiological Science and Technology, Japan, E-mail: shimizu.yuko@qst.go.jp

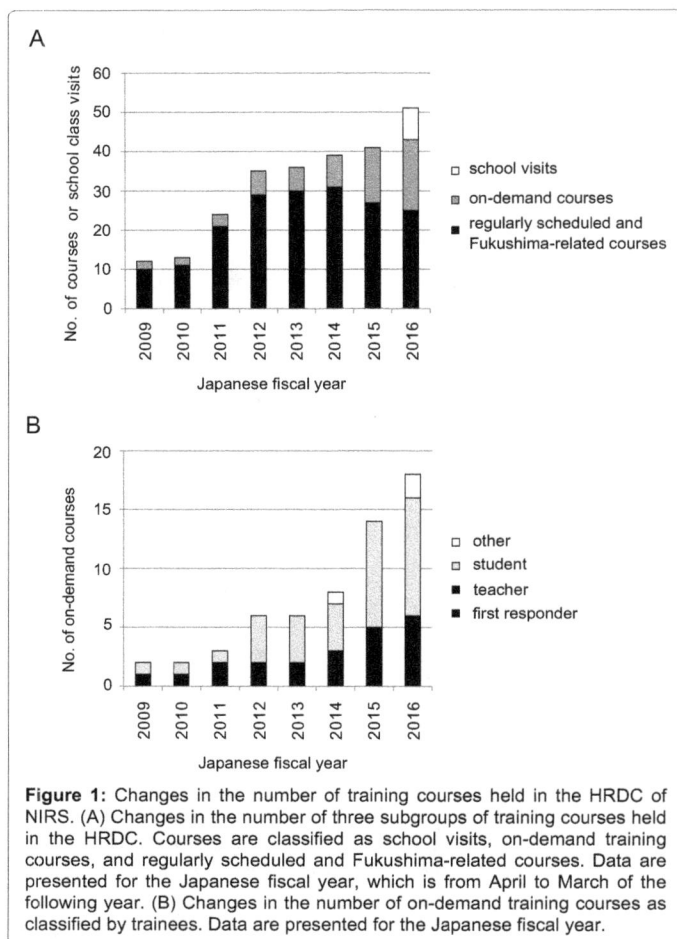

Figure 1: Changes in the number of training courses held in the HRDC of NIRS. (A) Changes in the number of three subgroups of training courses held in the HRDC. Courses are classified as school visits, on-demand training courses, and regularly scheduled and Fukushima-related courses. Data are presented for the Japanese fiscal year, which is from April to March of the following year. (B) Changes in the number of on-demand training courses as classified by trainees. Data are presented for the Japanese fiscal year.

Trial of systematic school visits for radiation education

NIRS started to visit schools from 2016 to support education on radiation basics in cooperation with the Chiba city education board and to improve the contents of radiation education. NIRS staff visited two schools in 2016, and 258 students took the class. A 45-minute-class on radiation basics was taken by almost all of the ninth-grade students at two public junior high schools in Chiba city. Each class consisted of less than 40 students so that we could devote our attention to all of the students, and NIRS conducted 8 classes in total. The class covered the characteristics of radiation, natural radiation in the environment, its effects on humans, and its application in medicine and industry. These contents have been included in the school curriculum guidelines. To make sure the students understood well, NIRS explained radiation in plain words and phrases without using scientific or technical words. To arouse the students' interest, a cloud chamber was used. Although radiation cannot be detected directly by using our senses, it can be detected indirectly. A cloud chamber is a detector that allows visualization of the tracks of charged particles. We used a large-scale cloud chamber (Toda-type desk cloud chamber B-112, RADO) to show the tracks of the radiation and radioactive decay (Figures 2A-2C). Moreover, using a survey meter, the students could detect natural radiation in mineral deposits under the supervision of experts. In addition, a live experiment in a radiation-controlled area at NIRS was shown to students via a TV phone.

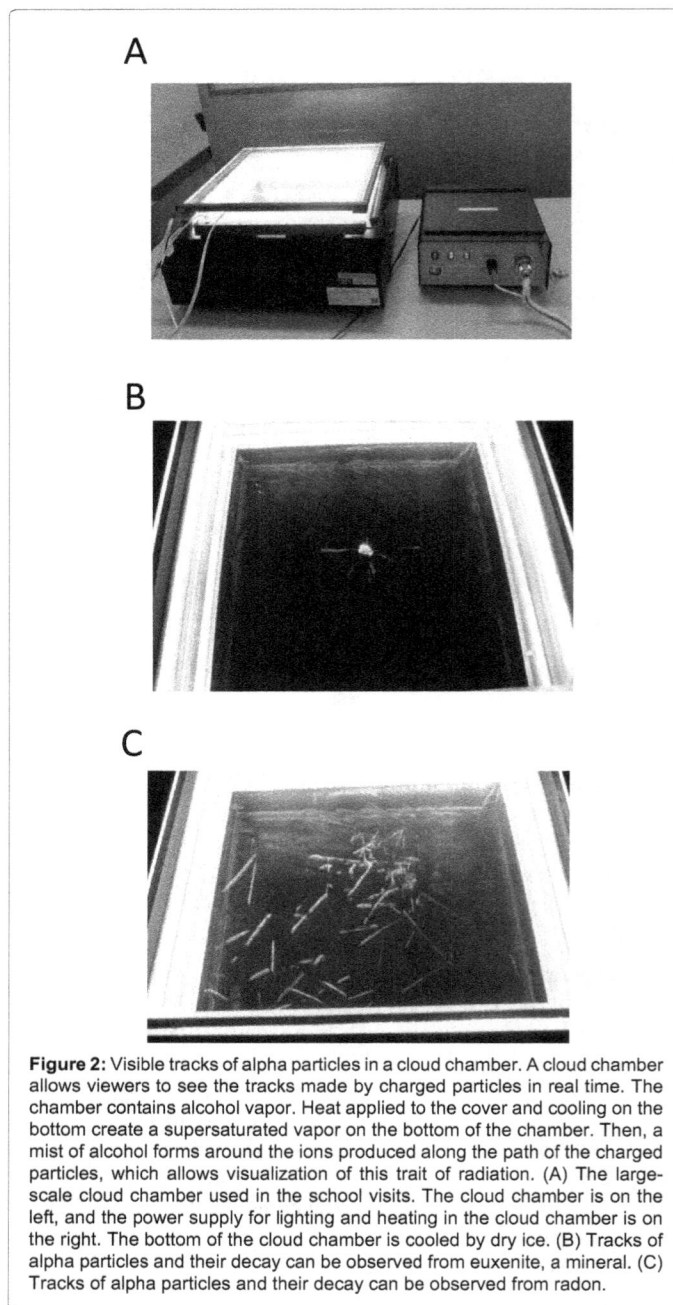

Figure 2: Visible tracks of alpha particles in a cloud chamber. A cloud chamber allows viewers to see the tracks made by charged particles in real time. The chamber contains alcohol vapor. Heat applied to the cover and cooling on the bottom create a supersaturated vapor on the bottom of the chamber. Then, a mist of alcohol forms around the ions produced along the path of the charged particles, which allows visualization of this trait of radiation. (A) The large-scale cloud chamber used in the school visits. The cloud chamber is on the left, and the power supply for lighting and heating in the cloud chamber is on the right. The bottom of the cloud chamber is cooled by dry ice. (B) Tracks of alpha particles and their decay can be observed from euxenite, a mineral. (C) Tracks of alpha particles and their decay can be observed from radon.

Questionnaire about the class

At the end of the course, all 258 students were asked to complete the questionnaire to evaluate the effect of the school visits. Figure 3 shows the responses to the questions. The response rate was 100%. Science or mathematics was the most favorite subject of only 23% of the students and the least favorite subject of 39% (Figure 3A and 3B). Almost half of the students thought that the content of the class was rather difficult to understand, and more than half though that the content was rather easy or appropriate (Figure 3C). Of most interest was the live experiment: half of the students were interested in the live experiment shown on the TV phone (Figure 3D). Slightly more than 42% of the students answered that the cloud chamber experience was interesting (Figure 3D). Before taking this class, more than 50% of the students had felt somehow scared of radiation (Figure 4A), but after the class, that percentage had decreased to almost 20% (Figure 4B). Over 65% of the students answered that knowledge of radiation was useful for their life (Figure 4C).

Discussion

Radiation cannot be felt, smelled, or tasted, nor does it induce immediate signs or symptoms after exposure. Because there have been few chances to be exposed to radiation at a significant level, opportunities for learning about radiation have been limited.

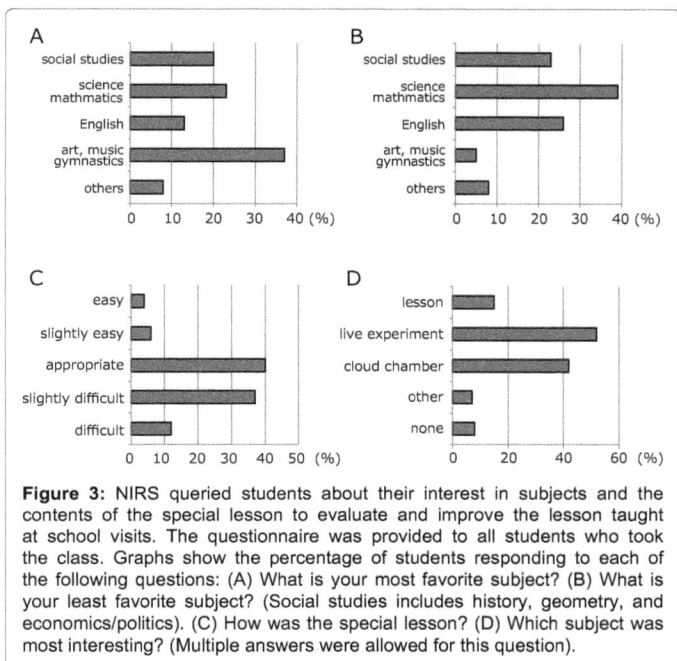

Figure 3: NIRS queried students about their interest in subjects and the contents of the special lesson to evaluate and improve the lesson taught at school visits. The questionnaire was provided to all students who took the class. Graphs show the percentage of students responding to each of the following questions: (A) What is your most favorite subject? (B) What is your least favorite subject? (Social studies includes history, geometry, and economics/politics). (C) How was the special lesson? (D) Which subject was most interesting? (Multiple answers were allowed for this question).

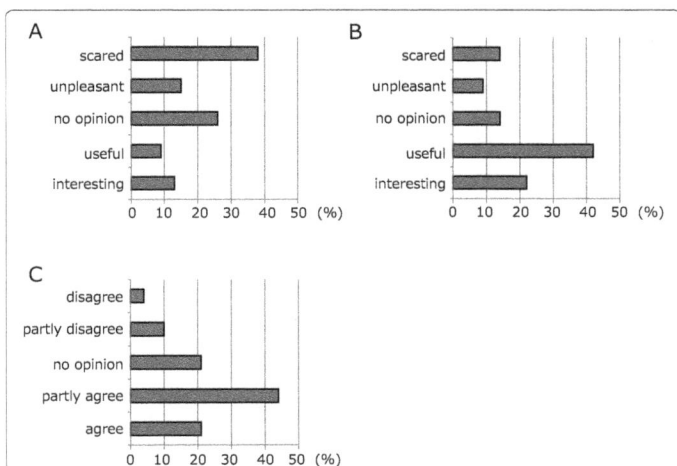

Figure 4: A questionnaire survey was carried out to examine the effects of the special class on the students. NIRS queried the students about their impression of radiation before and after taking the class and about their knowledge of radiation in life. The questionnaire was provided to all students who took the class. Graphs show the percentage of students responding to each of the following questions: (A) Before you took the special lesson, how had you felt about radiation? (B) After you took the special lesson, how do you feel about radiation? (C) Is knowledge about radiation useful for your life?

Therefore, the public did not have adequate knowledge on radiation and its effects. With the Fukushima accident, however, large amounts of radioactive materials were released into the atmosphere, and a lot of information of various quality was spread among the public. Although society started to realize that education on radiation basics should be required in schools, the problem was that there was no human resources or materials/equipment for teaching radiation basics in schools. Furthermore, teachers in schools were too busy. Thus, NIRS started a trial to visit schools teach a class on radiation basics in 2016.

After the Fukushima accident, NIRS increased its number of regularly scheduled courses, and the number of people who attended these courses reached a plateau. However, NIRS also conducted more on-demand courses especially for teachers and students. NIRS has been involved in the education and training of experts or professionals for 57 years. However, providing these opportunities to teachers and students is a big challenge because providing information in a certain way sometimes can lead to confusion among them, and the NIRS staff has to study communication countermeasures to avoid this risk.

Most of the on-demand training courses were for students who voluntarily participated in and, apparently, were interested in radiation before taking the courses. The remaining courses were for students who had studied science or medicine. However, the NIRS school visit targeted all ninth-grade students in public junior high school, which means almost all of the children at the specific ages in a district, including those who are not good at science nor those who are willing to participate in a special activity to learn science. In fact, at the school visits, less than 23% of the student stated that they liked science, and 39% answered that science or mathematics was their least favorite subject. Thus, school visits can promote students in various course and classes to gain knowledge on radiation, leading to mitigation of the misunderstandings about radiation in society.

It appeared that more than half of the students understood the contents of the lesson. However, because almost half of the students also thought that the class was somewhat difficult, further improvement is required, such as by using more instruments and easier explanations, to describe radiation concepts more clearly. Moreover, it might be helpful to use fictional characters and events to attract more classroom attention.

The students were interested in the live experiment by TV phone and the cloud chamber, indicating that obtaining knowledge through visual examples was readily acceptable and that this technique, although well known in society but unfamiliar to the younger age, was a good tool with which to arouse the students' interest. These instruments helped to promote the understanding of radiation by the students. The use of a survey meter was also well accepted by the students (data not shown). These results indicate that the appropriate use of instruments will increase their understanding. After taking the class, the students' feelings about radiation dramatically changed from "scared" to "interesting", indicating that effective education can decrease fear and increase scientific interest. Moreover, 65% of the students thought that knowledge of radiation was useful for their life.

The Fukushima disaster has caused many people to relocate from Fukushima to other prefectures. Recently, there are still reports of children from Fukushima becoming targets of school bullying in other prefectures [2,3]. In fact, one case of bullying in Yokohama city was recognized as a grave concern by a third party, the local education board in 2016. It is generally thought that school bullying is caused mainly by stress from the heavy burden at school. However, in this case, one main cause was thought to be harmful rumors or misinformation in society. Children's behavior might reflect anxiety in society. Thus, education is the most powerful tool to improve this situation, to decrease the damage to one's reputation, and to promote restoration of normal life following the accident.

In summary, we learned that it is necessary to support and sustain school education on radiation. NIRS has conducted classes and has distributed a mini-textbook at school visits. We believe that these are helpful for school teachers because these schools do not have devices for radiation detection and the teachers do not have enough knowledge about radiation to teach it. In addition, we are planning a service to lend a survey meter to the schools. This sustainable support will lead to the promotion of recovery from the Fukushima Daiichi NPP accident.

References

1. Website of the Ministry of Education, Culture, Sports, and Science and Technology (2017) Japan.

2. Wilson T, Funakoshi M (2017) Six years on, Fukushima child evacuees face menace of school bullies. Reuters.

3. University Teacher Harassed Fukushima Student (2017) NHK WORLD.

4. Hachiya M, Akashi M (2016) Lessons learned from the accident at the Fukushima Dai-ichi nuclear power plant – more than basic knowledge: education and its effects improve the preparedness and response to radiation emergency. Radiat Prot Dosimetry 171: 27-31.

5. Shimizu Y, Iida H, Nenoi M (2016) Trends of training courses conducted in Human Resources Development Center of National Institute for Quantum and Radiological Science and Technology after the Fukushima Dai-ichi nuclear power plant accident. Health Physics.

11

Knowledge Extraction for Sleep Apnea Medical Diagnosis

Hung-Hsiang Chiu* and Bing-Jun Wang

Department of Electrophysics, National Chiao Tung University, Hsinchu 30010, Taiwan

Abstract

This research aimed to extract medical diagnostic knowledge about sleep apnea by applying theories from process control management, library science, and knowledge management. We interviewed the President of the International Sleep Science Technology Association (ISSTA), a medical doctor, on the subject of sleep apnea, and validated the research findings with four other sleep apnea experts to achieve the following: A formal knowledge extraction procEduccre was established for sleep apnea. All medical knowledge pertaining to sleep apnea was mapped out.

Keywords: Sleep apnea; Knowledge management; Knowledge extraction; Library science

Introduction

Many sleep disorders have been documented, such as insomnia, obstructive and central sleep apnea, restless legs syndrome, and periodic limb-movement disorder. Sleep apnea is one of the most common sleeping disorders. According to the American Academy of Sleep Medicine (2005), approximately 4%-6% of adults in the United States are deeply troubled by sleeping disorders, this being the case especially for men, the elderly, and the obese (BMI $\geq$ 30 kg/m^2). Risk factors for sleep apnea include large neck circumference (male>17 inches; female>16 inches), and craniofacial or upper airway structure abnormalities. Without medical treatment, the recurrent sleep disruption and lack of oxygen, which characterizes sleep apnea, increases heart load and susceptibility to fatal diseases and causes hypertension, myocardial infarction, and angina pectoris.

Therefore, the authors of the present article believe that the appropriate and effective treatment of sleep apnea stands to benefit broadly from the health of patients with this disorder. Thus, it is critically important that physicians have at their disposal a correct and complete resource of sleep apnea diagnostic knowledge. By observing physicians specialized in sleep medicine, and validating results with the input of four other sleep medicine experts, this study aimed to map the theoretical and practical knowledge relating to sleep apnea in its entirety.

Literature Review

Theory of knowledge management

Gilbert and Cordey [1] demonstrated the importance of operational procEduccres and processes management in knowledge management. Quintas, Lefrere, and Jones [2] further noted eight categories about an organization knowledge: (1) market and customer information, (2) product information knowledge, (3) expert, (4) human resource information, (5) core business processes, (6) transaction-related information, (7) management information, and (8) vendor information. Borghoff [3] believed that a knowledge management framework should contain four elements: (1) knowledge flow, (2) a knowledge map, (3) knowledge workers, and (4) a repository of knowledge. In addition, Holsapple [4] proposed that a knowledge map should contain two parts: knowledge contents (e.g., keywords), and the relevant elements (e.g., experts, project teams, processes, articles, courses, etc).

The knowledge extraction process applied in the present study was therefore designed to include the following three elements of organization: (1) the organizational procEduccres/process, (2) the operator, and (3) the output documents. However, although much of the literature advises the inclusion of four elements, this literature fails to describe in detail how to use the tools espoused to extract knowledge. We therefore used methods developed in process management and library science to construct a knowledge extraction method for sleep apnea.

Theory of process management

The Work Breakdown Structure (WBS) deconstructs work through the application of top-down logic, rEducccing work to smaller and more manageable and controllable unitary systems. The International Project Management Institute believe that one can breakdown tasks by the following steps: first, one must clearly identify the major deliverables of the process. Second, one must ensure that each deliverable has reached a level of detail sufficient to estimate the cost and time. Third, the deliverables must be verifiable results.

In the basic requirements of Create WBS, the following are specified: (1) a particular task should appear as only one place in the WBS; (2) the WBS of a task is the sum of all items under the WBS; (3) a WBS item only by a liability, and even though many people are likely to work on it, just one takes principle responsibility for it, all others are only participants; (4) a WBS must be consistent with the actual work of implementation; (5) the project team should be allowed to actively participate in creating the WBS, and consistency must be ensured; (6) each WBS item must be documented in detail, in order to ensure that all project stakeholders can understand them fully. Additionally, when an organization creates a WBS, they must consider the following: (1) the appropriate WBS level, corresponding to the lowest level WBS elements requiring tangible deliverables; (2) the WBS lifecycle and the development of activities at different stages of the project, including project management; (3) planning, performance reporting, integrated change control, and range management needs; (4) resource planning and risk management needs [5].

*Corresponding author: Hung-Hsiang Chiu, Department of Electrophysics, National Chiao Tung University, Hsinchu 30010, Taiwan, E-mail: oldchu1972@gmail.com

We believe the WBS to be well suited to the separation and analysis of activities, and it can also reinforce the knowledge extraction process. In addition, because the topic of this study, sleep medicine, is a highly specialized area of medicine, this research aimed to bring together the classification methods from library science to improve knowledge extraction.

Theory of library science

In general, the classification element of library science includes three design elements: the category table, category tag, and index. The category table is the table refers to all categories of classification in accordance with a system in order to show them out. An effective classification table should contain the following elements: (1) a category covering all knowledge; (2) systematic categories; (3) flexibility and scalability; (4) the category clearly. The category tag is composed of the category number and author number. It main purpose of the order is sorted by category tag. As the index is a tool, which to label content material to facilitate data query out.

The medical classification method employed in the present study is that of the US National Library of Medicine Classification (NLM; NLM, 2016) [6], which in 1951 was officially dedicated to the Medical and Health Sciences. The US National Library of Medicine Classification is divided into two parts, namely, the classification code (QS-QZ) for Medical Science (Preclinical Sciences), pre-classification number (W-WZ) for Medicine and Related Subjects. For example, the WB classification category is used for medical practice. It begins with WB1-177 for reference data, and thereafter comprises the following: WB120-130, family health; WB141-293, diagnosis; and WB300-962, therapy for 4 major categories. Each category starting with a WB class under 0-9 has a decimal classification number. Table 1 below describes the classification system applied to forensic science and related disciplines.

Sleep medicine

According the International Classification of Sleep Disorders Second Edition, general common sleep disorders can be divided into the following categories: (1) insomnia: the inability to fall asleep, stay asleep, or to feel fatigue even after sleeping; (2) obstructive and central sleep apnea: upper respiratory tract muscle relaxation and/or obesity resulting in a repeated obstruction of the airway, causing apnea; (3) loss of airflow within the upper respiratory tract for at least ten seconds; (4) restless legs syndrome and periodic limb movement disorder: common neurological diseases characterized by urgency and constant movement of the feet, especially during sleep, these symptoms will be more obvious. Three diagnostic modalities are typically applied to sleep problems: scale analysis, measuring instruments, and medical history assessment. Sleep disorders are generally treated by the following methods: (1) continuous positive airway pressure during sleep; (2) snoring mouthpiece during sleep; (3) upper respiratory tract reconstructive surgery [7].

The medical profession is one rich with knowledge. Good knowledge management can rEduccce the uncertainty of medical services and improve the quality of medical care [8]. Wennberg reported that the way of physicians to treating or surgical, which have significant exist between different hospitals [9]. Hence, if one were to build an extraction mechanism, which from physicians diagnose process, to collate, sharing and exchange knowledge, it would likely have a significant impact upon the medical profession.

Research Methods

The research framework

Based on the previous chapters, the research architecture of this study is represented by Figure 1 and described in detail in Table 2. Those two used theories from knowledge management, process management, and library science to complete the following four knowledge extraction procEduccres as applied to the sleep apnea medical diagnosis: (1) expert interviews and content analysis; (2) knowledge of the construction work description table; (3) knowledge classification; (4) verification of results by other experts in the field.

Description of interviewee background

We were permitted by Dr. Chiang Rayleigh Ping-Ying, a sleep medicine expert of Taiwan, to interview him and extract his sleep apnea diagnostic knowledge. Dr. Chiang Rayleigh Ping-Ying graduated from the Institute of Clinical Medicine of National Taiwan University, and

W-WB (General Health and Medicine)	
Classification Number	**English Name**
W	Health Professions
WA	Public Health
WB	Practice of Medicine
WC-WD (Diseases of the Whole Body)	
Classification Number	**English Name**
WC	Communicable Diseases
WD100	Nutrition Disorders
WD200	Metabolic Diseases
WD300	Immunologic and Collagen Diseases, Hypersensitivity
WD 400	Animal Poisons
WD 500	Plant Poisons
WD 600	Disorders and Injuries of Environmental Origin
WD 700	Aviation and Space Medicine
WE-WL (Systems of the Body)	
Classification Number	**English Name**
WE	Musculoskeletal System
WF	Respiratory System
WG	Cardiovascular System
WH	Hemic and Lymphatic Systems
WI	Digestive System
WJ	Urogenital System
WK	Endocrine System
WL	Nervous System
WM-WZ (Specialty Areas of the Health Science)	
Classification Number	**English Name**
WM	Psychiatry
WN	Radiology, Diagnostic Imaging
WO	Surgery
WP	Gynecology
WQ	Obstetrics
WR	Dermatology
WS	Pediatrics
WT	Geriatrics, Chronic Disease
WU	Dentistry, Oral Surgery
WV	Otolaryngology
WW	Ophthalmology
WX	Hospitals and Other Health Facilities
WY	Nursing
WZ	History of Medicine

Table 1: The united states national library of medicine [6].

ProcEduccre	Significance and Description	Tools/Theory Used	Outputs/Achievements
Expert Interviews	We used an interview outline designed for the present study to interview physicians specializing in sleep apnea while recording their responses verbatim.	1. Interview outline for organization knowledge Expert (Appendix A) 2. In-depth interviews for qualitative research	1. Interview outline for medical experts 2. Interview record 3. Analysis of interview records
Knowledge Worksheet Construction	Through construct of interview records to do knowledge operation process description table.	1. Interview record 2. Record analysis 3. Tools of process control management	1. Sleep apnea medical diagnostic work description table 2. Sleep apnea diagnostic process and medical knowledge correspondence table
Knowledge Classification	Knowledge classification through the use of the following four tools: NLM, WBS, sleep apnea medical diagnostic work description table, sleep apnea diagnostic process, and medical knowledge correspondence table	1. NLM 2. WBS 3. Sleep apnea medical diagnostic work description table 4. Sleep apnea diagnostic process and medical knowledge correspondence table	The clinical diagnosis of sleep apnea knowledge classification structure table
Other Expert Verification	Four sleep medicine physicians provided expert opinions on the research results listed in the next column	1. Interview outline for organization knowledge expert 2. Sleep apnea medical diagnostic work description table 3 Sleep apnea diagnostic process and medical knowledge correspondence table 4. The clinical diagnosis of sleep apnea knowledge classification structure table	Medical expert verification table

Table 2: Research architecture.

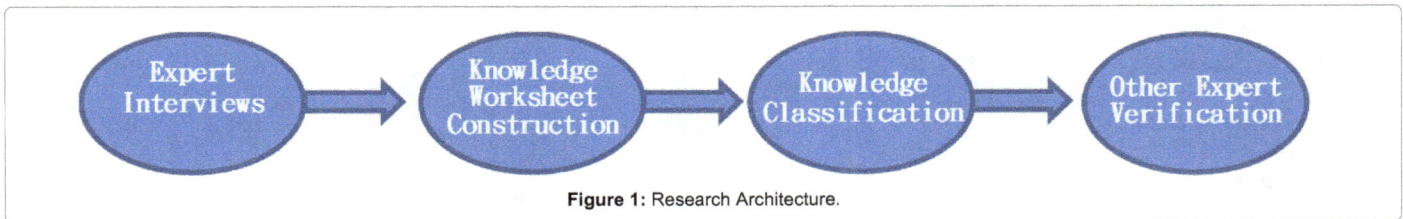

Figure 1: Research Architecture.

was a researcher at the Sleep Medicine Center of Stanford University. He is the Deputy executive director of the sleep medicine center of Taipei Veterans General Hospital, the Grandparent Somnologist of European Union and the President of ISSTA [10,11]. His specialties include poor sleep quality (including insomnia), snoring and sleep apnea, etc. In 2016, Dr. Chiang became the President of ISSTA.

After 45 working days, we finished the collection of two datasets: first, using the proprietary "knowledge feature set and extraction interview outline" (Appendix A) in-depth interview, and second, the interview records and all knowledge charts, tables, and discussion meeting. Each meeting lasted 2.5 hours, and meeting data were recorded by a stenographer. The following is an excerpt from Dr. Chiang's interview manuscript:

Interview paragraph A

Interviewer: I would like to ask you in the implementation of the medical diagnosis process, such as the bottleneck or obstacles, what are the ways or the activity can help you to solve those difficult problem?

Dr. Chiang: Most of the patients is sleep special outpatient. When sleep specialist physicians believe that the case shall need the other doctor consultation, or referral. It will held a consultation meetings to discuss how to carry out the subsequent treatment decisions. In addition to we will also participate in the global sleep medicine annual meeting or seminar to study new knowledge or ask to my teachers: Professor Nelson B. Powell and Professor Christian Guilleminault in Stanford.

Interview paragraph B

Interviewer: When patients completed clinic and sleep screening process, which will output what document?

Dr. Chiang: It were be outcome an inspection report after the sleep examination process. And then, we will make treatment recommendations, which based on inspection data from this report and other medical history of the disease.

Verification method

In this research, we invited four sleep medicine physicians, all of whom had otolaryngology and sleep medicine experience in difference general hospitals. They verified four research results:

(1) the interview outline for sleep apnea experts; (2) the sleep apnea medical diagnostic work description table; (3) the sleep apnea diagnostic process and medical knowledge correspondence table; (4) the clinical diagnosis of sleep apnea knowledge classification structure table.

Verification began by requesting the four doctors' agreement to participate by telephone. We then sent all of our research data to them by e-mail. Table 3 tabulates the comments of the four doctors:

According to the verification results provided by these four sleep medical specialists, several verification conclusions were drawn. Firstly, the "Sleep apnea medical expert interview outline" provides structured sleep apnea diagnosis knowledge; secondly, the four expert physicians unanimously agreed that the contents of two forms can clearly express

ProcEduccre	Significance and Description	Tools/Theory Used	Outputs/ Achievements
Expert Interviews	We used an interview outline designed for the present study to interview physicians specializing in sleep apnea while recording their responses verbatim.	1. Interview outline for organization knowledge Expert (Appendix A) 2. In-depth interviews for qualitative research	1. Interview outline for medical experts 2. Interview record 3. Analysis of interview records
Knowledge Worksheet Construction	Through construct of interview records to do knowledge operation process description table.	1. Interview record 2. Record analysis 3. Tools of process control management	1. Sleep apnea medical diagnostic work description table 2. Sleep apnea diagnostic process and medical knowledge correspondence table
Knowledge Classification	Knowledge classification through the use of the following four tools: NLM, WBS, sleep apnea medical diagnostic work description table, sleep apnea diagnostic process, and medical knowledge correspondence table	1. NLM 2. WBS 3. Sleep apnea medical diagnostic work description table 4. Sleep apnea diagnostic process and medical knowledge correspondence table	The clinical diagnosis of sleep apnea knowledge classification structure table
Other Expert Verification	Four sleep medicine physicians provided expert opinions on the research results listed in the next column	1. Interview outline for organization knowledge expert 2. Sleep apnea medical diagnostic work description table 3 Sleep apnea diagnostic process and medical knowledge correspondence table 4. The clinical diagnosis of sleep apnea knowledge classification structure table	Medical expert verification table

Table 3: Research architecture.

Categories / Task Name	Principal	Tools Used	Delivery	Outcome Document	Users
1. Preliminary Interrogation	Sleep Doctor	Outpatient tool	Patient record system	Outpatient records	Sleep Doctor
2. Executive Sleep Inspection	Sleep Doctor, Examiner, Nurse	Sleep inspection report	Patient record system	Sleep inspection report	Sleep Doctor
3. Diagnose Sleep Apnea	Sleep Doctor	Sleep inspection report	Patient record system	Diagnosed proof	Sleep Doctor
4. Treatment	Sleep Doctor	1. Continuous positive airway pressure 2. Snoring mouthpiece 3. Surgical equipment	Patient record system	Treatment records	Sleep Doctor
5. Subsequent Visit	Sleep Doctor	Outpatient tool	Patient record system	Treatment records	Sleep Doctor

Table 4: Sleep apnea clinical diagnostic protocol.

the corresponding processes and related knowledge and concepts; thirdly, it is easy to read, although two of the four experts suggested merging two forms; finally, the four sleep doctors accepted that using classification principles is a good way to represent the entirety of the disorder. Besides using WBS and NLM, it provides information on medical professional relationships and cases to enrich the reader's knowledge of the field.

The verification opinions of the four sleep experts are positive. The work reflects effective knowledge extraction from the medical professionals, and covers all aspects of sleep apnea.

Results

After finishing this research, which is based on the literature review, Figure 1 and Tables 2 and 3 of research procEduccre design, it completed several research results. Table 4 which is based on the interviews content, shows five categories that correspond to the patient treatment process. Those categories are the responsible officer, use of tools, delivery, output documents, and users. In this form, it demonstrates a relationship between the diagnostic procEduccres for

sleep apnea and the "Persons, Tools, and Documents" categories. It was order to become an important simple job description table, which use for clinical references to the sleep apnea medical diagnosis process.

Table 5 shows the correspondence between the three categories: (1) the process task of sleep apnea diagnosis; (2) the principal who executive sleep apnea diagnostic processes; (3) the medical theoretical knowledge and medical clinical knowledge in the process of the diagnosis of sleep apnea. For example, the sleep doctor accountable process task in process 1 is called "newly diagnosed". This process used theories related to the respiratory system, sleep medicine, otolaryngology, and patient observation, as well as the Pittsburg Sleep Quality Index to define "newly diagnosed." A detailed description of sleep apnea diagnostic processes and related knowledge is provided below in Table 5.

This research also separates sleep apnea medical diagnostic knowledge into two categories, transverse and straight, and used Table 6 to show mutual correspondence between these categories. The transverse category, which for this research was defined as the "clinical knowledge category," comprised three subcategories: interrogation knowledge, detection knowledge, and treatment knowledge. These

Process Task	Principal	Theoretical Knowledge	Clinical Knowledge
1. Newly diagnosed			
1.1 Ask patients: Do you have daytime Fatigue? How frequently do you doze?	Sleep Doctor	Respiratory system, sleep medicine, otolaryngology, clinical medicine, sleep disorders (sleep apnea, snoring, limb hyperactivity disorder)	Patient observation and dialogue
1.2 Ask patients and their families: have sleep snoring, snoring interrupted, Sleep up half will, apnea stop?			
1.3 Ask patients: have heart disease, diabetes, or hypertension?			
1.4 Ask patients: Do you have limb pain when you get up?			
1.5 Observation of the patient: have not focus on the spirit, fatigue?			
1.6 Pittsburgh Sleep Quality Scale (PSQI) [Note 1] measurement			PSQI Completion instructions
1.7 Interpretation of typical sleep apnea and arrange inspection of sleep			PSQI Indicator interpretation
2. Inspection			
2.1 Blood test, radiography, issuing inspection cover, alternate instructions, teaching	Sleep Specialist Physicians, Examiner, Nurse	Respiratory system sleep medicine, otolaryngology, clinical medicine, metabolomics, neuroscience, endocrinology, respiratory physiology, nursing, sleep disorders (sleep apnea, snoring, limb hyperactivity disorder)	SaO2 indicator interpretation [Note 2]
2.2 Inspection of vital signs, neck circumference, body type, facial bone type, upper respiratory detailed theoretical inspection, craniofacial X-ray measurements, fiber endoscopy			PNC indicator interpretation [Note 3]
2.3 Inspection of upper respiratory tract stenosis or collapse extent (nasal cavity, oropharynx, hypopharynx, larynx)			Upper respiratory tract Stenosis or subsidence of the respiratory tract as a whole accounted for more than 50%
2.4 Inspectors detected multifunction overnight sleep physiology Nursing care during the night shift			Patient care knowledge, detection equipment operational knowledge
2.5 Physicians confirmation			1. RDI Indicator interpretation [Note 4] 2. AHI Indicator interpretation [Note 5]
3. Diagnosed as sleep apnea	Sleep Specialist Physicians	Sleep Medicine	Inspection data interpretation knowledge
4. Treatment			
4.1 Wearing snoring mouthpiece	Sleep Specialist Physicians, Dentist	Otolaryngology, respiratory system science, dentistry	Snoring mouthpiece using knowledge
4.2 Wearing continuous positive airway pressure (CPAP) device	Sleep Specialist Physicians	Otolaryngology, respiratory system science, pediatrics	CPAP using knowledge
4.3 Upper airway reconstructive surgery [Note 6]			
4.3.1 Uvulopalatopharyngoplasty surgery + hydroxylamine genioglossus advancement surgery			Upper airway reconstructive surgery capacity
4.3.2 Upper/lower jaw forward surgery			
4.3.3 Removal of hypertrophic tonsils and adenoids jaw surgery (obstructive sleep apnea for children)			
5. Return to outpatients			
5.1 Observation of the patient: have focus on the spirit, good spirit?	Sleep Specialist Physicians	Clinical Medicine	Patient observation and dialogue
5.2 Ask patients: still have daytime fatigue? Dozing how frequently?			
5.3 Ask patients: the status wear respirator/ snoring braces/postoperative			
5.4 Comparison with initial outpatient records - Significant improvement?			
5.5 Continued return to outpatients 2-3 times			

[Note 1] PSQI: Pittsburg Sleep Quality Index. PSQI>5 (good quality of sleep), PSQI ≤ 5 (poor quality of sleep).
[Note 2] SaO2: oxygen saturation index. SaO2>85 (low), 65 ≤ SAO2 ≤ 85 (moderate), SAO2<65 (severe).
[Note 3] PNC: perimeter of neck circumference. PNC<43 cm (low probability), 43-48 cm (moderate probability), PNC>48 cm (high probability).
[Note 4] RDI: respiratory disturbance index. RDI<5 (normal), 5 ≤ RDI<15 (low), 15 ≤ RDI<30 (moderate), RDI ≥ 30 (severe).
[Note 5] AHI: apnea-hypopnea index. AHI>5 (sleep disorder).
[Note 6] First type of surgery: uvulopalatopharyngoplasty surgery+ hydroxylamine genioglossus advancement surgery (for adults), second type of surgery: removal of hypertrophic tonsils and adenoids jaw surgery (for children).

Table 5: Sleep apnea diagnostic processes and related knowledge.

Clinical Knowledge Category / Theory Knowledge Category	Interrogation Knowledge	Detection Knowledge	Treatment Knowledge
WB (Practice of Medicine)			
WB200 (Physical Diagnosis)	Foundation interrogation methods		
WB305 (Instructions for devices)		Sleep detector operation method	
WF (Respiratory System)			
WF39 (Handbooks. Resource guides)	1. PSQI [Note 1] 2. The medical records		
WF141 (Diagnostic Methods)			
WV (Otolaryngology) WV150 (Diagnostic Methods)	Ask patients: have sleep snoring, snoring interrupted, sleep up half will, apnea stop?	1.RDI indicator [Note 2] 2.AHI indicator [Note 3] 3.PNC indicator [Note 4] 4. Upper respiratory tract stenosis or subsidence of the respiratory tract as a whole accounted for more than 50%	
WG (Cardiovascular System) WG141 (Diagnostic Methods)	Ask patients: Do you have hypertension or heart disease?	SaO2 indicator [Note 5]	
WK (Endocrine System) WK810 (Diabetes mellitus)	Ask patients: Do you have diabetes?	SaO2 indicator [Note 5]	
WL (Nervous System) WL141 (Diagnostic Methods)	Ask patients: Do you have limb pain when you get up?	Patients involuntarily jitter in the thumb, foot, ankle, knee, or when bending more than 15 times per hour during monitored sleep	
WF145 (Therapeutics)			Using snoring mouthpiece/continuous positive applied pressure device
WV (Otolaryngology) WV168 ENT Surgery WS (Pediatrics) WS366			Upper airway reconstructive surgery capacity [Note 6]
WY(Nursing)			
WY163 (Respiratory System Nursing		Night care for patient	

[Note 1] PSQI: Pittsburg Sleep Quality Index. PSQI>5 (good quality of sleep), PSQI ≤ 5 (poor quality of sleep).
[Note 2] RDI: respiratory disturbance index. RDI<5 (normal), 5 ≤ RDI<15 (low), 15 ≤ RDI<30 (moderate), RDI ≥ 30 (severe).
[Note 3] AHI: apnea-hypopnea index. AHI>5 (sleep disorder).
[Note 4] SaO2: oxygen saturation index. SaO2>85 (low), 65 ≤ SAO2 ≤ 85 (moderate), SAO2<65 (severe).
[Note 5] PNC: perimeter of neck circumference. PNC<43 cm (low probability), 43-48 cm (moderate probability), PNC>48 cm (high probability).
[Note 6] First type of surgery: uvulopalatopharyngoplasty surgery+ hydroxylamine genioglossus advancement surgery (for adults), second type of surgery: removal of hypertrophic tonsils and adenoids jaw surgery (for children).

Table 6: Clinical diagnosis of sleep apnea knowledge classification schema [6].

subcategories were used in the classification tools from the work breakdown structure and the sleep apnea diagnosis process, which from interview records to do category classification. For example, newly diagnosed patients must complete the Pittsburgh Sleep Quality.

Scale test to measure the quality of their sleep. The interpretation knowledge of the patients filled out answers and fractions for scale. This was classified as diagnostic knowledge in the present study.

The straight category, which for this research was defined as the "medical theoretical knowledge category," comprised three subcategories: WB (Practice of Medicine), WF (Respiratory System), and WY (Nursing). These subcategories were used in the classification tools from the US National Library of Medicine Classification to separate the medical knowledge of sleep apnea. Every subcategory based on actual condition to do some small category, which still follows the principle of US National Library of Medicine Classification. For example, the WF classification is based on three components: handbooks and reference materials, diagnostic knowledge, and

therapeutic knowledge regarding WF39 (Handbooks and Resource guides), WF141 (Diagnostic Methods), WF145 (Therapeutics). In WF141 of this category, it would be provided with required medical theoretical, which basis on US National Library of Medicine Classification, into the more detailed categories. Those categories are WV (Otolaryngology), WG (Cardiovascular System), WK (Endocrine System), and WL (Nervous System).

Table 6 shows the interactions between the transverse category (clinical knowledge) and straight category (theoretical knowledge).

Conclusions and Contribution

A comprehensive preceding chapters contents, this research base on the research executive producer of Table 2, to present complete sleep apnea medical diagnosis knowledge. This study also provides a complete and readily applicable knowledge extraction mechanism, and the associated procEduccres, for use in the field of sleep medicine.

Knowledge Extraction Questions Table
01. What are the "critical activity processes" in your field of specialization?
02. Which complementary "critical knowledge" do you need to complete these key activitely processes?
03. What ich "predisposing knowledge" do you think needs to be first learned to possess the critical knowledge?
04. Which "extended knowledge learning" do you think is needed to improve your specialty after obtaining the critical knowledge?
05. In the aforementioned critical activity processes, which complementary "critical resources (project scope) do you think you need to complete these processes?
06. Do you think there are areas of concern or to pay attention to regarding "the acquisition of critical resources (project scope)?
07. In critical activity processes, which "critical partners (people scope) do you think are needed to complete the processes through collaborative efforts?
08. When executing critical activity processes, which methods ways or activities will help you "solve problems" when bottlenecks or obstacles are encountered (such as seminars, participating in expert forums, searching for data online, etc.)?
09. When engaging in the abovementioned problem-solving activities or methods, which method do you use to contact or communicate (such as e-mail, telephone, etc.)? What are the content, form, and format?
10. Which "result and relevant record document files" are produced after executing and completing the critical activity processes?
11. "Where within the organization do you store" your the results and document files? What "retrieval mechanisms and tools" are provided by the organization?
12. Further In continuation to question Q10, what do you think is the "retrieval process" of the results and document files? Is there a control program? If so, what is it?
13. Further to question in continuation to Q10, which "subsequent processes" within the organization do you think will access these results and document files?
14. Further to question in continuation to Q10, which "personnel" within the organization do you think will subsequently use these results and document files? How do they use them?
15. To what What do you think is "the degree is of integration between the knowledge and the organization interior integrated"? Has the knowledge been "fully integrated into our products and services"? What is are "lacking?" "What can be improved?" "How can we start providing what are needed?"

Appendix A: Knowledge extraction questions table.

We successfully extracted sleep apnea medical diagnosis knowledge from the interview data of a sleep medicine specialist, Dr. Chiang Rayleigh Ping-Ying, and verified our results with the input of four other sleep medicine doctors. This confirms that one can use the theories of process management, library science, and knowledge management in the organization of medical knowledge. More importantly, we believe our research results provide a general principle of knowledge extraction applicable to other medical specialties, and one which medical experts may use for such purposes.

Finally, the results tabulated in the present article not only present knowledge in a clear and digestible fashion, but also represent a more systematic process by which to display whole subjects of knowledge. We believe that our findings will assist in the Educcation of medical professionals, improving the teaching, dissemination, and sharing of sleep apnea medical diagnosis knowledge.

Recommendations for Future Research

In the present study, based on in-depth interviews and qualitative research, and supported by project management, library science, and knowledge management, sleep apnea diagnostic knowledge was successfully extracted. However, in this field of medical diagnostic knowledge, there are still many different types of sleep disorders upon which knowledge extraction is yet to be conducted. The present study did not concern itself with the storage and sharing of knowledge via computer systems. Therefore, further research is warranted in the following areas.

(1) Knowledge extraction for medical diagnosis illustrations

The present study was conducted to collect knowledge and extraction work, while output corresponding to the relevant chart. However, is it can apply to other institutions? Are there different industry knowledge extraction differentiation exist? What is it variable? It shall be the relevant research can extend the follow-up.

(2) Innovation research in knowledge management computer systems

In this study, only do the existing knowledge extraction of research. And construction the various types of schematic diagram, which is the structure knowledge type by this research.

The knowledge document for organization process outcome, can also use metadata tables, which design by this research, to construction can easy automated document search mechanism. However, this research did not explore the use of computer systems for knowledge management. For example, while this research presented knowledge in the form of charts, nowadays the computer system, is it design computer auto showing corresponding knowledge document or knowledge graph when the computer point refers to the knowledge operation process? And then, when the user double click the knowledge document or the knowledge graph, which can auto link or open corresponding screen content (like some web site, some knowledge explanation document, etc.) This design should not have technical problems. But it can let computer systems make friendly and more automation to do knowledge management be showing for users. It should be a very meaning full extended research issue.

References

1. Gilbert M, Cordey-Hayes M (1996) Understanding the process of knowledge transfer to achieve successful technological innovation. Technovation 16: 301-312.

2. Quintas P, Lefrere P, Jones G (1997) Knowledge management: A strategic agenda. Long Range Plann 30: 385-391.

3. Borghoff UM, Pareschi R (1998) Information technology for knowledge management, Springer, Berlin.

4. Holsapple CW (2002) Handbook on Knowledge Management 1: Knowledge Matters, Springer, Berlin.

5. Project Management Institute (2004) A Guide to the Project Management Body of Knowledge (PMBOK Guide), Project Management Institute, Newtown Square, PA.

6. National Library of Medicine Classification (2016) NLM, U.S. National Library of Medicine.

7. International Classification of Sleep Disorders (2005) (2nd Edition), AASM.

8. Bose R (2003) Knowledge Management - Enabled Health Care Management Systems: Capabilities, Infrastructure and Decision-Support, Expert Syst Appl 24: 59-71.

9. Wennberg JE, Freeman JL, Culp WJ (1987) Are hospital services rationed in new haven or over-utilized in Boston? Lancet 329: 1185-1189.

10. Introduction to Modern Sleep Technology (2012) (1nd Edition), Springer, Berlin.

11. Leavitt HJ, Pondy LR (1964) Readings in managerial psychology, University of Chicago Press, Chicago, IL.

12

Medical Music Therapy Knowledge among Medical Students of Jimma University, Ethiopia

Kumera Negash Amente*

School of Music, College of Social Sciences and Humanity, Jimma University, Ethiopia

Abstract

The use of music therapy as an adjunct medical treatment option is well established. However, there is no evidence on the knowledge of music therapy among medical practitioner in Ethiopia. Hence, this institutional based cross-sectional study was conducted to assess the knowledge and practices of Jimma University medical students on music therapy as an adjunct medical treatment option. A total of 349 medical students were involved in the study. More than half (51%) of the medical students had heard about the music therapy. However, majority (56.7%) of the medical students had lower mean knowledge (low knowledge) on the application of music therapy in specific medical condition and quality of life. The major source of information is internet. There is also higher interest (83.4%) on music therapy training and education among the study participants. Majority (75.4%) of the medical students were show interest in referring patients to a music therapy. The mean knowledge of the medical students was significantly associated to age, ethnicity and level education in medical school. Therefore, effort should be done to in cooperate the music therapy in formal curriculum of medical education and also continues professional development program is need for medical practitioners to ensure the integration of music therapy program on medical system in the country

Keywords: Music therapy; Knowledge; Medical students; Jimma university

Background

Music therapy is one type of complementary and alternative medicine therapy. It is gaining increasing recognition for its benefit in medical settings. It has been defined by the World Federation of Music Therapy as the professional use of music and its elements, to intervene in the medical, educational and everyday environments with individuals, groups, families or communities seeking to optimize their quality of life and improve their physical, social, communicative, emotional conditions, intellectual, and spiritual health and wellness' research, education, clinical education and practice in music therapy are based on professional standards according to cultural, social and political contexts [1].

Music therapy is an allied health profession and one of the expressive therapies, consisting of a process in which a music therapist uses music and all of its facts-physical, emotional, mental, social, aesthetic, and spiritual-to help clients improve their physical and mental health [2,3]. Music therapists have an ethical and professional responsibility to provide the highest quality care possible to their patients [4]. Music therapy has been shown to be an efficacious, non-invasive and valid treatment option for medical patients with unique outcomes possible [5]. Music therapy can be used to address patient needs related to respiration, chronic pain, physical rehabilitation, diabetes, headaches, cardiac conditions, surgery, and obstetrics, among others. Out of these, the three common areas in which music therapy is used widely are pain management (most common), the reduction of anxiety, and the treatment of depression; each of which are common acute and chronic medical conditions [6].

Music therapy is part of various services that provided in patient care in a wide variety of medical settings such as hospitals, cancer treatment centers, rehabilitation centers, skilled and intermediate care facilities, hospices and more [7-11].

Despite the increasing use of medical music therapy, many medical practitioners seem to remain largely uninformed of the efficacy and applications of music therapy to meet patient needs. A positive perception and understanding results in increased referrals to the music therapist, and more opportunities for direct patient care. Contrariwise, if the medical practitioners do not have an adequate understanding of the music therapist's role or capabilities, they can easily create a barrier between the patient and music therapist because of medical practitioners have a powerful impact on the kinds of treatments their patients choose [6].

Understanding the knowledge of medical practitioner regarding music therapy is paramount in successful integration of music therapy into the treatment team. However, there is no evidence on the music therapy knowledge among medical practitioner in Ethiopia. Hence, this study was done to fill these information gaps.

Methods and Materials

Study design and population

This institutional based cross-sectional study was carried out between August and September 2016 among Jimma University Medical Students using a self-administered questionnaire. The study includes a randomly selected medical student from 1st to 6th year.

Data collection process

The questionnaire used was prepared by the researcher after detail review of the relevant international literature, and finalized following

---

***Corresponding author:** Kumera Negash Amente, School of Music, College of Social Sciences and Humanity, Jimma University, Ethiopia,
E-mail: kumera2012@gmail.com

a pilot application prior to data collection. Students completed the questionnaires during class hours after obtaining necessary permits from the official faculty administrations. The questionnaire was verbalized in English language and was not translated to other languages as English is the medium of instruction at universities in Ethiopia.

The questionnaire consisted of three parts. The first part consisted of questions on socio-demographic characteristics of the students, second part on the knowledge and the last part was on the practice of the study respondent on the music therapy.

To ensure quality of the study, trained data collector administered data collection. The completeness each part of the questionnaire used were check by principal investigator.

Sample size

The sample size was calculated using a sample size determination formula for a single population proportion with the following assumptions: 50% expected prevalence of knowledge and practices of the study participants at 95% confidence level with 5% degree of desired precision. The final calculated sample size was 384. However, only 349 randomly selected voluntary medical students of Jimma University in Ethiopia were included in the study. The study participants were from first year to internship level (fifth and sixth years).

Data management and analysis

The collected data were entered to Microsoft Excel and then, cleaned. The clean data were transported and analyzed using SPSS version 20. The data were analyzed using descriptive statically tool and presented using table. The strength of association between dependent and independent variables was assessed using multiple regression model at 95% conference interval.

Ethical issue

The study protocol was approved by Jimma University Institutional Research Review Committee. Official permission was obtained from School of the Medicine. Informed consent was also obtained from the study participants before administering the data collection. The data were collected kept confidential.

Results

Socio-demography of the study participants

A total of 349 medical students were participated in this study with respondent rate of 91.0%. More than half of 189 (54.2%) the respondents were urban dwellers before joining the university, and 201 (57.6%) protestant followers. Majority 271 (77.7%) of the respondents were in the age group of less than or equal to 24 years old, with the mean and Median age of 22.97 and 23.0 years, respectively. Great majority 327 (93.7%) were single marital status. Two hundred sixteen (61.9%) participants were on medical intern study level (Table 1).

Source of information and knowledge of music therapy

Half of responds were heard about the music therapy. The Internet was found to be the most commonly used source of information on music therapy from the ten options provided in the questionnaire, followed by Television/Radio and books. However, few 6 (1.7%) report the contribution of medical school (Table 2).

Majority of the study respondents were known as music therapy is help patient condition and safe. However, they have low understanding on the contribution music therapy on improving pain, anxiety,

nausea, restless, agitation, distress, relaxation, spiritual comfort, self-expression, autonomy, communication, socialization and self-expression. Majority of the participants had less than mean knowledge score (bad knowledge) on the application of music therapy in medicine and quality of life (Table 3).

Particles of medical students on music therapy

Majority of the study participants were show interest in refer patients to a music therapy but they intension to support the program is decline because their knowledge gaps on the area and its application in medical practices. In addition, lack of music therapy course in the education system of medicine in the institute is one of the major hindrances for the support of the program. However, most of the responds has high interest in education and training on music therapy (Tables 4 and 5).

Factor affecting the music knowledge among medical students

The knowledge of the medical students was determined by age, ethnicity and level of education of the student in medical school when controlling their confounding variables. Where the study participant with more than 24 year olds [AOR=0.367 (95% CI, 0.21-0.64)] had less mean knowledge than their counter part. The oromo [AOR=0.14 (95% CI, 0.029-0.69)], Amahra [AOR=0.18 (95% CI, 0.036-0.88)], and Tigeray [AOR=0.07 (95% CI, 0.01-0.44)] ethnic groups study participants had less mean knowledge comparing to the Somali ethic students. In contrary medical Intern [AOR=0.34 (95% CI, 0.21-0.57)] study participants had low mean knowledge that shows low contribution medical education level on the music knowledge.

Discussion

Music therapy has been shown to be an efficacious and valid treatment option for medical patients with a variety of diagnoses. Music is a form of sensory stimulation, which provokes responses due to the familiarity, predictability, and feelings of security associated with it. Inspite of music therapy has limited side effect on the patients and more economical to be practical in developing countries like Ethiopia, it practices is reserved to palliative care for patients who have an incurable illness in Africa [12].

The level of incorporation of music therapy in modern medicine influenced by the knowledge of health care provider to refer patient to the music therapy center and promote its implementation as part of health care system. Accordingly, the aim of this explorative study mainly focuses on the knowledge and practices of medical students of Jimma University in Ethiopia.

More than half of the medical student's participants in the study heard about the music therapy. However, majority of the participants had less than mean knowledge score (bad knowledge) on the application of music therapy in medicine and quality of life. This observed because of lack of formal course in the curriculum of medicine in the study instruction. This is clearly found as medical school has low contribution as sources of information and the major sources of information is internet in present study. This similar with other studies done in different countries [13-16].

Majority of the medical students had low understanding on the contribution music therapy on specific medical and social condition like in improving pain, anxiety, nausea, restless, agitation, distress, relaxation, spiritual comfort, self-expression, autonomy, communication, socialization and self-expression. This could be attributed to the presence limited knowledge on music therapy among the study participants. Surprisingly, majority of the study respondents

Variable	Frequency	Percentage
Sex		
Male	263	75.4
Female	86	24.6
Age (Mean=22.97 and median=23.0)		
<or=24	271	77.7
>24	78	22.3
Address before university		
Rural	160	45.8
Urban	189	54.2
Ethnic		
Somali	13	3.7
Oromo	152	43.6
Ahmara	121	34.7
Tigeray	23	6.6
other	40	11.5
Religion		
Muslim	38	10.9
Orthodox	201	57.6
Protestant	90	25.8
Catholic	12	3.4
other	8	2.3
Marital status		
married	12	3.4
Single	327	93.7
Divorced	8	2.3
Windowed	2	0.6
Level of year		
1st year	6	1.7
2nd year	24	6.9
3rd year	31	8.9
4th year	72	20.6
5th & 6th year	216	61.9

Table 1: Socio-demography of the study participants (n=349).

Variables	Frequency	Percentage
Source of information		
Personal experience using music therapy	10	2.9
Family and friends	9	2.6
Newspapers/Magazines	16	4.6
Television/Radio	53	15.2
Internet	55	15.8
Books	21	6.0
Journals	7	2.0
Medical school (University)	6	1.7
Other health care professionals	1	0.3
Not heard music therapy	171	49.0

Table 2: Source of information on music therapy knowledge among Medical students of Jimma University, Ethiopia (n=349).

were reported as music therapy is help patient condition and safe. They also showed higher interest in referring patients to a music therapy but their intension to support the program is decline because their knowledge gaps on the area and its application in medical practices. In addition, lack of music therapy course in the education system of medicine in the institute is one of the major hindrances for the support of the program.

Most of the medical students had high interest on music therapy education and training. This support report from other studies [13,14].

Variable	Frequency	Percentage
Music therapy would help the patient's condition		
Yes	248	71.1
No	101	28.9
Music therapy is safe		
Yes	224	64.2
No	126	35.8
Music therapy can be used to address or improve pain		
Yes	93	26.6
No	256	73.4
Music therapy can be used to address or improve anxiety		
Yes	188	53.9
No	161	46.1
Music therapy can be used to address or improve nausea		
Yes	52	14.9
No	297	85.1
Music therapy can be used to address or improve restless		
Yes	132	37.8
No	217	62.2
Music therapy can be used to address or improve agitation		
Yes	113	32.4
No	236	67.6
Music therapy can be used to address or improve distress		
Yes	170	48.7
No	179	51.3
Music therapy can be used to address or improve relaxation		
Yes	142	40.7
No	207	59.3
Music therapy can be used to address or improve spiritual comfort		
Yes	101	28.9
No	248	71.1
Music therapy can be used to address or improve self-expression		
Yes	95	27.2
No	254	72.8
Music therapy can be used to address or improve socialization		
Yes	96	27.5
No	253	72.5
Music therapy can be used to address or improve overall quality of life		
Yes	67	19.2
No	282	80.8
Music therapy can be used to address or improve family support		
Yes	51	14.6
No	298	85.4
Music therapy can be used to address or improve communication		
Yes	104	29.8
No	245	70.2
Music therapy can be used to address or improve autonomy		
Yes	61	17.5
No	288	82.5
Mean knowledge		
Good (≥ mean knowledge)	151	43.3
Bad (<mean knowledge)	198	56.7

Table 3: Music therapy knowledge among Medical students of Jimma University, Ethiopia (n=349).

This could be a great opportunity to incorporate the music therapy in the national health system through continues professional development program.

The age is significantly associated with the mean knowledge of the study participants where medical students more than 24 year olds had 0.37 less good mean knowledge. This is could be associated to the higher

Variable	Frequency	Percentage
Would you refer patients to a music therapy		
Yes	263	75.4
No	86	24.6
Reason for not support a music therapy program		
I do not have enough know on music therapy	131	37.5
I do not think music therapy is effective in the medical environment	144	41.3
I think music therapy would be too expensive	28	8.0
I do not think patients would benefit from music therapy	12	3.4
I do not think a music therapist is work in the medical environment	7	2.0
Other	2	0.6
Support a music therapy	25	7.2
Studied Music Therapy		
As part of the core coursework at your medical school	13	3.7
As an elective at your medical school	4	1.1
Outside of your medical school	15	4.3
Never Studied	317	90.8
Like to know more about Music Therapy		
Yes	291	83.4
No	58	16.6
Rate your interest in education and training on Music Therapy		
Very interested	80	22.9
Interested	168	48.1
Equivocal	64	18.3
Uninterested	37	10.6

Table 4: Music therapy practices among Medical students of Jimma University, Ethiopia (n=349).

use of internet services among the younger which is major sources of information in the present study. The presence of mean knowledge significant difference on the of the music therapy among the ethnic groups of the study participants will need further study.

Surprisingly, the Medical Intern Students had 0.34 less likely had good mean knowledge than Pre Medical Intern. This observed difference could be attributed to medical intern had more knowledge and practices in medicine and they had less likely to support music therapy where they did not have formal education in the medical school.

Concussion

More than half of the medical students had heard about the music therapy. However, majority of the medical students had low mean knowledge on the application of music therapy in specific medical condition and quality of life. The major source of information is internet and the medical school has low contribution on the knowledge and practices of music therapy. There is also higher interest on music therapy training and education among the study participants. The mean

knowledge of the medical students was affected by age, ethnicity and level education in medical school.

Therefore, effort should be done to in cooperate the music therapy in formal curriculum of medical education and also continues professional development program is need for medical practitioners to ensure the integration of music therapy program on medical system in the country.

Acknowledgements

I would like to appreciate support provided by College of Social Sciences and Humanity of Jimma University. I am grateful to Department of Medicine, College of Health Sciences, Jimma University for facilitated the data collection. The author also would like to appreciate the study participants for their commitment during data collection. Lastly not the least, I would like to thank Mr. Eyasu Ejeta for his comment and support in writing the manuscript.

Funding Sources

The study was conducted from materials support from College of Social Sciences and Humanity of Jimma University.

Variable	Good knowledge, n%	COR(CI)	P-value	AOR(CI)	P-value
Sex					
Male	146(55.5)	1			
Female	52(60.5)	1.23(0.75-2.01)	0.421		
Age					
<or=24	170(62.7)	1		1	
>24	28(35.9)	0.33(0.20-0.56)	0.000*	0.367(0.21-0.64)	0.000*
Address before university					
Rural	92(57.5)	1			
Urban	106(56.1)	0.94(0.62-1.44)	0.790		
Ethnic					
Somali	11(84.6)			1	
Oromo	78(51.3)	0.19(0.04-0.89)	0.035*	0.14(0.029-0.69)	0.016*
Ahmara	71(58.7)	0.26(0.05-1.22)	0.087	0.18(0.036-0.88)	0.035*
Tigeray	9(39.1)	0.01(0.12-0.65)	0.015*	0.07(0.01-0.44)	0.004*
Other	29(72.5)	0.48(0.10-2.52)	0.385	0.43(0.08-2.37)	0.335
Religion					
Muslim	25(65.8)	1	0.448		
Orthodox	119(59.2)	0.75(0.36-1.56)	0.104		
Protestant	45(50.0)	0.52(0.23-1.14)	0.330		
Catholic	6(50.0)	0.52(0.14-1.94)	0.149		
Other	3(37.5)	0.31(0.06-1.51)	0.448		
Marital status					
Single	189(57.8)	1			
Other	9(40.9)	0.50(0.21-1.22)	0.128		
Level of education					
Pre-Medical Intern	93(69.9)	1		1	
Medical Intern	105(48.6)	0.41(0.26-0.64)	0.000*	0.34(0. 21-0.57)	0.000*

COR=Crude Odds Ratio; AOR=Adjusted Odds ratio; CI=Confidence interval; 1=Reference; *=statistically significant

Table 5: Factor affecting on music knowledge among Medical students of Jimma University, Ethiopia (n=349).

Author's Contribution

KNA conceived and designed the protocol, supervise the data collection, contributed for data analysis, and wrote the paper. I read and approved the final paper.

Disclosures and Ethics

I declare there is no conflict of interest and the study was conducted after obtaining ethical approval and permission from concerned bodies.

References

1. World Federation of Music Therapy (2016).

2. Jump Up (2013) American Music Therapy Association.

3. Jump up (2011) "About Music Therapy & AMTA". American Music Therapy Association.

4. Davis WB, Gfeller KE, Thaut MH (2008) An introduction to music therapy theory and practice. Silver Spring MD: American Music Therapy Association.

5. McCaffrey R, Locsin RC (2002) Music listening as a nursing intervention: a symphony of practice. Holist Nurs Pract 16: 70-77.

6. American Music Therapy Association (2005) Medical music therapy.

7. Humpal ME (1990) Early intervention: The implications for music therapy. Music Ther Perspect 8: 30-35.

8. Hilliard RE (2004) A post-hoc analysis of music therapy services for residents in nursing homes receiving hospice care. J Music Ther 41: 266-281.

9. Taylor DB (1981) Music in general hospital treatment from 1900 to 1950. J Music Ther 18: 62-73.

10. Choi B (1997) Professional and patient attitudes about the relevance of music

therapy as a treatment modality in namt approved psychiatric hospitals. J Music Ther 34: 277-292.

11. Silverman MJ (2006) Psychiatric patients' perception of music therapy and other psychoeducational programming. J Music Ther 43: 111-122.

12. Ruth MS (2005) Music in West Africa: Experiencing Music, Expressing Culture. New York, USA.

13. Mathur A, Duda L, Kamat DM (2008) Knowledge and Use of Music Therapy Among Pediatric Practitioners in Michigan. Clinical Pediatrics 47: 155-159.

14. Emily JG (2013) Medical Music Therapy: Medical and Nursing Student Perceptions and Barriers to Program Implementation. Master's Thesis. Florida State University, USA.

15. Haque AE, Lan ACS, Abdul Kadir FHB, Abdul Rahman NAB, Segaran TS, et al. (2015) Complementary and Alternative Medicine: Knowledge and Attitude of Medical Students of the UniKL-RCMP, Perak, Malaysia. Research J Pharm Tech 8: 1189-1196.

16. Hasan SS, Yong CS, Babar MG, Naing CM, Hameed A, et al. (2011) Understanding, perceptions and self-use of complementary and alternative medicine (CAM) among Malaysian pharmacy students. BMC Complement Altern Med 11: 95.

13

Nutritional Assessment and Consumer Trends in Women University Students of Health Sciences in Madrid, Spain

Teresa Iglesias M*

Universidad Francisco de Vitoria, Spain

Abstract

Objective: The aim of the study was to know dietary habits and nutritional knowledge of women nursing students.

Material and methods: Participants of the study were a random sample composed of 200 female students of health sciences. This sample represented the 95% of total, and the 5% was excluded (men and chronic illness). We studied three-day record study, including a weekend. At the same time, we measured the weight, the height, diameter of hip and diameter of waist.

Results: The energy intake was 1720 Kcal/day, and as in similar studies the % energy from fat and proteins was higher than % energy from carbohydrates. Statured fatty acid intake was statistically significant higher than recommendations. Body mass index (BMI) was normal in 81.1% of women (21.3 Kg/m²). The rest was 10% underweight and 8.9% had overweight/obesity.

Conclusions: This information provided by this study, should be used in order to improve Nutritional studies in nursing schools.

Keywords: Nutritional assessment; Nutritional trends; University students; Women

Introduction

The adulthood period, over 18 years, is increasingly recognized as an important period of health behavior formation. Assessment of nutritional status is important in order to identify potential risk groups. Today it is possible, with the modification of the diet, to delay the appearance of diseases caused by both deficiency and above all by excess. We know that there is an increasing prevalence of related pathologies, such as obesity, diabetes, dyslipidemia, high blood pressure, different types of cancer or heart disease, etc. The location of fat seems to be more important than its total amount, thus studies have shown that there is a good correlation between the waist circumference and the intra-abdominal fat and of this one with the cardiovascular risk [1,2].

Spain has traditionally been a country where the dietary pattern was a healthy diet, Mediterranean diet, which has been abandoned by a less healthy, as the Anglo-Saxon, because of changes in living habits [3,4]. Currently young people are concerned about their image and body weight, and a high percentage follow varied guidelines aimed at weight loss, with inappropriate behaviors. The quality of diet in young people and university students is important to be studied, since it coincides with changes in their lifestyle, being also a vulnerable stage by the power of advertising (miracle diets, healthy foods, etc.), which causes them to modify their eating habits, which will sometimes be for life [5]. As for the female population, it will go through different physiological situations throughout its life that will cause its recommended intakes to be modified [6]. Characterizing the prevalence of health behaviors in university students may help to identify useful targets for health promotion. There are authors [7] that indicate that the dietary model presents an imbalance in the percentage contribution of the immediate principles, being necessary to promote the consumption of fruits, vegetables, legumes and olive oil. The WHO (1985; 1997) emphasizes the need to develop methodological strategies capable of promoting positive attitudes towards healthy habits and long-lasting behaviors [8,9]. Quantifying the knowledge (risk awareness), attitudes, and behaviors in this population may inform interventions that improve health behaviors and ultimately mitigate chronic disease risk.

The objective is to know in future health professionals the dietary habits assessed through a 3-day recall survey and frequency of food consumption, as well as their anthropometric measures and their physical activity.

Materials and Methods

A group of 200 students from health sciences at Universidad Francisco de Vitoria was studied, 100% of the students enrolled in this course accepted to participate voluntarily in this study after giving their informed consent, not having dropped out during the study. But 5% were excluded due to gender (mainly of the students are women, so the few men was rejected) or chronic illness. The age of participants was between 18 to 35 years, representing those over 25 years old 4%. Those who did not suffer from chronic diseases and who were not pregnant were selected after passing a questionnaire/medical record.

Anthropometric data (weight and height) were carried out by a nurse and following WHO standards (1999) (World Health Organization) [10]. The weight / size was made dressed and without shoes with a scale Tanita TBF 300 GS. The body mass index (BMI) allows classification according to the different categories [11] and was calculated from the weight and height data using the equation: BMI=Weight (kg)/size² (m).

The waist and hip diameter was measured with a metric tape of inextensible material (range 0-150 cm). Values higher than 0.85 in women was considered in risk.

***Corresponding author:** Teresa Iglesias M, Universidad Francisco de Vitoria, Spain, E-mail: m.iglesias.prof@ufv.es

A questionnaire was used for this study that included: life habits; frequency of food consumption (fruits, vegetables, vegetables, meat and fish), alcoholic beverages and salt and 3-day recall, including weekend. The DIAL program was used to evaluate the 3-day recall [12]. During the study period, all students were given blood to determine total plasma cholesterol and vitamin D.

Statistical package SPSS 21.0 was used to analyze the results, standard statistical software available at the Francisco de Vitoria University. Differences between groups were assessed using Student's t-tests and ANOVA, with statistically significant differences being considered for p<0.05

Results and Discussion

The average age of students was 20.4 ± 2.9 years, 96% is represented by students between 18-25 years and the remaining 4% is made up of students between 26-35 years old. As the latter percentage was so small, it was not considered to influence the final results.

BMI is the most frequently used indicator in obesity studies. The average energy intake of students is 1720.7 kcal, energy that is mainly provided by 3-4 meals (Table 1). For example, if we performed a comparative study of BMI versus energy intake of the students, we see that the differences are significant (p<0.05). 80% of the participants had a BMI within normal (21.3 ± 2.5 kg/m²), while 11.1% had low weight, 8.9% were overweight and none had obesity. The waist hip ratio is an indicator of cardiovascular risk, is also within the normal range 0.75 ± 0.06 (0.66-0.92).

When the students were asked, do you eat breakfast every day? the answer was that they mostly do it daily (Table 1) and the question "Number of meals a day? most make 3-4 meals/day, meals that 90% of the students do outside the home. The differences found were significant (p<0.01). If we related daily BMI-breakfast, the results are not significant (Table 1), in two studies, one conducted in Dubai and in the AVENA study, these were significant, and in them girls who did not eat breakfast tended to consume more food the rest of the day and therefore they gain weight [13,14], we have not been able to relate the omission of the breakfast with the greater BMI of the students. There are no significant results when comparing the number of daily meals with BMI, however, if there is a significant (p<0.05) relationship between BMI and students that reduce the amount of food eaten.

The growing sedentary of the society is becoming a public health problem [15], thus 43% of the population between 15-24 years of age does not practice any sport [16]. This sedentary lifestyle is greater in the female sex (82.9%) similar values to those observed in Granada students [17]. In a study carried out in different students [18-25] it has been observed that coronary diseases, dyslipemias and diabetes, directly related to the high levels of sedentary of young people, are emerging at an early stage. As for the activity they did daily, and as can be seen in Table 2, the differences are significant when students were asked about daily exercise, walking at least 30 minutes/day, efforts made and time spent watching TV. Among the students who watched TV (data not shown), when asked if they ate or drank while they watched, 50% (n=91) responded affirmatively and the differences observed were significant (p<0.05), this was observed by Zaal et al. [13].

In terms of macronutrient intake (Table 3), it was observed a high protein intake of 85.8 g/day compared to the recommended daily intakes (1.48 g/kg/day versus 0.8 g/kg/day recommended) and consequently the caloric intake (21.2%) almost doubles the recommended value (10-15%). The caloric intake of lipids was 42.3% of the energy intake, a figure that is above the recommended value, so a lower intake of energy from carbohydrates was detected (43%), which represents only the 85% of the recommended daily intake. The caloric profile is therefore unbalanced with a high percentage of calories provided by proteins and lipids and a lower percentage contributed by carbohydrates. This coincides with other studies, and even in some studies it has been observed that women present worse eating habits than men [26,27] although other authors such as Fernández et al. [21] report that men had a lower diet quality. The energy provided by these macronutrients is obtained mainly from 3-4 meals, which are the ones that are mostly carried out by the students (Table 1). With regard to where they eat during the week, 95% claim to do it outside the home (University), feeding mostly on precooked foods, high protein foods rich in fats, potato chips, industrial pastries and sugary soft drinks (data not shown).

Regarding the quality of the fat (Table 3), it was observed that 18% comes from saturated fatty acids (SFA), a value that doubles the recommended value (<7%), 19% of monounsaturated (MUFA), the same was observed in other studies [24,26-30], and 8% of polyunsaturated fatty acids (PUFA). Which respect to PUFA, 88.9% of the student's present values within adequate limits, while 11.1% exceed them (p<0.01).

Cholesterol intake was 304.9 mg/d, slightly higher than recommended (<300 mg/day). This could be related to the elevation of blood lipids that in recent decades have been observed in Spanish adolescents [22,23].

The low intake of fiber (Table 3) could be associated with the low consumption of fruits and vegetables in the students, consumption that has a protective effect against cancer and at the cardiovascular level [24]. We did not observe significant differences between their consumption and BMI (data not shown).

Conclusion

Although the size of the sample may reduce the possibilities of

BMI	Energy intake (kcal/day)	Have breakfast every day			Number of meals		Intake reduction of food		
		N	F	S	3-4 comidas	5-6 comidas	N	F	S
Underweight 11.1% (n=18)	1250.87 ± 571.6	4(2.2%)	6(3.3%)	10(5.6%)	19(10.5%)	1(0.6%)	2(1.1%)	12(6.7%)	6(3.3%)
Normalweight 80% (n=146)	1736.6 ± 533.5	33 (18.3%)	36 (20%)	75 (42.7%)	120 (66.7%)	24 (13.3%)	53 (29.4%)	71 (39.4%)	20 (11.1%)
Overweight 8.9% (n=16)	2153.6 ± 663.7	5 (2.8%)	5 (2.8%)	6 (3.3%)	13 (7.3%)	3 (1.7%)	6 (3.3%)	10 (5.6%)	0
Total (n=180)	1719.7 ± 583.6	42 (23.3%)	47 (26.1%)	91 (50.6%)	152 (84.4%)	28 (15.6%)	61 (33.9%)	93 (51.7%)	26 (14.4%)
P * F*	0.000 12.321	0.563 0.576			0.090 2.443		0.014 4.411		

N: Never; F: Frequently; S: Always; *ANOVA

Table 1: BMI, energy intake, number of meals and reduction in food intake in students.

BMI	I spend the day without activity			I walk every day 30 minutes			Physical exercise daily			I see every day TV		
	N	F	S	N	F	S	N	F	S	N	F	S
Underweight	7(3.9%)	12(6.7%)	1(0.6%)	8(4.5%)	7(3.9%)	5 (2.8%)	12(6.7%)	6(3.4%)	2(1.1%)	10(5.6%)	9(5%)	1(0.6%)
Normalweight	76(42.2%)	52(28.9%)	16(8.9%)	51(28.5%)	56(31.3%)	37 (20.7%)	71(39.7%)	47(26.3%)	25(14%)	114(63.3%)	27(15%)	3(1.7%)
Overweight	9(5%)	6(3.3%)	1(0.6%)	6(3.4%)	7(3.9%)	2 (1.1%)	8(4.5%)	8(4.5%)	0	13(7.2%)	3(1.7%)	0
Total	92(51.1%)	70(38.9%)	18(10%)	65(36.3%)	70(39.1%)	45 (24.6%)	91(50.8%)	61(34.1%)	27(15.1%)	137(76.1%)	39(26.7%)	4(2.2%)
P*F	0.656 0.422			0.710 0.343			0.427 0.854			0.018 4.125		

N: Never; **F**: Frequently; **S**: Always; *ANOVA

Table 2: BMI and physical activity in students.

N=180	Media ± DE	IDR[14]
Energy (kcal)	1720.7 ± 546.4	2200
Proteins (%E)	21.2 ± 8.6	10-15%
Proteins (g)	85.8 ± 37.7	41
Fat (%E)	42.3 29.4	<35%
SFA (%E)	18.5 22.2	<7%
MUFA (%E)	19.0 9.4	13-18%
PUFA (%E)	8 ± 6.8	<10%
Carbohydrates (%E)	42.6 ± 25.3	>50%
Fiber (g/day)	18.52	>25
Fiber (%RDA)	74.1 ± 5.2	
PUFA/SFA	0.6 ± 0.84	>0,5
(PUFA+MUFA)/SFA	1.9 ± 1.0	>2
Cholesterol (mg/day)	304.9 ± 146.5	<300

RDA=Recommended Daily Intake; SFA=Satutared Fatty Acids; MUFA=Monoinsatutared Fatty Acids; PUFA=Poliinsaturated Fatty Acids

Table 3: Mediun energy intake, proteins, lipids, carbohydrates, colesterol and fiber, after 3 days recall.

generalizing the results obtained, we believe that it provides descriptive information, which could be useful from the point of view of preventive medicine. Our results coincide with that reported by other studies on the change in eating habits of young people, characterized by a high intake of saturated fats and proteins at the expense of a low consumption of cereals, fruits, vegetables and vegetables, and consequently a low intake of fiber.

Given that in addition the group studied were students from health sciences, we believe that it is essential an adequate nutritional training that can contribute to improve their own dietary habits, and arouse their sensitivity to the errors or nutritional deficits of patients who in the future be in their charge.

Is already known the increase in cardiovascular risk in the population of western countries, and even reaches young people and adolescents, due to the increase in overweight, obesity and sedentary lifestyle. We consider that the health professionals are a very suitable group to promote a nutritional education that helps to prevent inadequate behaviors and can contribute to better prevention of cardiovascular diseases and all those in which good dietary habits are clearly implied.

The data obtained from this study have allowed us to demonstrate to the students themselves their dietary errors and have contributed to increase their interest in clinical nutrition and healthy habits. It is also useful to promote teaching in Health Sciences at our University.

References

1. Han TS, McNeill G, Seidell JC, Lean ME (1997) Predicting intra-abdominal fatness from anthropometric measures: the influence of stature. Int J Obes Relat Metab Disord 21: 587-93.

2. Snell-Bergeon JK, Hokanson JE, Kinney GL, Dabelea D, Ehrlich J, et al. (2004) Measurement of abdominal fat by CT compared to waist circumference and BMI in explaining the presence of coronary calcium. Int J Obes Relat Metab Disord 28: 1594-9.

3. Neumark-Stainer D, Hannan PJ, Story M, Croll J, Perry C (2003) Family meal patterns: associations with sociodemographic characteristics and improved dietary intake among adolescents. J Am Diet Assoc 103: 317-322.

4. Sánchez-Villegas A, Delgado-Rodríguez M, Martínez-González MA, Irala-Estévez J (2003) Gender, age, socio-demographic and lifestyle patterns in the Spanish Project SUN (Seguimiento Universidad de Navarra). EJCN 57: 285-292.

5. Riba I, Sicart M (2002) Estudio de hábitos alimentarios en población universitaria y sus condiciones. Universidad Autónoma de Barcelona, p: 289.

6. Ortega R (2007) Nutrición en la población femenina: Desde la infancia a la edad avanzada. Editorial Ergón, p: 158.

7. Bollat Montenegro P, Durá Travé T (2008) Modelo dietético de los universitarios. Nutric Hosp 23: 619-629.

8. WHO (1985) Requerimientos de energía y proteínas. Technical Report Series, Ginebra 724: 71-80.

9. WHO (1997) Programme of Nutrition, Family and Reproductive Health. Obesity Preventing and Managing the Global Epidemic, Geneva, pp: 3-5.

10. WHO (1999) Salud para todos en el siglo XXI. Madrid: Ministerio de Salud y Consumo.

11. Rankinen T, Kim SY, Perusse L, Despres JP, Bouchard C (1999) The prediction of abdominal visceral fat level from body composition and anthropometry: ROC analysis. Int J Obes Relat Metab Disord 23: 801-9.

12. Ortega Anta R, López Sobaler AM, Andrés Carvajales P, Requejo Marcos AM, Molinero Casares LM (2007) DIAL 1.0. Programa de evaluación de dietas y gestión de datos de alimentación. Alce Ingeniería, p: 107.

13. Bin Zaal AA, Musaiger AO, D'Souza RD (2009) Dietary habits associated with obesity among adolescents in Dubai, United Arab Emirates. Nut Hosp 24: 437-444.

14. Moreno LA, Kersting M, Henauw S, González-Gross M, Sichert Hellert Matthys C, et al. (2005) How to measure dietary intake and food habits in adolescence: the European perspective. Int J Obes 29: 566-577.

15. Edwards B (2005) Childhood obesity: A school-based approach to increase nutritional knowledge and activity levels. Nurs Clin N Am, pp: 661-669.

16. García Fernando M (2001) Los españoles y el deporte: prácticas y comportamientos en la última década del siglo XX. Madrid, CSD, MECD.

17. Muros Molina JJ, Som Castillo A, Zabala Días M, Oliveras López MJ, López García de la SH (2009) Evaluación del estado nutricional en niños y jóvenes escolarizados en Granada. Nutr Clin Diet Hosp 29: 26-32.

18. Ollat Montenegro P, Durá Travé T (2008) Modelo dietético de universitarios. Nutr. Hosp 23: 626-627.

19. Valdés J, Grau M, Subirana I, Marrugat J, Covas MI, et al. (2009) Secular trends in energy intake and diet quality in a Mediterranean population. Ann Nutr Metab 54: 177-183.

20. Serra-Majem I, Ribas-Barba L, Salvador G, Jover L, Raidó B, et al. (2007) Trends in energy and nutrient intake and risk of inadequate intakes in Catalonia, Spain (1992-2003). Public Health Nutr 10: 1354-1367.

21. Fernández Morales I, Aguilar Vilas MV, Mateos Vega CJ, Martínez Parra MC (2007) Ingesta de nutrientes en una población juvenil, prevalencia de

sobrepeso y obesidad. Nutr Clin Diet Hosp 3: 148-158.

22. Carrero I, Rupérez E, Tejero JA, Pérez-Gallardo L (2005) Ingesta de macronutrientes en adolescentes escolarizados en Soria capital. Nutr Hosp XX 3: 204-209.

23. Izaga Arroyo M, Pablo Rocandio AM, Alday Ansostegui L, Apalauza Pascual E, Beti Salces I, et al. (2006) Calidad de la dieta, sobrepeso y obesidad en estudiantes universitarios. Nutr Hosp 21: 673-679.

24. Oliveras López MJ, Nieto Guindo P, Agudo Aponte E, Martínez F, López García H, et al. (2006) Evaluación Nutricional de una población universitaria. Nutr Hosp 21: 179-183.

25. Wright M, Adair L, James C, Amuleru-Marshall O, Peltzer K, et al. (2015) The association of nutrition behaviors and physical activity with general and central obesity in Caribbean undergraduate students. Rev Panam Salud Publica 38: 278-285.

26. Martínez Roldán C, Veiga Herreros P, López de Andrés A, Cobo Sanz JM, Carvajal Azcona A (2005) Evaluación del estado nutricional de un grupo de universitarios mediante parámetros dietéticos y de composición corporal. Nutr. Hosp XX 3: 197-203.

27. Velasco J, Mariscal-Arcas M, Caballero ML, Hernández-Elizondo J, Olea-Serrano F (2009) Valoración de la dieta de escolares granadinos e influencia de factores sociales. Nutr Hosp 24: 193-199.

28. Martins Bion F, de Castro Chagas MH, de Santana Muñiz G, Oliveira de Sousa LG (2008) Estado nutricional, medidas antropométricas, nivel socioeconómico y actividad física en universitarios brasileños. Nutr Hosp 23: 234-241.

29. Van Duyn MA, Pivonka E (2000) Overview of the health benefits of fruit and vegetable consumption for the dietetics professional: selected literature. J Am Diet Assoc 1000: 1511-1521.

30. Moreno LA, Sarriá A, Popkin BM (2002) The nutrition transition in Spain: a European Mediterranean country. Eur J Clin Nutr 56: 992-1003.

14

Pakistani Healthcare Practitioners' Understanding of the *Zika* Virus Disease

Wajiha Iffat[1], Sadia Shakeel[1]* and Fatima Fasih[2]

[1]*Dow College of Pharmacy, Dow University of Health Sciences, Karachi-Sind, Pakistan*
[2]*Dow International Medical College, Dow University of Health Sciences, Karachi-Sind, Pakistan*

Abstract

The current study aims to assess the knowledge of healthcare practitioners regarding Zika virus disease in Karachi, Pakistan. A cross sectional descriptive study was conducted from January 2016 to April 2016. The study population were physicians selected by non probability convenience sampling technique and were rendering their services in different hospitals and clinics of Karachi. Among the study participants, 41.4% considered themselves not very conversant about Zika virus. Medical literature (50%) and mass media (32%) were the major sources of health information. Approximately 75% did not know the availability of vaccine against Zika virus disease whereas 72.07% were not well versed with the availability and mode of treatment. Around 78% and 22% believed that mosquito bite and body fluid and secretions are the major source of infection respectively. It is concluded that our physicians are not well versed with the Zika virus disease. There is a need to advance the knowledge and understanding of Zika virus disease among physicians as they symbolize a well-informed component of society and healthcare structure. Furthermore, well-organized educational programs are necessary to expand appropriate awareness of public as regards Zika virus disease.

Keywords: Healthcare practitioner's knowledge; Pakistan Zika virus disease

Introduction

The Zika virus (ZIKV), a vector borne virus is affecting a large number of people around the world and has become a major public health hazard [1]. The virus belongs to a family of flavivirus was first identified in Monkeys in year 1947 in Zika forest of Uganda [2,3]. From the 1950s to 1981 numerous studies conducted in the African countries such as Uganda, Egypt, Tanzania, Sierra Leon, Central African Republic and also different parts of Asia showed evidence of ZIKV in humans [4-8]. These results were not a cause for worry due to its low prevalence. Since then sporadic cases have been observed in different parts of the world without ringing alarm bells. Since the ZIKV's identification it has been isolated from different species of Aedes but researchers were not been able to establish any connection between these breed and animals infected with ZIKV. In 1956 for the first time Boorman and Porterfield were able to confirm the transmission of ZIKV from *Aedes ageypti* (Figure 1) to animal especially in mice and monkey [5,9,10]. First documented human ZIKV transmission case was by Simpson who occupationally acquired Zika virus in 1964 [4]. Only one out of five infected patients develop symptoms of ZIKA disease [11].

Neither severe presentation, nor death had been reported before the current epidemic in French Polynesia. Since October 2013, French Polynesia has experienced the largest documented outbreak of ZIKV infection. From November 2013 to February 2014:42(3%) of 1,505 blood donors, although asymptomatic at the time of blood donation, were found positive for ZIKV by PCR [12]. Lorenzo Zammarchi reported the first two cases of laboratory confirmed ZIKV infections imported into Italy from French Polynesia. Both patients presented with low grade fever, malaise, conjunctivitis, myalgia, arthralgia, ankle oedema, and axillary and inguinal lymphadenopathy. One patient showed leukopenia with relative monocytosis and thrombocytopenia [13]. In October 2015 an outbreak of microcephaly cases were observed in the new born babies that led to the amniotic fluid analysis of pregnant women in the country [14]. The results from this test pointed towards the presence of ZIKV. According to a W.H.O. report on April 28, Brazil normally has an average of 163 cases of microcephaly each year, with only about 40 in the less populous northeast. Since October, officials have confirmed about 1,200, nearly 900 of them in the northeast and more than 13 countries have reported sporadic cases of ZIKV. Due to its rapid spread from Brazil in matter of months, it now requires a quick assessment and management of this communicable disease [15]. This virus has the probability to extend to vicinities where the Aedes mosquito vector is presented and could be a risk for our country. So

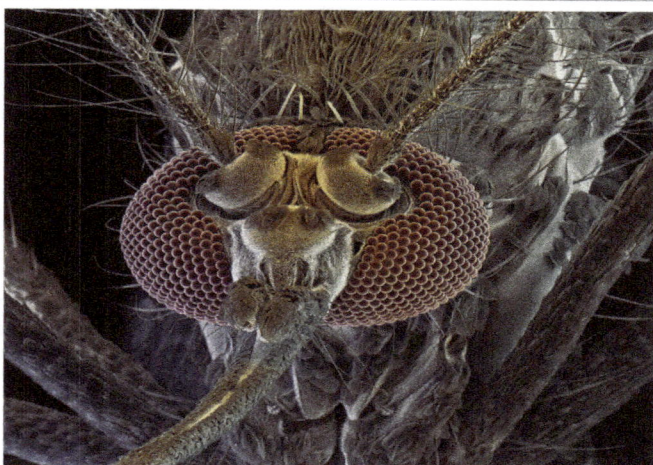

Figure 1: *Aedes ageypti*; Source of ZIKV disease.

*Corresponding author: Sadia Shakeel, Dow College of Pharmacy, Dow University of Health Sciences, Karachi-Sind, Pakistan,
E-mail: sadia.shakeel@duhs.edu.pk

it is important for physicians to have sufficient knowledge so they can screen potential carriers in clinical settings and thus this study aims to assess the knowledge of healthcare practitioners on ZIKV in Karachi, Pakistan.

Methods

A cross sectional descriptive study was conducted from January 2016 to April 2016. The study population were physicians selected by non probability convenience sampling technique and were rendering their services in different hospitals and clinics of Karachi. Physicians were surveyed with a 22 items questionnaire to assess their current knowledge regarding ZIKV disease. The questionnaire consisted of the demographic information of the physicians, items that explored their knowledge towards the recent outbreak, major source and route of transmission of infection, symptoms, diagnosis and potential complications of ZIKV disease. Prior to initiate the study consent was obtained from the concerned authorities in the hospitals and clinics. The purpose of research was explained to the physicians and their consent was obtained before the questionnaires were distributed. The questionnaires recovered were entered into Statistical Package for Social Sciences (SPSS 20.0, Chicago, IL) for study. The frequencies and percentages were used to analyze the demographic data of the participants. Descriptive statistics were employed to observe the response of physicians to survey items. The correlation of the independent characteristics with the responses of participants towards ZIKV disease was determined by means of a chi-square, at 0.05 level of significance.

Results

In current study, two hundred survey forms were distributed through direct correspondence and left for a period of one week. On subsequent collection only one hundred and eleven forms were returned back. Hence the response rate was 55.5%. Majority of the physicians (64.86%) were male. Mass population (83.78%) of study was rendering their services in public sector hospitals (Table 1).

Medical literature (50%) and mass media (32%) were the major sources of health information. On inquiring about the knowledge towards ZIKV, 41.4% of physicians considered that ZIKV is a nationally notifiable condition however they did not considered themselves very up to date. Around 65% knew about the current status of ZIKV in the world, 80% stated that Africa was the place of recent outbreak. Male physicians were more likely to believe that mosquito bite and body fluid and secretions are the major source of transmission of ZIKV (p=0.034). More than 70% deemed that ZIKV disease is vector-borne and the chiefly observed clinical features of ZIKV were fever (90.09%), myalgia (86.49%), retro-orbital pain (84.68%), headache (80.18%) and arthralgia (74.7%) (Figure 2). More than half (58.56%) did not know that ZIKV is fatal and only 5.41% assumed that symptoms of ZIKV are similar to those of dengue and chikungunya whereas 45% linked ZIKV with Guillain Barré syndrome (GBS). Majority (59.5%) of the male respondents (p<0.0001) considered that the symptoms normally last for 1-10 days whereas 28.8% believed that the symptoms normally last for 7-15 days.

The responses of physicians regarding their knowledge of ZIKV are stated in Table 2. Approximately 75% did not know about the availability of vaccine against ZIKV whereas 72.07% were not well versed with the availability of treatment. Merely 39.63% and 45.95% knew the potential complications of ZIKV and how ZIKV is diagnosed respectively. Greater part (61.26%) did not know that ZIKV can be either sexually

Demographic Characteristics	Percentages (%)	p value
Gender		
Male	64.86	p=0.045
Female	35.13	
Age (Years)		
Less than 30	16.22	
30-39	37.84	p<0.001
40-49	25.23	
50 and above	20.72	
Organization		
Public Sector	83.78	p=0.429
Private	16.22	
Field		
Clinical	56.76	p=0.200
Academics	42.34	
Position		
Consultant/Surgeon	9.91	
Head of department	7.21	
RMO	28.83	p<0.0001
Professor	15.32	
Lecturer	38.74	
Experience (Years)		
Less than 5	61.26	
5-10	17.12	p<0.0001
15-20	18.02	
20 and above	3.60	

Table 1: Characteristics of Study Population.

Statement	Yes (%)	No (%)	Don't know (%)
ZIKV is a nationally notifiable condition	41.44	30.63	27.93
ZIKV disease is fatal	19.82	21.62	58.56
Symptoms of ZIKV are similar to those of dengue and chikungunya	5.41	46.84	47.75
Know the potential complications of ZIKV?	39.63	22.52	36.03
Know that how ZIKV is diagnosed?	45.95	21.62	31.53
Is there any vaccine available against ZIKV?	24.32	0.90	74.77
Is there any treatment available against ZIKV disease?	2.70	25.23	72.07
Is there any link between ZIKV and Guillain Barré syndrome (GBS)?	45.05	29.73	24.32
Is ZIKV sexually transmitted?	18.92	19.82	61.26
Do you know that what can you recommend your patients to protect them from ZIKV?	47.75	18.02	33.33

Table 2: Physicians Knowledge of ZIKV Disease.

transmitted. Nearly half of the study population (47.75%) knew what to recommend the patients and general public to protect from ZIKV.

Around 40% opined that pregnant women are more likely to develop symptoms of ZIKV as compared to the general population (Table 3). More than half (52.25%) believed that ZIKV during pregnancy may be linked to microcephaly in newborns. Forty-four percent thought that women can transmit ZIKV to their fetuses during pregnancy or childbirth whereas 36.94% opined that mothers with ZIKV can breastfeed their baby.

Discussion

New Caledonia reported imported cases of ZIKV from French Polynesia in 2013 and reported an outbreak in 2014 [16]. The profusion of mosquito vectors of flavivirus and accessibility of air travel in the Pacific region elevated concern for the stretch of ZIKV disease to other

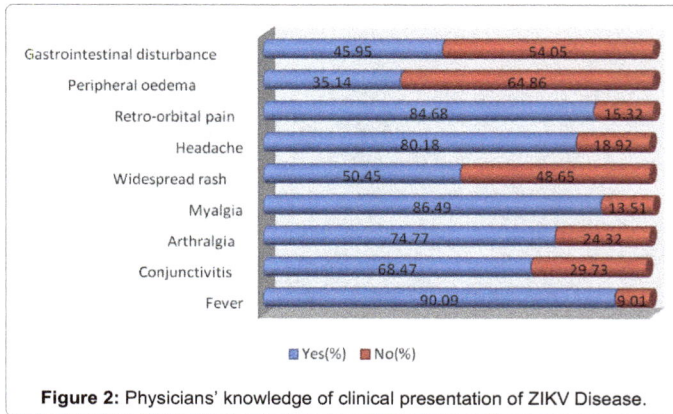

Figure 2: Physicians' knowledge of clinical presentation of ZIKV Disease.

Statement	Yes (%)	No (%)	Don't know (%)
Pregnant women are more likely to develop symptoms of ZIKV as compared to the general population	37.84	33.33	27.93
Can women transmit ZIKV to their fetuses during pregnancy or childbirth?	44.14	0.00	55.86
ZIKV during pregnancy may be linked to microcephaly in newborns?	52.25	28.83	16.22
Can mothers with ZIKV breastfeed their baby?	36.94	45.95	15.32

Table 3: Physicians Knowledge of Association among ZIKV Disease and Pregnancy.

islands in Oceania and yet to the America [15]. ZIKV is transmitted via mosquitoes, particularly Aedes species [17]. In current study, 41.4% physicians considered themselves not very conversant. Around 78% believed that mosquito bite is the major source of infection. Greater part (61.26%) did not know that ZIKV can be sexually transmitted or not. However, direct inter-human transmission, most probably by means of sexual intercourse, has been depicted [18].

The clinical symptoms become visible after few days of the infected mosquito bite and last around 3 to 12 days. Frequencies of asymptomatic presentations are common. However, ZIKV infection can cause wide range of symptoms similar to dengue like syndrome [19]. The symptoms range from mild fever, edema of extremeties headaches, retro-orbital pain, conjuctival hyperremia and maculopapular rashes [20]. Our research report that fever (90.09%), myalgia (86.49%), retro-orbital pain (84.68%), headache (80.18%) and arthralgia (74.7%) were the chiefly observed clinical features of ZIKV observed by the physicians. Approximately 75% did not know that is there any vaccine available against ZIKV whereas 72.07% were not well versed with the availability of treatment. The typical clinical representation of ZIKV infection bear a resemblance to that of dengue fever and chikungunya apparent by headache, myalgia, arthralgia, fever, and maculopapular rash, a multifaceted symptom that hinders differential diagnosis [21]. Though the infection is self-limiting, cases of neurologic manifestations and the Guillain Barré syndrome were depicted in French Polynesia and in Brazil during ZIKV epidemics [14]. In this study, 45% linked ZIKV with Guillain Barré syndrome (GBS). There is no known effective drug or vaccine available drug to fight against ZIKV. Patients infected with ZIKV are generally advised to rest and drink lots of water [22]. Treatment, if required, is mainly supportive, including intravenous fluids and antipyretics. Anti-inflammatory drugs like Ibugesic need to be avoided till dengue positivity is completely ruled out [17].

In current study 37.84% opined that pregnant women are more likely to develop symptoms of ZIKV as compared to the general population.

More than half (52.25%) believed that ZIKV during pregnancy may be linked to microcephaly in newborns. ZIKV was observed in amniotic fluid of two fetuses having microcephaly, revealing the intrauterine transmission of virus [14]. Patrícia reported a significant increase in cases of neonatal microcephaly amongst pregnant women that delivers in northeastern Brazil, and a consecutive increase was accounted in southeast Brazil in September 2015 [23]. ZIKV has been isolated from the amniotic fluid of pregnant women with infants having microcephaly and from the brain of a fetus with central nervous system (CNS) abnormalities [19]. In this study, 44% thought that women can transmit ZIKV to their fetuses during pregnancy or childbirth whereas 36.94% opined that mothers with ZIKV can breastfeed their baby. Besnard reported that the possible routes of perinatal transmission were trans placental, for the period of delivery, for the duration of breastfeeding and by close contact involving the mother and her baby [17]. He reported that sera from the mothers were RT-PCR positive in post-delivery two days and those of their baby within post-delivery four days suggestive of the fact that she was viraemic or at least incubating ZIKV at the moment of delivery [17].

The limitations of current research are the small sample size and constraint to the population of few institutions in Karachi. As with any retrospective study, our study faces the probable influence of problems with recall and social desirability response bias. Other limitations include lack of research and survey studies in the concerned field, so difficult to generalize the findings in Pakistan. Time duration and lack of funds directly reduces the survey sampling as well as further extension of this work.

Conclusion

It is concluded that our physicians are not well versed with the ZIKV disease. There is a need to advance the knowledge and understanding of ZIKV disease among physicians as they symbolize a knowledgeable component of society and healthcare structure. Furthermore, well-organized educational programs are necessary to expand appropriate awareness of public as regards ZIKV disease.

References

1. Gulland A (2016) Zika virus is a global public health emergency, declares WHO. BMJ 352: 657.

2. Dick G, Kitchen S, Haddow A (1952) Zika virus (I). Isolations and serological specificity. Transactions of the Royal Society of Tropical Medicine and Hygiene 46: 509-520.

3. Dick G (1952) Zika virus (II) Pathogenicity and physical properties. Transactions of the Royal Society of Tropical Medicine and Hygiene 46: 521-534.

4. Hayes EB (2009) Zika virus outside Africa. Emerg Infect Dis 15: 1347-1350.

5. Fagbami A (1979) Zika virus infections in Nigeria: virological and sero epidemiological investigations in Oyo State. Journal of Hygiene 83: 213-219.

6. Robin Y, Mouchet J (1974) Serological and entomological study on yellow fever in Sierra Leone. Bulletin de la Societe de Pathologie Exotique et de ses Filiales 68: 249-258.

7. Saluzzo J, Ivanoff B, Languillat G, Georges A (1981) Serological survey for arbovirus antibodies in the human and simian populations of the South-East of Gabon (author's transl). Bulletin de la Societe de Pathologie Exotique et de ses Filiales 75: 262-266.

8. Jan C, Languillat G, Renaudet J, Robin Y (1977) A serological survey of arboviruses in Gabon. Bulletin de la Societe de Pathologie Exotique et de ses Filiales 71: 140-146.

9. Marchette N, Garcia R, Rudnick A (1969) Isolation of Zika virus from Aedes aegypti mosquitoes in Malaysia. American Journal of Tropical Medicine and Hygiene 18: 411-415.

10. Boorman J, Porterfield J (1956) A simple technique for infection of mosquitoes with viruses transmission of Zika virus. Transactions of the Royal Society of Tropical Medicine and Hygiene 50: 238-242.

11. Elachola H, Gozzer E, Zhuo J, Memish ZA (2016) A crucial time for public health preparedness: Zika virus and the 2016 Olympics, Umrah, and Hajj. The Lancet 387: 630-632.

12. Musso D, Nhan T, Robin E, Roche C, Bierlaire D, et al. (2014) Potential for Zika virus transmission through blood transfusion demonstrated during an outbreak in French Polynesia, November 2013 to February 2014. Euro Surveill 19: 20761.

13. Zammarchi L, Stella G, Mantella A, Bartolozzi D, Tappe D, et al. (2015) Zika virus infections imported to Italy: clinical, immunological and virological findings, and public health implications. Journal of Clinical Virology 63: 32-35.

14. Mlakar J, Korva M, Tul N, Popović M, Poljšak-Prijatelj M, et al. (2016) Zika virus associated with microcephaly. New England Journal of Medicine 374: 951-958.

15. Duffy MR, Chen TH, Hancock WT, Powers AM, Kool JL, et al. (2009) Zika virus outbreak on Yap Island, federated states of Micronesia. New England Journal of Medicine 360: 2536-2543.

16. Campos GS, Bandeira AC, Sardi SI (2015) Zika virus outbreak, Bahia, Brazil. Emerging infectious diseases 21: 1885.

17. Besnard M, Lastere S, Teissier A, Cao Lormeau V, Musso D (2014) Evidence of perinatal transmission of Zika virus, French Polynesia. Euro Surveill 19: 20751.

18. Foy BD, Kobylinski KC, Chilson FJL, Blitvich BJ, Travassos DRA, et al. (2011) Probable non-vector-borne transmission of Zika virus, Colorado, USA. Emerg Infect Dis 17: 880-882.

19. Brasil P, Pereira J, Jose P, Raja GC, Damasceno L, et al. (2016) Zika virus infection in pregnant women in Rio de Janeiro preliminary report. New England Journal of Medicine.

20. Ioos S, Mallet HP, Goffart IL, Gauthier V, Cardoso T, et al. (2014) Current Zika virus epidemiology and recent epidemics. Medecine et maladies infectieuses 44: 302-307.

21. Oehler E, Watrin L, Larre P, Leparc GI, Lastere S, et al. (2014) Zika virus infection complicated by Guillain-Barre syndrome--case report, French Polynesia. December 2013. Euro Surveill 19: 20720.

22. Benelli G, Mehlhorn H (2016) Declining malaria, rising of dengue and Zika virus: insights for mosquito vector control. Parasitology research 115: 1747-1754.

23. Calvet G, Aguiar RS, Melo AS, Sampaio SA, Filippis DI, et al. (2016) Detection and sequencing of Zika virus from amniotic fluid of fetuses with microcephaly in Brazil: a case study. The Lancet Infectious diseases 16: 653-660.

15

Perception of Pediatric Physicians' Attire by Children and Parents within General Pediatrics Practice in Saudi Arabia

Yossef Alnasser[1]*, Habeeb AlSaeed[1], Nourah Z Al-Beeshi[2], Hadeel Al-Sarraj[1], Haya Alotaibi[2], Rawabi Algahmdi[2], Kholoud AlAmari[2] and Ayshah Jaber[2]

[1]Department of Pediatrics, King Saud University, Riyadh, Saudi Arabia
[2]Depatment of Medicine, King Saud University, Riyadh, Saudi Arabia

Abstract

Background: Physicians' attire can play a critical factor in patient-doctor relationship. Such relationship is necessary to improve healthcare outcomes and eventually lead to healthier children.

Objective: This study aims to assess perceptions of Saudi children and parents toward physicians' attire within inpatient general pediatrics settings. To our knowledge, no such assessment has been presented until now.

Methods: A questionnaire was adopted and evaluated by pilot study. Then, data were collected from parents along with certain demographic data within inpatients general pediatrics settings.

Results: Perceptions of attire differ according to physician's gender. Wearing scrubs was found more professional, approachable, and trust-worthy for male physicians by parents while wearing conservative long black skirts with lab coat perceived similarly for female physicians. However, wearing summer dress and Saudi traditional attire thought to jeopardies infection controls. Furthermore, children found these attires more intimidating. Although majority of parents thought wearing lab coat is necessary, most of children disagreed. Also, discordance in perception of decorated stethoscopes was observed. Surprisingly, tennis shoes were the preferred shoes for both male and female physicians.

Conclusion: Physicians' attire can be interpreted as indicator of professionalism which could impact patient-doctor relationship. Moreover, children can perceive physician attire differently from their parents.

Keywords: Physician attire; Scrubs; Formal attire; Lab coat; Tennis shoes

Introduction

Physicians' attire can play a critical factor in patient-doctor relationship [1]. Such relationship is necessary to improve healthcare outcomes and eventually lead to healthier children. It means more than a fashion statement. It could be interpreted as indicator of professionalism, competency and trust-worthiness [2].

Physicians' attire and styles might be subject to cultural sensitivity [3]. Moreover, they also could be perceived differently according to gender and clinical practice [4,5]. In pediatrics, those attires have to consider not only the main patients, children, but also their caregivers [6]. In addition, those attires have to be less intimidating and child friendly [7].

In Saudi Arabia, assessment of physician-attire within adult outpatient clinics had un-expected results [8]. Formal Western attires were perceived most professional, even more than Saudi traditional costumes with no gender difference. To our knowledge, no such assessment has been presented to Saudi pediatrics society.

In this study, we aimed to assess perceptions of Saudi Arabia children and parents of physicians' attire within inpatient general pediatrics. This study explored traditions involvement, cultural norms and gender's role in such perceptions. The study stressed on which attire can improve child-doctor rapport and bonding in addition to their parents and caregivers.

Our hypothesis focused on three main domains. First domain: physician-attire might be perceived differently by children and their parents in Saudi Arabia's general pediatrics practice. Second domain: Such perceptions might be dependent on physician gender. Third domain of our hypothesis focused on importance of lab coat in child healthcare and how it might be alarming to children and their parents.

Methods

Data collection and study population

Two questionnaires were adopted and evaluated initially by a pilot study of 20 participants from King Saud University Medical City's (KSUMC) General Pediatrics wards. First questionnaire was designed for surveying parents while the second utilized simpler language to meet children conceptual ability. The questionnaires were analyzed from clearness and easiness measures. Meanwhile, inclusion and exclusion criteria were finalized (Table 1).

Questionnaires employed pictures to demonstrate five different attires for each gender (Surgical Scrub, formal western for male, smart-casual western for male, two traditional male dresses with different headwear, female conservative and formal attire, female formal suite-pants, colored skirt and female summer dress) (Figure 1). Mainly, eight variables were employed as measures of perceptions (professionalism, trust-worthiness, likely to follow recommendations, knowledgeable, approachable, pose risk of infection, confidant, and amenable). Additionally, perceptions of wearing a lab coat were scrutinized in

*Corresponding author: Yosef Alnasser, Pediatric Resident, Pediatric Department, King Saud University Medical City, King Saud University, Riyadh, Saudi Arabia, E-mail: yossef.alnasser@gmail.com

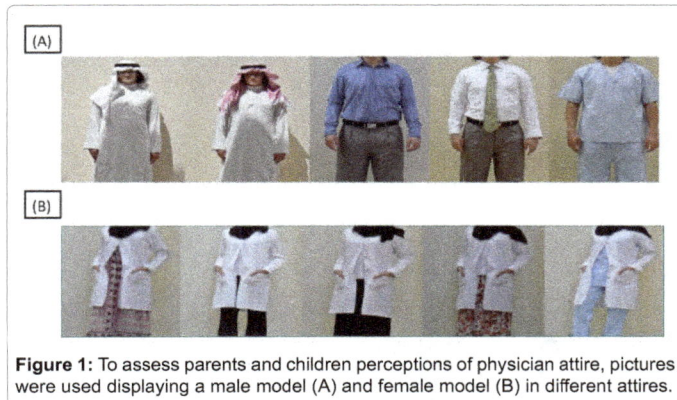

Figure 1: To assess parents and children perceptions of physician attire, pictures were used displaying a male model (A) and female model (B) in different attires.

Inclusion Criteria	Exclusion Criteria
Parents of any child admitted to general pediatric wards	Any child younger than 6 years
Child has to be six years or older	Non-communicative children
Informed consent obtained from caregivers with children's asset	Children with improper cognitive function
Patient of Saudi citizenship	Exclude any child who his/her caregivers were interviewed first

Table 1: Shows used inclusion and exclusion criteria in the presented study.

both parents and children populations. Effect of wearing jewelries and type of footwear in both gender were included in the designed questionnaires. Furthermore, role of decorating stethoscope with toys was inspected.

Parents and children were allowed to choose pictures that best express their opinions. Other questions asked them on a 3-point scale (0=do not bother, 1=no, 2=yes) to advise whether lab-coats, shoes, and specific types of stethoscopes were favored for physicians.

Statistical analysis

A simple convenience sample were targeted allowing the children and their parents to enroll themselves electively into the study using an electronic survey designed online by using dedicated iPad for this purpose. Data were compiled into an excel sheet and were analyzed using commercial software SPSS, IBM version 20. Percentages and counts were used to describe categorical variables, and a chi-squared (χ^2 goodness-of-fit test) was used to explore our hypothesis. We assumed that participants would select each type of attire, footwear, stethoscope, and lab coat equally. So, no prior assumption on how selections would be distributed. Thus, an equal opportunity of selection was presumed for each question and the test were carried out accordingly.

Research ethics

An informed consent was sought from each respondent adult and guardian with children's assent to answer the questionnaire completely and the study has an IRB approval. All authors disclosed no conflict of interest during study design, data collection, results analysis, and manuscript preparation.

Results

Parents and children population

Most of participated parents were females (91.9%). All of surveyed women were biological mothers. Majority aged between 20-30 years (45.5%). Their Educcations were almost equally distributed between less than high school, high school diploma and university degree or

higher (Table 2). Children aged between 6-12 years. Boys were double the number of girls (Table 3).

Male physicians' attire perceptions

Scrub was selected by majority of parents as favorable attire in general pediatrics settings. It was perceived as most professional, trust-worthy, likely to follow recommendations, knowledgeable, approachable, confidant, and amenable. Additionally, children selected scrub as most friendly, trust-worthy, amenable, least to pose risk of infection, likely to follow recommendation and best doctor in general. However, children saw official western attire as least intimidating. Surprisingly, traditional attire with red headwear (shamag) was the most intimidating and carried highest risk of infection in eyes of children. In contrast, casual western attire was presumed to affect infection control by parents (Figure 2).

Female physicians' attire perceptions

Conservative formal attire including simple long black skirt with a lab coat was chosen by most of parents as favorable attire by all measured variables. Instead, children thought wearing scrub by female physicians is an indicator of being a better doctor, more trust-worthy, amenable and the friendliest. However, children were more likely to follow recommendation of conservative formal attire. Summer dress was selected to pose highest risk of infection by both parents and children. Furthermore, children saw it as most intimidating attire for female physicians (Figure 3).

Importance of lab coat

Most parents admitted that wearing lab coat by their child's doctor is preferred (88.9%). However, majority did not care if lab coat was buttoned or not (54.5%). Dissimilarly, children believed lab coat is not necessary (71.9%).

Jewelries, stethoscope, shoes, and nametags

Although parents were more accepting of female physicians' jewelries, they were less tolerant to male physicians' jewelries especially bracelets (Table 4). While parents appreciated, physicians decorating their stethoscope with toys, children preferred standard stethoscope. Unexpectedly, parents and children favored Tennis shoes for both male and female physicians (Figure 4). Majority of parents valued having nametags by physicians (92%).

Discussion

Patient-doctor relationships are essentials in building partnerships to reach a common goal: healthier children [9]. Such relationships can be established by trust and certain competencies. Indeed, physician attire can serve as an indicator of those desired competencies and improve patient-doctor relationship [10].

Unpredictably, scrubs were perceived as favorable attire for male physicians by parents and children in inpatient general pediatric settings. These surprising results have not been documented before in such settings as far as we know. Undeniably, scrubs were desired dress code in other setting and specialty [11]. Nonetheless, such attire was not chosen in previous researches involving general pediatric settings [6]. But, physician attire perception differs according to geography and culture [12]. However, adult perceptions in surgical and non-surgical settings in Saudi Arabia showed formal western attire is preferred [8,13]. This study is the first to document pediatric physician attire perceptions within Saudi Arabia to our knowledge. As practice settings

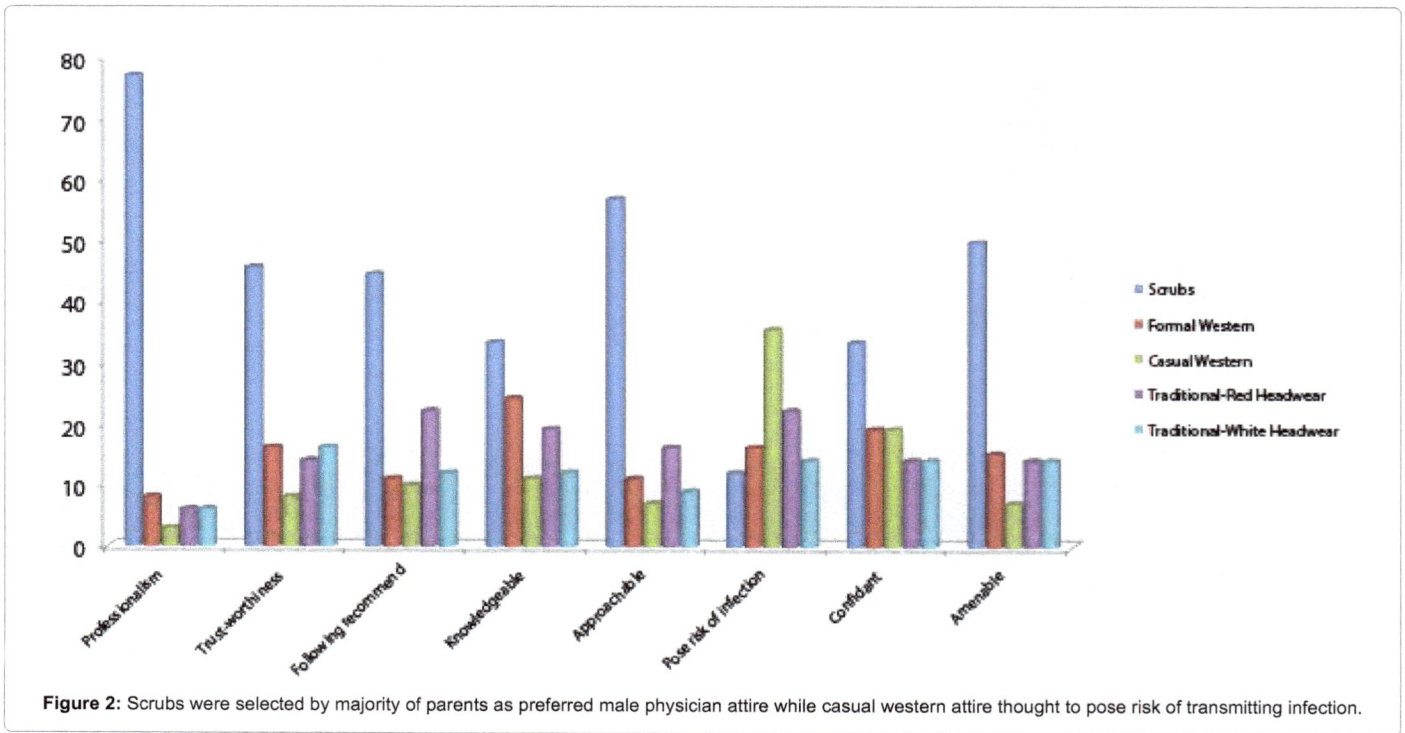

Figure 2: Scrubs were selected by majority of parents as preferred male physician attire while casual western attire thought to pose risk of transmitting infection.

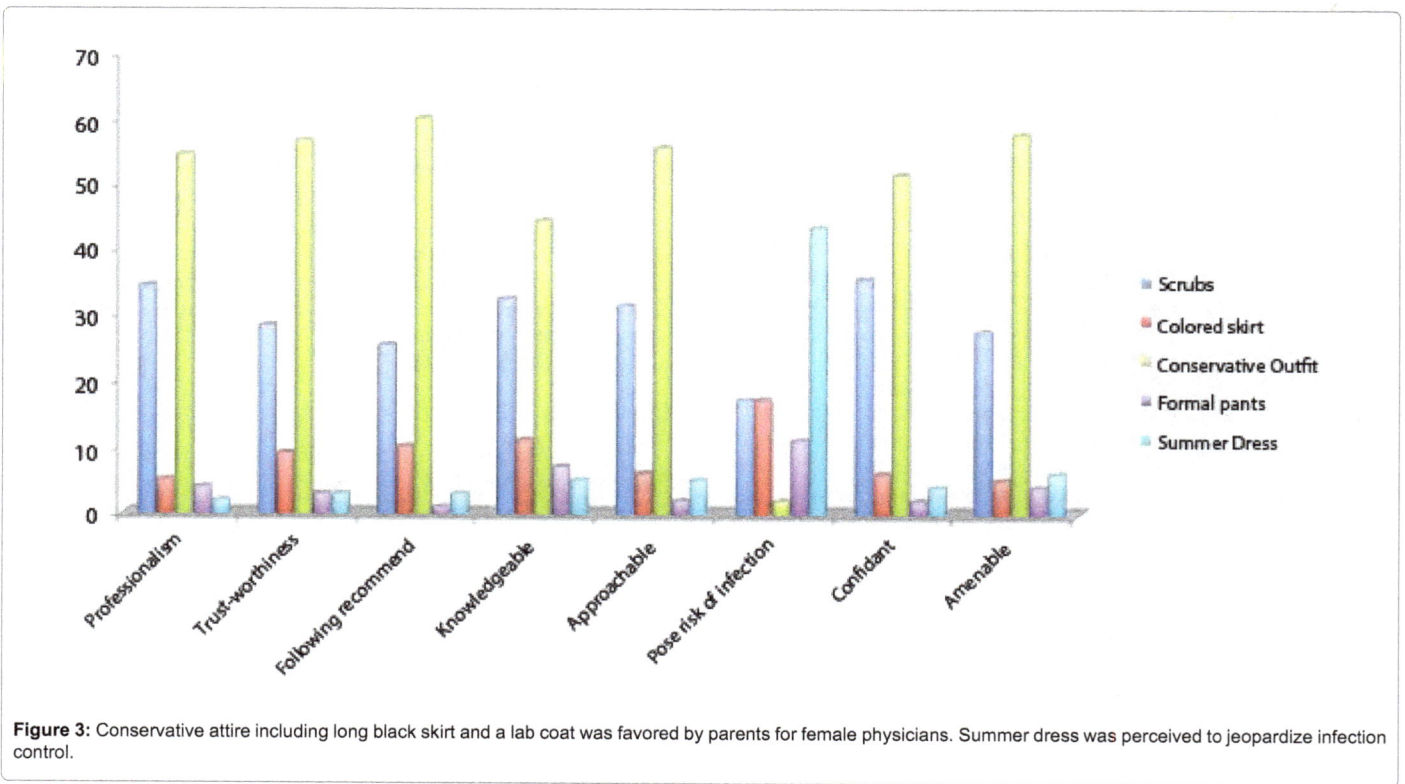

Figure 3: Conservative attire including long black skirt and a lab coat was favored by parents for female physicians. Summer dress was perceived to jeopardize infection control.

play critical role in such perceptions [14], this could explain our unanticipated findings.

Female physicians were perceived as more competent if they wear formal conservative attire by parents. This supports earlier results in outpatient adult settings in Saudi Arabia [8]. When children were asked, they choose scrubs as indicator of best female doctors. Also, children found summer dress attire and male traditional attire with red headwear most intimidating for female and male physicians, respectively. Although these were statistically significant results, it

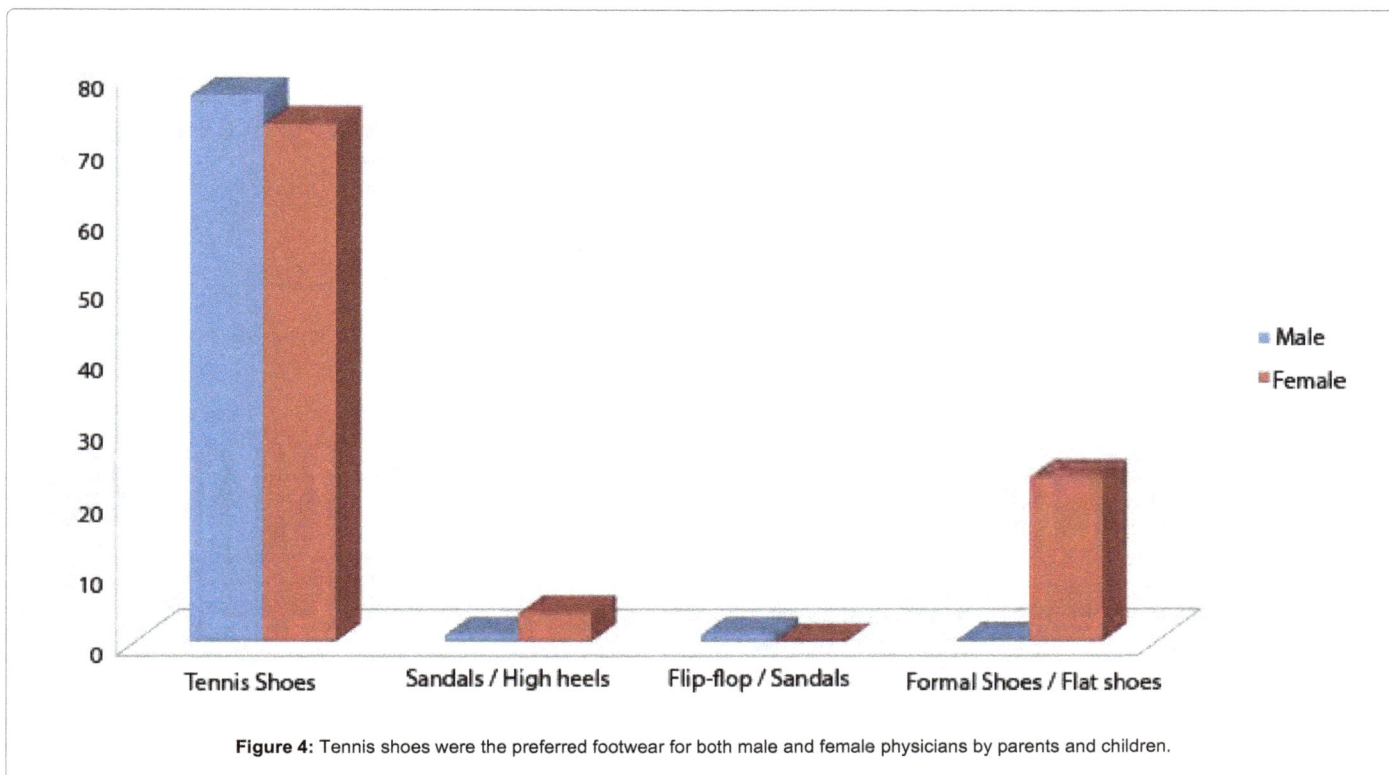

Figure 4: Tennis shoes were the preferred footwear for both male and female physicians by parents and children.

	Count	Percentage
Gender		
Mother	91	91.9
Father	8	8.1
Age		
Less than 20	3	3
20-30 years	45	45.5
30-40 years	32	32.3
More than 40 years	19	19.2
Educcation		
Less Than High School	32	32.3
High School	32	32.3
University Degree and Higher	35	35.4

Table 2: Distribution of Educcation between less than high school, high school diploma and university degree or higher.

	Count	Percent
Age		
6-8 Years	13	39.4
9-10 Years	11	33.3
11-12 Years	9	27.3
Sex		
Male	22	66.7
Female	11	33.3
Educcation		
First to Third Class	19	57.6
Fourth to Sixth	7	21.2
Intermediate	7	21.2

Table 3: Children characteristics. N=33 child.

is hard to rationalize such selections. We speculate that preferred male and female physicians' attire were elected based on being the commonest used attire by physicians in our hospital.

Parents selected male casual western attire as posing highest risk for transmitting infections. Entertainingly, such attire without a lab coat has been recommended as best attire to minimize nosocomial infections [15]. On the contrary, children nominated traditional attire with red headwear and summer dress to jeopardize infection controls for male and female physicians, respectively. This could be explained by how children found these particular attires the most intimidating.

Lab coat was important attire in parents' views while children thought it is not necessary. Lab coat has been thought to terrorize children by many pediatricians [7]. Nevertheless, previous researches showed that parents and children prefer it [16,17]. This study reported new evidence of discordance of parents and children opinions on value of lab coat in child healthcare.

Parents and children agreed that tennis shoes are favored in general pediatrics settings for both male and female physicians. This finding does not support earlier perceptions of surgical and non-surgical adult physician's footwear in Saudi Arabia [8,13]. Even perceptions of pediatric physicians in other countries were in contrast to our findings [7]. This is another proof of cultural and geographical impacts on perceptions of physicians' attire. Additionally, cultural, and geographical sensitivities were evident in perceptions of wearing jewelries by physicians. Although wearing jewelries is not recommended as they pose risk of transmitting infections [15], parents were more accepting of male physicians' rings and female physicians' jewelries in general. When asked about nametags, majority of parents expressed their necessity. This finding supports earlier finding by Najafi et al. [3].

	Not True	I Don't Bother	True	χ2 (df=2)	p
A Male Physician Wearing rings affects quality of care?	25(25.3%)	28(28.3%)	46(46.5%)	7.82	0.02
A Male Physician Wearing Bracelets affects the quality of care?	15(15.2%)	24(24.2%)	60(60.6%)	34.36	<0.001
A Female Physician Wearing rings affects the quality of care?	35(35.4%)	20(20.2%)	44(44.4%)	8.91	0.012
A Female Physician Wearing Bracelets affects quality of care?	31(31.3%)	20(20.2%)	48(46.5%)	12.1	0.002
It is preferred that a Physician wears a lab coat?	4(4%)	7(7.1%)	88(88.9%)	137.64	<0.001
Lab coat's buttons are preferred to be always tucked.	7(7.1%)	54(54.5%)	38(38.4%)	34.61	<0.001
An ID badge is necessary to wear?	3(3%)	4(4%)	92(92.9%)	158.24	<0.001
Physicians Shoes affect his /her appearance.	15(15.1%)	18(18.2%)	66(66.7%)	49.64	<0.001
A Stethoscope with a toy icon is friendlier for children.	44(44.4%)	10(10.1%)	45(45.5%)	24.1	<0.001
The Physicians type of shoes affects the child's comfortability.	44(44.4%)	28(28.4%)	27(27.3%)	49.64	0.063

Table 4: Perceptions of physicians' jewelries by parents differed according to physicians' gender. Nametags, shoes, and type of stethoscope thought to play a factor in physicians' professional image.

Conclusion

Perception of Physicians attire can be used as indicator of several competencies of pediatric physicians to improve child-doctor and parent-doctor relationships. There is a cultural impact on these perceptions in Saudi Arabia. Male physicians were found more competent if they wear scrub with tennis-shoes by both parents and children. Female physicians were perceived as better doctor if they wear conservative formal attire with tennis-shoes by parents while children saw scrub is more suitable attire for their female physicians within inpatient general pediatric settings. Although parents emphasized importance of lab coat, children did not find it essential in their care.

Limitations

This study reports physician attire perception by parents and children in one teaching hospital. To generalize our data to cover Saudi Arabia, multicenter study needs to be employed. Another limitation was apparent in encouraging fathers to participate which was very challenging and not feasible. Moreover, displaying a picture of female physician model without a lab coat was not accepted by adult participants which demonstrates indirect evidence of importance of lab coat in parents' views especially for female physicians.

References

1. Kaser M, Bugle LW, Jackson E (2009) Dress code debate. Nurs Manag 40: 33-38.

2. Darby J (2008) Thinking about changing your dress code. Gastroenterol Nurs 31: 295-296.

3. Najafi M, Khoshdel A, Kheiri S (2012) Preferences of Iranian patients about style of labelling and calling of their physicians. J Pak Med Assoc 62: 668671-668695.

4. Aitken SA, Tinning CG, Gupta S, Medlock G, Wood AM, et al. (2014) The importance of the orthopaedic doctors' appearance: A cross-regional questionnaire based study. The Surgeon 12: 40-46.

5. Wilson A, Moudraia O (2003) Interactive effects of shoe style and verbal cues on perceptions of female physicians' personal attributes. Cogprints.

6. Del Rey JAG, Paul RL (1995) Preferences of parents for pediatric emergency physicians' attire. Pediatr Emergency Care 11: 361-364.

7. Matsui D, Cho M, Rieder MJ (1998) Physicians' attire as perceived by young children and their parents: the myth of the white coat syndrome. Pediatr Emergency Care 14: 198-201.

8. Al-Ghobain MO, Al-Drees TM, Alarifi MS, Al-Marzoug HM, Al-Humaid WA, et al. (2012) Patients' preferences for physicians' attire in Saudi Arabia. Saudi Med J 33: 763-767.

9. Levinson W, Roter DL, Mullooly JP, Dull VT, Frankel RM (1997) Physician-patient communication: the relationship with malpractice claims among primary care physicians and surgeons. JAMA 277: 553-559.

10. Chung H, Lee H, Chang DS, Kim HS, Lee H, et al. (2012) Doctor's attire influences perceived empathy in the patient–doctor relationship. Patient Educc Couns 89: 387-391.

11. Cha A, Hecht BR, Nelson K, Hopkins MP (2004) Resident physician attire: does it make a difference to our patients? Am J Obstetr Gynecol 190: 1484-1488.

12. Petrilli CM, Mack M, Petrilli JJ, Hickner A, Saint S, et al. (2015) Understanding the role of physician attire on patient perceptions: a systematic review of the literature-targeting attire to improve likelihood of rapport (TAILOR) investigators. BMJ open 5: e006578.

13. Batais MA (2014) Patients' attitudes toward the attire of male physicians: a single-center study in Saudi Arabia. Ann Saudi Med 34: 383-389.

14. Rowland PA, Coe NP, Burchard KW, Pricolo VE (2005) Factors affecting the professional image of physicians. Curr Surg 62: 214-219.

15. Bearman G, Bryant K, Leekha S, Mayer J, Munoz-Price LS, et al. (2014) Healthcare personnel attire in non-operating-room settings. Infect Control Hosp Epidemiol 35: 107-121.

16. Ellore VPK, Mohammed M, Taranath M, Ramagoni NK, Kumar V, et al. (2015) Children and Parent's Attitude and Preferences of Dentist's Attire in Pediatric Dental Practice. Int J Clin Pediatr Dent 8: 102-107.

17. Kazory A (2008) Physicians, their appearance, and the white coat. Am J Med 121: 825-828.

16

Perceptions of Becoming Personal Physicians within a Patient-Centered Medical Home

Patricia A Carney[1]*, Elizabeth Jacob-Files[2], Susan J Rosenkranz[3], Deborah J Cohen[4], Larry Green[5], Samuel Jones[6], Colleen T Fogarty[7], Elaine Waller[4] and M Patrice Eiff[4]

[1]*Department of Family Medicine and Public Health and Preventive Medicine, Oregon Health and Science University, Portland, Oregon, USA*
[2]*BJF Research, Seattle, Washington, USA*
[3]*School of Nursing, Oregon Health and Science University, Portland, Oregon, USA*
[4]*Department of Family Medicine, Oregon Health and Science University, Portland, Oregon, USA*
[5]*Department of Family Medicine, Epperson-Zorn Chair for Innovation in Family Medicine and Primary Care, University of Colorado, Denver, Colombia, USA*
[6]*Fairfax Family Medicine Residency Program, Fairfax, Virginia, USA*
[7]*Department of Family Medicine, University of Rochester, Rochester, New York, USA*

Abstract

Objective: Residency training is transforming how to teach residents about practicing as a personal physician in a Patient Centered Medical Home [PCMH], but little is known about how trainees experience these responsibilities.

Methods: This study used an online survey with open-ended questions to assess residents experiences with curricular innovations as part of learning to practice as physicians in a PCMH. The survey questions were distributed every six to 12 months. This analysis focuses on responses to a single question administered once, "What does being a personal physician working in a medical home mean to you?" Two independent researchers analyzed text responses using an immersion-crystallization approach. The full research team met to discuss emerging themes.

Principal findings: Sixty-two residents representing 78.6% of participating training programs responded to the online survey question that is the focus of this analysis. Overwhelmingly, resident respondents reported finding meaning in the humanistic and interpersonal aspects of medicine. In particular, residents reported that being a personal physician in a PCMH meant being the go-to person for patients' healthcare needs. This included delivering patient-centered, continuous care in the context of a physician-patient relationship that broke down the traditional physician-patient hierarchy. Being a personal physician also included an important role for the physician and clinical team members in orchestrating the referral and care coordination process. To accomplish this, residents recognized that personal physicians needed to learn the art of practice.

Conclusion: Physicians trained in newly redesigned residencies understand and embrace their role and relationships with patients and health care teams that emerge as part of the PCMH. Residency redesign efforts can inculcate new family physicians with key practice ideals and knowledge about how to achieve these in practice.

Keywords: Graduate medical education; Patient centered medical home; Personalized physician

Introduction

The allopathic and osteopathic primary care professional disciplines, including the American Academy of Family Physicians, the American Academy of Pediatrics, the American College of Physicians and the American Osteopathic Association, are committed to providing comprehensive primary care for children, youth and adults in a health care setting that facilitates partnerships between individual patients, their personal physicians, and when appropriate, the patient's family via the Patient Centered Medical Home [PCMH] [1]. Within the PCMH, the term "personal physician" has been defined as a person with an ongoing patient relationship who is trained to provide first contact, continuous and comprehensive care [1]. With healthcare reforms continuing to move toward the PCMH [1-7], much research has focused on the potential benefits such an approach could make toward improving quality of care while containing costs [3-6]. The idea of being a personal physician and the need for educational redesign to address being a personal physician are not new. In 1926, Dr. Francis Peabody underscored the need for the good physician to know his/her patients completely, as in many cases both appropriate diagnosis and treatment can depend on a personal relationship between patients and physicians [8]. Similarly, in 1960, Dr. Fox [9] indicated that, "The more complex medicine becomes, the stronger are the reasons why everyone should have a personal doctor who will take continuous responsibility for him… the doctor treats people, not illnesses…".

The role of the physician continues to expand in the current decade with additional physician directives as part of the PCMH movement, such as [1] leading a team of individuals who collectively take responsibility for the ongoing care of patients; [2] taking responsibility for all of the patient's healthcare needs rather than just illness needs, such as providing preventive services and end of life care; [3] integrating care across all elements of complex health care systems and the patient's community; and [4] providing care that is facilitated by registries, information technology, health information exchange and other means to assure that patients get the indicated care when and where they need and want it in a culturally and linguistically appropriate manner [1]. With this movement, the types of competencies that physicians need within the context of PCMH are quite different from the competencies physicians have needed in the past.

*Corresponding author: Patricia AC, Professor of Family Medicine, Oregon Health and Science University, Portland, Oregon, USA,
E-mail: carneyp@ohsu.edu

How do family medicine residents think about these new directives during training? As part of the Preparing the Personal Physician for Practice [P⁴] initiative [10] data were collected from residents about their experiences with innovative curricula that embodied principles of the PCMH, including training about becoming a personal physician. We conducted a qualitative analysis to understand how these physicians early in their careers consider the meaning of being a personal physician.

Methods

The P⁴ project

The P⁴ project is described in detail elsewhere [11-13]. Briefly, P⁴ is a comparative case series of innovative redesigns in residency training, such as changes in the length, structure, and composition of training designed to prepare family medicine residents for practice in PCMHs. Innovations include use of information technology in patient care, a focus on training in teams, and fewer hospital-based rotations in favor of more continuity clinic time to provide more clinical experiences in the care of patients over time.

Fourteen programs were selected that represented the best innovations as determined by a peer-review committee. The programs included broad geographic representation from rural, urban and suburban areas as well as community and/or university-based or administered programs. All programs participated in core data collection activities as part of the project, including annual surveys completed by all residents, the program director and medical director and/or clinic staff at continuity clinics. Oregon Health and Science University's Institutional Review Board [IRB #3788] reviewed study activities and granted the study an educational exemption.

The online survey

The P⁴ online survey was specifically designed to collect qualitative data from P⁴ programs using a secure, web-accessible, survey application running on the Agency for Healthcare Research and Quality's [AHRQ] server. The customized software application was based on the commercial online survey product Checkbox [14] and ran on the Microsoft.Net framework [15]. The system provided flexible survey and questionnaire capabilities with email invitations and triggers, advanced logic and web services features with options to support online forms, evaluations and other functions.

Using this system, we disseminated four to five open-ended questions at six to nine-month intervals to assess the residents, program directors, and continuity clinic staffs reactions to clinical practice and training innovations they were implementing and testing. Responding to the online survey questions was voluntary and confidential. The system administrator at AHRQ assigned numeric codes to residents' responses to identify residents by residency program and program year. Only the P⁴ evaluation team could see survey responses [no one at the residents' sites, including other residents, staff, or directors and supervisors had access to the residents responses]. In the spring of 2010, one question directed to the residents was: "What does being a personal physician working in a medical home mean to you?" Our analysis focused on the responses to this question.

Data management and analysis

The P⁴ Evaluation Team received de-identified data files. The online survey data files were imported into QSR International NVivo v.8.0 software [16]. All of the responses to the open-ended question of interest

were stratified by program and year and analyzed by two members of the investigative team [authors EJF and SJR]. During a first immersion-crystallization cycle, the analysts independently read all of the data to identify emerging themes and met regularly to discuss patterns and develop a preliminary codebook. The codebook was revised and themes were refined during the second immersion-crystallization cycle until agreement was reached among the team [17,18]. At key intervals in the process, author PAC met with the analysts to review, independently audit and assess the face validity of the emerging findings.

We used quantitative data that we collected via resident surveys to compare the characteristics of respondents and non-respondents to the online survey question to assess potential sources of bias. Continuous variables, such as age, were analyzed using t-tests. Categorical data, such as gender, were analyzed using Chi square. All tests were two-tailed and alpha levels were set at 0.05. We used SPSS Statistics [18,19] for the statistical analysis.

Results

Our analysis is based on 62 residents responses to the study question of interest and included residents from 11 of the 14 [78.6%] programs (Table 1) and across all program years [PGY1: n=23, PGY2: n=20; PGY3: n=19]. The 62 residents represented 18.2% of the total number of residents who received the online survey [n=341]. While the majority of respondents were female, white and PGY1 residents, these characteristics were not statistically different between responders and non-responders (Table 2). Similarly, there were no differences in marital or parental status, the proportion that undertook medical school in the U.S., the influence of P⁴ in their ranking of residency or overall satisfaction with their training programs.

Our qualitative analysis revealed that some PGY1 residents [n=3] indicated they were not yet clear on the meaning of the PCMH. For example, one resident wrote:

"I don't know yet, as I have not had the opportunity to experience this yet since I spend most of my time as an intern in the hospital." [Resident #10; Site D]

However, the majority of responding residents reported that they found meaning in the humanistic elements of being a personal physician. This included the interpersonal aspects of medicine, such as relationship-building, communication, trust and collaboration and was not limited to valuing the relationship with patients. Residents also found meaning in their relationships with other physicians and clinic staff.

P⁴ Program	PGY1 n (%)	PGY2 n (%)	PGY3 n (%)	Total n (%)
Site A	2	1	0	3
Site B	1	3	2	6
Site C	0	0	3	3
Site D	3	1	1	5
Site E	3	2	1	6
Site F	2	1	1	4
Site G	1	1	0	2
Site H	6	2	1	9
Site I	0	2	4	6
Site J	0	2	4	6
Site K	5	5	2	12
Total by Year and Overall	23 (38.3%)	20 (33.3%)	19 (31.7%)	62 (100%)

Table 1: Overall responses to online survey question by program and training year.

Characteristics	Among Residents Who Contributed Online Survey Data (n=62)	Among Residents Who Did Not Contribute Online Survey Data (n=279)	p value
Mean Age in Years (SD)	30.5 (5.0)	31.1 (5.2)	0.39
Gender			
Male	45.0%	43.8%	0.48
Female	55.0%	56.2%	
Race			
White	72.9%	64.8%	0.15
Black	5.1%	10.1%	0.17
Asian/Pacific Islander	15.3%	17.4%	0.43
American Indian/Alaska Native	1.7%	1.0%	0.53
Other	6.8%	10.1%	0.30
Ethnicity (Hispanic Origin)	10.2%	6.7%	0.25
Residency Program Year			
PGY1	38.3%	33.2%	
PGY2	33.3%	30.8%	0.53
PGY3	31.7%	32.2%	
Marital Status			
Single (never married)	33.3%	32.8%	
Married/Partnered	65.0%	66.2%	0.86
Divorced/Separated	1.7%	1.0%	
Have Children			
Yes	30.0%	36.7%	0.20
No	70.0%	63.3%	
Attended Medical School in the U.S.			
Yes	78.3%	70.3%	0.14
No	21.7%	29.7%	
First Generation College Graduate			
Yes	23.3%	23.7%	0.55
No	76.7%	76.3%	
First Person in Family to become a Physician			
Yes	81.7%	72.8%	0.10
No	18.3%	27.2%	
Influenced by P[4] in Ranking this Program in the Match			
No - was in program before P[4]			
No - was neutral about P[4]	28.3%	40.8%	
Yes, P[4] was positive feature of program	25.0%	21.6%	0.31
	46.7%	37.3%	
Yes, P[4] was negative feature of program	0.0%	0.3%	
Overall, how satisfied are you with your residency training thus far?			
Very unsatisfied	3.4%	4.5%	
Somewhat unsatisfied	5.1%	4.5%	0.88
Neutral	10.2%	7.0%	
Somewhat satisfied	32.2%	29.7%	
Very satisfied	49.2%	54.2%	

Table 2: Characteristics of residents who contributed data to these analyses.

Residents identified three different but intertwined roles or activities associated with being personal physician (Table 3). First, they reported that being a personal physician in a medical home means being the go-to or point person for all of their patients healthcare needs. For example, one first year resident wrote:

"It means that the physician acts as the clearinghouse, gatekeeper and manager for all matters of a person's health and wellness: bio, psycho and social." [Resident #03, Site I]

This included the perspective that one's individual family doctor can provide for all of a patient's needs by serving as the patient's point-of-contact for referral recommendations and coordinating multidisciplinary health care services. While the response below

suggests that the intent of providing personalized care has been present for a while, perhaps it has not been as effective as it can be now within the context of a PCMH, and with a team approach to care delivery.

"I have always felt that we were trying to do this all along; but to me it means being a headquarters for patient's health, offering a variety of services through interdisciplinary care, and creating an atmosphere that is welcoming and that no question or concern is too small or at all inconvenient." [emphasis added; Resident #98; Site K]

Entwined with being the point person for patients' healthcare needs, residents expressed views that being a personal physician in a PCMH meant delivering patient-centered care, including respecting patients' requests, responding to patient concerns in a timely and socially sensitive manner, and believing that patient needs come before medical or system priorities. Residents also reported that delivering patient-centered care requires working to understand the whole person when caring for patients and that continuity of care over time is a key element of being a personal physician. For example, one first year resident wrote:

"I want to have a panel of patients that I follow from birth to death while also caring for their family members. I want to provide their acute care, prenatal and obstetrics, disease management and end of life care. I want to be coordinating their care with specialists as necessary to be sure they receive the best care and have a single point of contact for questions and concerns" [Resident #13, Site B].

These prior quotes suggest that while family physicians in training see themselves as a single point of contact, they express the need for teams working together to provide all the care that patients need. The practice is the headquarters for care while the delivery is the responsibility of more than one person so that more can be accomplished.

As other resident responses across all years of training show, providing care that has continuity includes checking-in with the patient regularly when needed, seeing the patient over an extended period of time, and making themselves available to patients beyond the clinical setting, such as by telephone or email when needed. We found that some first year residents, in particular, spoke about continuity of care over time in conjunction with being the go-to person, as the prior example illustrates.

Residents reported that this level of communication and continuity of care results in patients [and physicians] feeling a greater connection to each other. This connection was described as 'rapport' by a number of residents. Rapport, at a minimum, means to them that the personal physician is responsible for developing a deep understanding with patients and at the maximum that this relationship could allow the personal physician to transcend the traditional hierarchy of physician-patient roles. For example, a PGY1 resident wrote: "I am enjoying getting to know patients' medical issues, social issues and getting to know their families." [Resident #28, Site G]

A second year resident wrote: "Making our patients feel that they can come to us with any problems they have including social issues." [Resident #64; Site F]

Rapport building is also important to the 'art of medicine.' A number of residents expressed feeling the need to learn skills and knowledge that would allow them to practice empathy and compassion for patients well beyond their physical health needs. This response occurred more prominently among PGY1 residents than it did among PGY2 and PGY3 residents: "Being a knowledgeable, competent physician who takes

Theme/Subtheme	Definition	Exemplars
1. Go To Person	Point person for all their patients' healthcare needs.	It means that the physician acts as the clearinghouse, gatekeeper and manager for all matters of a person's health and wellness: bio, psycho and social.
Patient-centeredness	Respect for patient needs comes before any medical or systematic priorities.	It means that I am a provider for a patient's every need and if I cannot provide that need I will guide the patient in the direction they will need to go, but always have a path for them to return to their medical home.
Longitudinal continuity of care	The same provider repeatedly seeing the same patients over a long period of time.	I want to have a panel of patients that I follow from birth to death while also caring for their family members. I want to provide their acute care, prenatal and obstetrics, disease management and end of life care. I want to be coordinating their care with specialists as necessary to be sure they receive the best care and have a single point of contact for questions and concerns.
Physician-patient relationship	Physician-patient rapport building and breaking down the traditional physician-patient hierarchy.	...it means that there is a mutual commitment-The physician to the needs of the patient and the patient to that physician as their first and primary contact point for the address of these needs. It means that I am not just seeing patients randomly but I am able to be their personal physician and able to follow up regularly and able to develop a good rapport to maintain good health, prevent illnesses, inculcate good living habits and preventive medicine care.
2. Teamwork	Emphasis on helping and working with an interdisciplinary network of clinicians.	It means helping to coordinate multidisciplinary health care for any patient.... Family Physicians should be well equipped to help patients summarize their care plans, clarify all medication changes and guide future care. This requires, also, that the specialty physicians are timely with their clinic notes and forward these notes to the PCP. Patients are often not savvy enough to coordinate all this care on their own and many times they, and family members, are overwhelmed with managing their care. I've seen this many times, and within my own family, to know that Family Physicians need to be kept "in the loop," regarding their patients' care. ...allowing my patients access to seeing me developing an expectation that patient is cared for by a team of nurses, MA's, MD's working in a one-stop-shop that has labs, imaging, nursing, certain urgent care resources, DM educators, mental health, other specialists all in the same office.
Specialized patient care	Greater involvement in referral process, working closely with specialists, and improved PCP-specialist communications.	...They are part of a team (along side nurses, pharmacists, techs, therapists...). A medical home is not only a medical home for the patient but also for the doctor. It's not being part of a system that bounces you around to different offices..... It's a multidisciplinary approach to medicine. Many times patients see multiple specialty physicians with no central "medical home." Because of this, patients and doctors risk mismanagement of medications, misinterpretation of information and poor quality care.
3. Art	Learning the non-medical knowledge based characteristics of practice.	Personal physician means knowing the patient and family, pt feels they have a doctor they can trust and is familiar with their life story, joys, and challenges. I am enjoying getting to know patients medical issues, social issues and getting to know their families. Making our patients feel that they can come to us with any problems they have including social issues... Being a knowledgeable, competent physician who takes genuine interest in the care of one's patients working in an environment best equipped to help one accomplish excellent patient care.

Table 3: Thematic interactions between main and sub themes.

genuine interest in the care of one's patients working in an environment best equipped to help one accomplish excellent patient care" [Resident #63, Site H].

" ... A personal physician is one who sees the patient a majority of the time. The Physician knows the patient, and doesn't have to look in the chart to re-familiarize him or herself with the patient. The personal physician also does not see him or herself above the patient. They are part of a team [alongside nurses, pharmacists, techs, therapists"] [Resident #26; Site F].

Residents reported that teamwork and leading effective teams is a core task for the personal physician in the PCMH and has benefits for both patients and providers. A PGY2 resident wrote: "It means helping to coordinate multidisciplinary health care for any patient Family Physicians should be well equipped to help patients summarize their care plans, clarify all medication changes and guide future care. This requires, also, that the specialty physicians are timely with their clinic notes and forward these notes to the PCP [primary care physician].

Patients are often not savvy enough to coordinate all this care on their own and many times they, and family members, are overwhelmed with managing their care. I've seen this many times, and within my own family, to know that Family Physicians need to be kept "in the loop," regarding their patients' care." [Resident #80, Site B].

For some residents, the collaborative aspects of teamwork involved working with a network of interdisciplinary clinical staff, including but not limited to physicians, and making this interdisciplinary approach visible to patients by: "allowing my patients access to seeing me, developing an expectation that patient is cared for by a team of nurses, MA's, MD's...DM educators, mental health, other specialists all in the same office." [Resident #80, Site B].

Discussion

This study is the first to report on the reactions of residents who are experiencing newly redesigned curricula focusing on the PCMH. Findings from our analyses indicate that for residents the term "personal physician" connotes an ongoing relationship with a physician trained to provide first contact, continuous and comprehensive care that expands well beyond their physical needs to social and environmental contexts. These are ideals that residents appear to fully embrace, just as their well known predecessors Drs. Peabody and Fox did decades ago, though residents' responses suggest this may be easier to do within the context of Patient Centered Medical Homes. Not surprisingly, evolutions in medicine and health care systems may make the personal physicians' relationships with or perceptions of patients more complex than prior conceptualizations, and it may be that today's residents understand the importance of this vital relationship earlier during their training than has occurred in the past, though this is impossible to confirm as so little research has been published on this topic.

The residents we heard from reported an understanding of the meaning of the personal physician consistent with the definition set out in the Joint Principles [1]. Residents understood the personal physician to be the point person for patients' healthcare needs, and this required working as a team to coordinate and integrate care for patients, and getting to know patients over time. Residents' responses regarding what it means to be a "personal physician working in a medical home" also centered on the themes of "Physician-patient relationship" and "Art of medicine." The strength of this finding may indicate that these themes are important to any resident learning to hone their patient care skills, regardless of being involved in P[4]. It may also indicate that residents involved in P[4] training are either bringing these qualities of rapport building, compassion, trust and caring into their development as a personal physician or they are learning them from the P[4] curriculum.

Our findings are consistent with another qualitative study conducted in Canada. Beaulieu and colleagues [20] conducted a focus group study of French, Belgian and Canadian family medicine residents during the last year of training and found that key features of practice were the relationship built over time between the patient and physician; the capacity to take care of a variety of problems at the primary care level; and integration and coordination of the patient's care needs. Further, the scope of practice was further defined as being a first responder to the patient's complaints and coordinating and integrating the patient's care as well as considering the contextual issues of health and illness, such as familial, social and economic issues.

Interestingly, we found in our study that residents placed little to no emphasis on the role of information technology, registries and other systems that might be needed to assure that patients' healthcare needs get met in a timely way. This may reflect an emphasis that these residency programs place on interpersonal relations and/or a potential deficit in training residents to be systems thinkers capable of devising systems of care and using tools that support the care process. Alternatively, residents may be trained in systems approaches to care delivery, but not see this central to the meaning of being a personal physician, especially as it relates to their relationships with patients.

Some features related to the medical home were absent in these residents' reflections. For example, while quality of care was mentioned, safety was not. This may be because the residents are early enough in their careers to not have experienced medical errors or close calls. Also, they might not feel confident to write about this issue using an online survey. Another area not noted by residents was enhanced access and payment reform. Residents typically have little to do with setting clinic hours and billing, and in many cases, are so consumed with learning clinical skills that they may give less importance to practice management topics that are offered in residency curricula. In addition, residents, especially PGY1s and PGY2s, possibly have not had enough clinical experience to recognize access or payment issues.

We also expected to see more reflections or insights on adopting PCMH principles in this analysis, such as how enhanced access and differing patient communication mechanisms affect workload. However, we now believe this didn't occur because residents are not at a stage in their development where they can reflect on these changes. It is much more likely that faculty practicing in clinic settings undergoing PCMH transformation would identify these issues rather than residents. To the residents, what they are experiencing is simply the reality in which practice now occurs, as they are not familiar with the previous ways of doing things.

Strengths of this study include our use of an online survey designed specifically to collect qualitative information from residents participating in cutting-edge P[4] programs dispersed across the country. Another strength is the use of a standardized open-ended question that elicited residents' perspectives on being a personal physician within the context of the PCMH. Finally, this study includes residents' perspectives on training and emerging understanding of the PCMC. This is an understudied area in a rapidly changing field that is vitally important to understanding how to support the training needs of future physicians in the context of major practice transformation.

Limitations of the study include that the overall response rate was low, though nearly 80% of programs and all program years were represented in the data. The demographic characteristics of responders and non-responders were similar, which suggests that bias based on certain participant characteristics did not influence our findings. However, we cannot measure the extent to which our sample of responders represent "early adopters" of employing PCMH concepts into practice, which could represent an unmeasured bias in our study. Providing responses to the online survey was not mandatory, which may explain the low response rate. In addition, our analysis focused on text responses to a single open-ended question. Gaining access to the online survey was challenging for some sites [n=3], which necessitated that they be excluded from this study. Internal computer security systems may have played a role in this. In addition, residents' responses were sometimes brief, often including phrases or a few short sentences. The brevity in responses likely reflects the multiple clinical and administrative demands of training, with answering optional online questions low on a resident's list of priorities. Despite this, we saw stability across residents' perspectives as they undertake redesigned training.

In conclusion, these P[4] family medicine residents, training in programs engaged in redesigning training for new models of practice, revealed an understanding that being a personal physician entails relationship development that includes the PCMH features of team-based care, responsibility for all of the patient's health care needs and coordinating and integrating care both within a complex health system and in social and familial environments. Care that is facilitated by information technology and management was not identified as a feature of personal doctoring. How these new practice features help or hinder being a great personal physician is uncertain to these residents, which will be important to consider in further research.

Acknowledgements

This work was supported by the Preparing the Personal Physician for Practice [P⁴] Project, which is jointly sponsored by the American Board of Family Medicine Foundation, the Association of Family Medicine Residency Directors, and the Family Medicine Research Program at Oregon Health and Science University, Portland, OR. The online survey system was made available by the Agency for Healthcare Research and Quality [AHRQ].

References

1. American Academy of Family Physicians, American Academy of Pediatrics, American College of Physicians, American Osteopathic Association (2007) Joint Principles of the Patient-Centered Medical Home. March 2007.

2. Dartmouth Atlas of Health Care (2006) Variation among States in the Management of Severe Chronic Illness.

3. Wagner EH, Austin BT, Davis C, Hindmarsh M, Schaefer J, et al. (2001) Improving chronic illness care: translating evidence into action. Health affairs 20: 64-78.

4. Starfield B, Shi L, Macinko J (2005) Contribution of primary care to health systems and health. Milbank quarterly 83: 457-502.

5. Starfield B, Shi L, Grover A, Macinko J (2005) The effects of specialist supply on populations' health: assessing the evidence. Health Affairs 24: W5.

6. Starfield B (2006) Presentation to the Commonwealth Fund. Primary Care Roundtable: Strengthening adult primary care: models and policy options.

7. Beal AC, Doty MM, Hernandez SE, Shea KK, Davis K (2007) Closing the divide: how medical homes promote equity in health care. Commonwealth Fund New York.

8. Peabody FW (2015) The care of the patient. Jama 313: 1868-1868.

9. Fox TF (1960) The personal doctor and his relation to the hospital: observations and reflections on some American experiments in general practice by groups. The Lancet 275: 743-760.

10. Green LA, Jones SM, Fetter Jr, Pugno PA (2007) Preparing the personal physician for practice: changing family medicine residency training to enable new model practice. Academic Medicine 82: 1220-1227.

11. Carney PA, Eiff MP, Saultz JW, Douglass AB, Tillotson CJ, et al. (2009) Aspects of the patient-centered medical home currently in place: initial findings from preparing the personal physician for practice. Fam Med 41: 632-639.

12. Carney PA, Eiff MP, Green LA, Lindbloom E, Jones SE, et al. (2011) Site-Specific Innovations, Hypotheses, and Measures at Baseline. Family medicine 43: 464-471.

13. Carney PA, Eiff MP, Saultz JW, Lindbloom E, Waller E, et al. (2012) Assessing the impact of innovative training of family physicians for the patient-centered medical home. Journal of graduate medical education 4: 16-22.

14. Checkbox Survey Software. Accessed on: 9/26/11.

15. Microsoft.Net Framework. Accessed on: 9/26/11.

16. QSR International NVivo v.8.0 software. Accessed on: 9/26/11.

17. Crabtree BF, Miller WL (1999) Doing Qualitative Research in Primary Care: Multiple Strategies. Newbury Park CA, pp: 163-177.

18. Patton MQ (1999) Enhancing the quality and credibility of qualitative analysis. Health services research 34: 1189.

19. SPSS Statistics 18. Accessed on: 9/26/11.

20. Beaulieu MD, Dory V, Pestiaux D, Pouchain D, Rioux M, et al. (2009) What does it mean to be a family physician? Exploratory study with family medicine residents from 3 countries. Canadian Family Physician 55: 14-20.

17

Personal Disaster and Pandemic Preparedness of U.S. Human Resource Professionals

Terri Rebmann[1]*, Amy M Strawn[1], Zachary Swick[1] and David Reddick[2]

[1]Institute for Biosecurity, Saint Louis University, College for Public Health and Social Justice, St Louis, MO, USA
[2]Bio-Defense Network, 116 Embassy Lane, Kirkwood, USA

Abstract

Background: All citizens need to have a personal disaster plan, but past studies indicate poor preparedness. Predictors of preparedness need to be clearly defined so interventions can be developed.

Methods: Human resource (HR) professionals were sent an online survey in May-July, 2011 that assessed their personal/family disaster plan for natural disasters and pandemics, determinants of preparedness, and attitudes and beliefs regarding disaster preparedness. Linear regressions were used to describe factors associated with higher preparedness scores. Chi squares compared attitudes and beliefs about preparedness by whether or not their employer encouraged them to have a personal plan.

Results: 471 HR professionals from 33 states participated. Average scores for personal and pandemic preparedness were 12.6 (0 - 20 range) and 4.5 (0- 9 range), respectively.

One-third (35.3%, n = 100) had half or fewer preparedness measures, and half (47%, n = 133) had 4 or fewer of the 9 possible pandemic preparedness measures. Determinants of personal preparedness included high perception of personal preparedness for natural disasters and pandemics, having fewer years of work experience, being encouraged by the employer to have a personal preparedness plan, having received disaster preparedness training during the past two years, and not having children in the household. From linear regression, determinants of pandemic preparedness were high perception of personal preparedness for both natural disasters and pandemics, not having children in the household, being male, and having received disaster preparedness training during the past two years. HR professionals whose employer encouraged him/her to have a personal disaster plan had significantly higher perceived importance for family and business preparedness, and higher perceived preparedness compared to those whose employers have not encouraged them to have a personal plan (p<.001 for all).

Conclusion: HR professionals will play a critical role during a disaster, but many lack personal preparedness.

Keywords: Personal preparedness; Disaster planning; Pandemic; Influenza; Preparedness; Disaster; Plan

Introduction

Every year, disasters victimize millions of individuals, kill thousands worldwide, and cost billions of dollars [1]. Disaster preparedness can mitigate many of the negative consequences from disasters [2]. Disaster preparedness is essential for all organizations, agencies, and businesses [3], and is also vital for individuals and families or household members [4]. Although regional and federal resources will be made available following a declared public health emergency, deploying these resources will take time. Individuals and/or family/household members may need to be self-sufficient for up to 72 hours before supplies and provisions are made available within communities [5]. Individual/family/household preparedness (hereafter referred to as *personal preparedness*) is therefore essential to ensure the safety and health of individuals and families. Many organizations and federal agencies have released checklists and guidelines for developing a personal disaster plan for individuals and families/household members [4-7]. Personal disaster plans generally call for both creating stockpiles of tangible supplies, such as non-perishable food and water, as well as designing plans/procedures for emergency response, such as for evacuation and having a designated meeting place for family members who may be separated as a result of the disaster [8].

Many researchers have stated that it is essential that healthcare, public health, and emergency responders have a personal disaster plan so that they are able to continue working during and after a disaster strikes their community, while ensuring the safety of their family members [9-

14]. As a way of better ensuring that such plans are made, it has been suggested that healthcare agency administrators should encourage personnel to have a personal disaster plan [9], that this policy should be implemented on a systems basis [12], and that staff should be told about the policy upon being hired and then annually after that Despite this, multiple studies indicate that the majority of healthcare and public health personnel do not have adequate personal disaster plans [11,14-16]. A study of Missouri nurses found that 75% did not have at least half of the assessed disaster plan supplies, and 20% did not have any components of a personal disaster plan [16]. Infection prevention (IPs) professionals, many of whom are often on hospital disaster planning committees and involved in hospital disaster planning activities, were found to be similarly unprepared for a disaster; a 2007 study reported that about half of participating IPs did not have a personal disaster plan [15]. Researchers assessing personal preparedness of public health

---

*Corresponding author: Terri Rebmann, Institute for Biosecurity, College for Public Health & Social Justice Saint Louis University, 3545 Lafayette Avenue Room 463, Saint Louis, Missouri 63104, USA, E-mail: rebmannt@slu.edu

professionals found that 75% were minimally to not at all prepared in terms of having a personal disaster plan [14].

Similar findings have been identified in studies examining the personal preparedness of members of the general public [17-21]. A 2004 study from Los Angeles, CA reported that only 28% of individuals had stockpiled emergency supplies in preparation for a disaster [17]. A more recent study in 2006 found that while only 45% of the surveyed individuals met objective criteria for being prepared for a disaster, 78% reported that they believed that they were well prepared for such an event [18]. Researchers examining the factors that influence individuals to create a personal disaster plan have reported a number of predictors of better preparedness, including perceived preparedness [18]. However, the data regarding some predictor variables, such as race, is conflicting. One study reported that African Americans, Latinos, and Asian individuals were better prepared than whites [17], while another found the exact opposite [18]. Three studies have found that individuals with disabilities are more likely to have stockpiled supplies or have an evacuation plan compared to those without disabilities, while two other studies reported that those with disabilities are less likely to be prepared for disasters [17-21]. Although a study of public health professionals reported that risk perceptions of a disaster were not associated with better preparedness [14], a study of the general public found that those with higher risk perceptions of a terrorist attack were more likely to have a personal disaster plan than those with lower risk perceptions [17]. These conflicting findings regarding predictors of personal preparedness and the fact that the most recent study to examine personal preparedness was conducted using 2008 data indicate that more research needs to be done in this area. In addition, no study has examined personal preparedness related to biological events, such as bioterrorism, outbreaks of emerging infectious diseases, or pandemics. Biological disasters are longer-lasting than traditional terrorism or natural disasters and require an increase in supplies that need to be stockpiled (up to 2–3 weeks' worth) [7]. The purposes of this study are to examine the extent to which human resource (HR) professionals have a personal/family disaster plan for natural disasters and pandemics, and to describe the determinants of better preparedness. A secondary aim of the study is to describe HR professionals' attitudes and beliefs regarding disaster preparedness for natural disasters and biological disasters.

Methods

This study was part of a larger study that examined business continuity for biological events and U.S. businesses' experiences during the 2009 H1N1 pandemic; the results from that study have been described previously [5,22]. The sample consisted of HR professionals who were members of the Society for Human Resource Management (SHRM) organization and who worked for U.S. businesses in June – August, 2011. The survey was administrated through Qualtrics', an online research software program. Subjects were recruited through websites of state SHRM organizations, announcement at local SHRM meetings, or through SHRM newsletters. After completing the business continuity study, participants were asked if they would be willing to complete a second survey regarding their personal preparedness. If they agreed, they were directed to a second online survey administrated through Qualtrics'. The Saint Louis University Institutional Review Board approved this study.

Instrument

The instrument was based on existing studies examining personal preparedness as well as planning guides developed by governmental agencies [7,17,18,23]. Attitude and belief questions were based on questionnaires used in previous bioterrorism and/or pandemic research studies [16,24-26]. The 40-item survey consisted of 24 objective items measuring personal preparedness for a natural disaster or biological event, 2 assessing perceived personal preparedness, 5 measuring perceived importance of disaster planning, 4 questions related to risk perceptions for natural disasters and pandemics, 2 focused on perceived interest in disaster planning, and a single question related to disaster training sessions attended in the past two years, perceived cost barriers to personal disaster planning, and administrative encouragement to develop a personal disaster plan. In addition, participant demographics were assessed. A group of 10 U.S. business continuity and pandemic preparedness researchers provided feedback on content validity. A content validity index (CVI) was computed for each item [27]; no items had a CVI below 0.80, so no items were deleted. The final survey instrument contained 43 questions plus demographic items. Twenty human resources professionals from across the U.S. pilot tested the instrument. Feedback from pilot testing was used to further refine the instrument.

The 24 items that objectively measured personal preparedness were categorical items; most consisted of dichotomous *yes* or *no* answer options and were scored 1 or 0 points only. Examples of scoring for these indicators include having at least three days' supply of non-perishable food ($\geq$ 3 days' of stockpiled food: 1 point; less than 3 days' of stockpiled food: 0 points) and having a battery-operated radio with batteries (yes: 1 point; no: 0 points). Some items, such as having at least a 3 days' supply of prescription medication for everyone in the household, included a "not applicable" answer option that was re-coded into "yes" (1 point). Survey questions regarding risk perceptions, perceived importance, perceived preparedness, reported interest, and cost barrier to preparedness were measured using a 5-point Likert scale (strongly agree to strongly disagree).

Data Analysis

The Statistical Package for the Social Sciences (SPSS®) 20.0 was used for all analyses. Descriptive statistics were computed for each question and used to describe personal preparedness of HR professionals and HR professionals' risk perceptions and perceived importance of personal natural disasters and pandemics. A *personal preparedness* score was calculated by assigning one point for each of 20 possible objective measures of personal preparedness. A *pandemic preparedness* score was calculated by assigning one point for each of 9 possible objective measures of pandemic preparedness. Five indicators were shared between both personal preparedness and pandemic preparedness (Table 1). The highest possible score for personal preparedness was 20 and 9 for pandemic preparedness (one point for each preparedness-specific indicator).

Chi squares were used to compare HR professionals' attitudes and beliefs about disaster preparedness by whether their employer encouraged them to have a personal disaster plan. McNemar tests were used to compare HR professionals' attitudes and beliefs about disaster preparedness when comparing two attitudinal items, such as their perceived importance of preparing for a natural disaster versus their perceived importance of preparing for a pandemic. Linear regressions were used to describe factors associated with higher personal preparedness and pandemic preparedness scores. Univariate analyses were conducted prior to linear regression analyses, using demographic variables and attitude/belief items, such as age, number of household members, whether their employer encouraged them to have a personal disaster plan, amount of disaster preparedness training received in the

Table 1: Disaster and pandemic personal preparedness indicators.

Component of Personal Disaster Plan	Has Plan Component % (n) N = 283
Flashlight and batteries	97.5 (276)
Non-prescription medication (e.g. pain reliever, fever reducer)*	96.8 (270)
≥ 3-days' supply of prescription meds for household members	95.4 (270)
Smoke detectors on each level of home	95.1 (269)
Battery-operated radio and batteries*	83.7 (237)
≥ 3-days' supply of non-perishable food for household	77.9 (218)
Fire extinguisher	74.2 (210)
Family members have knowledge of fire extinguisher use	58.0 (164)
Back-up plan for child/family member care*	77.4 (219)
Emergency numbers posted near phone/in cell phone	64.3 (182)
All members of household familiar with family disaster plan*	58.7 (166)
Back-up pet care	56.2 (159)
≥ 3-days' supply of water for household	54.8 (155)
Designated safe location for self/family in case of evacuation	53.7 (152)
Household members know how to turn off water, gas, and electricity	47.3 (134)
Out-of-town contact person identified	44.2 (125)
Medical supplies (e.g. masks, gloves, needles, syringes)*	43.8 (124)
Sheltering-in-place procedures	38.2 (108)
Back-up transportation	34.6 (98)
Household regularly conducts emergency evacuation drills	8.5 (24)
Disaster Plan Components Specific to Biological Event	**Has Plan Component % (N)**
Non-prescription medication (e.g. pain reliever, fever reducer)*	95.4 (270)
Battery-operated radio and batteries*	83.7 (237)
Back-up plan for child/family member care*	77.4 (219)
All members of household familiar with family disaster plan*	58.7 (166)
≥ 14-days' supply of prescription meds for household members	53.7 (152)
Medical supplies (e.g. masks, gloves, needles, syringes)*	43.8 (124)
≥ 1 mask/respirator stored	20.5 (58)
≥ 14-days' supply of non-perishable food for household	14.8 (42)
≥ 14-days' supply of water for household	3.5 (10)

*Indicator part of both pandemic preparedness and personal preparedness

past two years, risk perceptions, and perceived importance of disaster planning. Only variables that were significant in univariate analysis (with a critical p-value of .05) were included in the multivariate analyses. Variables that were significant on univariate analysis, but non-significant on multivariate analysis were dropped from the model; only final models are reported. A critical p-value of .05 was used for all analyses.

Results

A total of 283 HR professionals from 24 states participated in the study, representing 60% of the original sample obtained for the larger business continuity study [5]. The majority of participants were female (83.4%, n=231) and over the age of 30, with most HR professional being between the ages of 31-40 (18.4%, n=51), 41-50 (37.2%, n=103), or over 51 (36.8%, n=102). Almost three-quarters of the participating HR professionals (72.4%, n=205) had either a bachelor's (43.0%, n=119)

or master's degree (31.0%, n=86). Almost all of the HR professional participants 87% (n=241) had significant work experience, with most having either 5-10 years' (28.9%, n=80) or 11 or more years' (58.1%, n=161) of HR work experience. They were most likely to live in either the South (48.0%, n=133) or Midwest (39.0%, n=108). The HR professionals reported working in a wide variety of business types, with the most frequently reported employer types including education (10.2%, n=29), healthcare (9.9%, n=28), or a governmental agency (13.8%, n=39). The majority of employers (77.7%, n=167) were for-profit agencies. Almost half of the HR professionals (46.2%, n=128) reported being a member of their company's disaster planning committee.

Personal preparedness and personal pandemic preparedness

The survey contained 20 indicators of personal preparedness and 9 indicators of pandemic preparedness, contributing to a maximum score of 20 and 9 for personal preparedness and pandemic preparedness, respectively. Scores for personal preparedness ranged from 0-20, with an average score of 12.6 (sd = 4.4). Approximately one-third of participants (35.3%, n=100) had half of fewer of the objective measures of personal preparedness. Pandemic preparedness scores ranged from 0-9, with an average score of 4.5 (sd=1.8). Almost half of the HR professionals (47%, n=133) reported having 4 or fewer of the 9 possible objective measures of pandemic preparedness. Indicators of personal preparedness and pandemic preparedness, as well as the frequency with HR professionals had each component of preparedness are outlined in Table 1. The most frequently reported indicators of personal preparedness (excluding shared indicators with pandemic preparedness, (Table 1) were having a flashlight and batteries (97.5%, n=276), at least 3-days' supply of prescription medication for each person who takes prescribed medicine in household (95.4%, n=267), and smoke detectors on each level of home (95.1%, n=269. The least frequently reported indicators of personal preparedness included having procedures for sheltering-in-place for the household (38.2%, n=108), having back-up transportation plans (34.6%, n=98), and conducting regular household emergency evacuation drills (8.5%, n=24). From linear regression, determinants of personal preparedness were as follows: high perception of personal preparedness for both natural disasters and pandemics, having fewer years of work experience, being encouraged by the employer to have a personal preparedness plan, having received disaster preparedness training during the past two years, and not having children in the household (Table 2). Age, gender, race, education level, number of people living in household, having a disabled person living in the household, risk perceptions related to natural disasters or pandemics, perceived importance of or interest in personal preparedness or business continuity of employer, perceived cost of personal planning as a barrier, being a member of their employer's disaster planning committee, type of employing agency (healthcare, retail, food, utilities, etc), size and location (urban, suburban, or rural area) of employing agency were not significant predictors of HR professionals' personal disaster plans.

The most frequently reported indicators of pandemic preparedness (including shared indicators with personal preparedness, (Table 1) were having a supply of non-prescription medication (95.4%, n=270), having a battery-operated radio and batteries (83.7%, n=837), and having back-up childcare/eldercare plans (77.4%, n=219). The least frequently reported indicators of pandemic preparedness included having at least one mask or respirator stored (20.5%, n=58), a two-weeks' or longer supply of non-perishable food (14.8%, n=42), and a two-weeks' or longer supply of water stockpiled in the home (3.5%, n=10). From linear regression, determinants of pandemic preparedness were as follows: high perception of personal preparedness for both natural disasters and pandemics, not having children in the household, being male, and having received disaster preparedness training during the past two years (Table 2). Age, education level, years of work experience in human resources, number of people living in household, having a disabled person living in the household, risk perceptions related to natural disasters or pandemics, perceived importance of or interest in personal preparedness or business continuity, perceived cost of personal planning as a barrier, being a member of their employer's disaster planning committee, type of employing agency, size and location of employing agency were not significant predictors of HR professionals' personal disaster plans.

Attitudes and beliefs about disaster preparedness

Almost all HR professionals reported that preparing for natural disasters is important, with more agreeing that it is important to them that their family be prepared compared to having their employer be prepared (94.3% versus 89%, p<.001). HR professionals also reported that preparing their family for natural disasters is more important to them than preparing their family for a pandemic (94.3% versus 80.6%, p<.001). Perceived importance of employer preparedness for natural disasters was reported to be higher than perceived importance of company pandemic preparedness (89% versus 80.6%, p<.01). HR professionals whose employer encouraged him/her to have a personal disaster plan were significantly more likely to report that disaster planning is important for their family and their employer, that they are interested in disaster planning for family and their employer, and that they are well prepared to face either a natural disaster or pandemic compared to those whose employers have not encouraged them to have a personal plan (Table 3).

Almost 70% (68.2%, n=193) HR professionals reported being interested in personal disaster planning; significantly fewer (54.4%, n=154; p<.001) reported being interested in business preparedness for disasters. About half (53.7%, n=152) reported that they and their family are well prepared to face a natural disaster; significantly fewer (33.6%, n=95) reported that their family is prepared for a pandemic. As mentioned earlier, perceived preparedness was associated with objective

Table 2: Factors related to disaster and pandemic personal preparedness.

Factor	Disaster Preparedness			Pandemic Preparedness		
	β	S.E.	p value	β	S.E.	p value
Perception of personal preparedness						
Natural disaster	3.1	.48	**< .001**	1.0	.24	**< .001**
Pandemic	1.8	.51	**< .001**	.70	.25	**< .01**
Years working in HR*						
1-2 years	3.0	1.4	**< .05**	NIM	NIM	NIM
No children in household	1.2	.20	**< .01**	.64	.10	**= .001**
Employer encouragement to have plan	.92	.39	**< .05**	NIM	NIM	NIM
Disaster preparedness training in last two years	.32	.10	**= .001**	.13	.05	**< .01**
Gender (male)	NIM	NIM	NIM	.61	.25	**< .05**

S.E. = standard error; NIM = Not in Model
*Years' experience referent: ≥ 3 years

Table 3: Human resource professionals' attitudes and beliefs about disaster preparedness by employer encouragement to have plan.

Statement	All Respondents N = 283		Encouragement to Have a Personal Plan N = 283				
			Encouraged N =		Not Encouraged N =		Enc. vs. Not Enc.
	% That Strongly Agreed or Agreed	n	% That Strongly Agreed or Agreed	n	% That Strongly Agreed or Agreed	n	P value*
It is important that me/my family be prepared for a natural disaster	94.3	267	97.9	137	90.9	130	**= .01**
It is important that my company be prepared for a natural disaster	89.0	252	94.3	132	83.9	120	**< .01**
It is important that I/my family have/has a personal disaster plan	86.9	246	94.3	132	79.7	114	**< .001**
It is important that me/my family be prepared for a pandemic	80.6	228	87.9	123	73.4	105	**< .01**
It is important that my company be prepared for a pandemic	80.6	228	86.4	121	74.8	107	**= .01**
I am interested in personal disaster preparedness	68.2	193	75.7	106	60.8	87	**< .01**
I am interested in business continuity planning	54.4	154	65.7	92	43.4	62	**< .001**
I/my family are well prepared to face a natural disaster	53.7	152	70.0	98	37.8	54	**< .001**
A natural disaster will likely affect my company's business in the next 5 years	52.7	149	59.3	83	46.2	66	**< .05**
I/my family are well prepared to face a pandemic	33.6	95	47.9	67	19.6	28	**< .001**
A natural disaster will likely affect my company's business in the next year	29.9	84	42.1	59	17.5	25	**< .001**
A pandemic will likely affect my company's business in the next 5 years	20.1	57	21.4	30	18.9	27	NS
Developing and/or maintaining a personal disaster plan is too expensive	13.4	38	12.9	18	14.0	20	NS
A pandemic will likely affect my company's business in the next year	6.7	19	12.1	17	1.4	2	**< .001**

NS = Not significant
*Determined by the X^2 test

measures of preparedness for both natural disasters and pandemics (Table 2). Very few HR professionals (13.4%, n=38) reported that developing and maintaining a personal disaster plan is too expensive, and there were no differences in this attitude, regardless of whether the employer encourages staff to have a personal disaster plan (Table 3).

Risk perceptions about natural disasters and pandemics

HR professionals were asked how strongly they agreed or disagreed that a natural disaster or pandemic was likely to affect their employer's business during the next year or next five years. About half of the HR professionals (52.7%, n=149) reported that they believe it is likely that a natural disaster will affect their company's business during the next five years; significantly fewer (29.9%, n=84; p<.001) reported that one will occur in the next year (Table 3). Perceived risk of a pandemic was far lower compared to that of a natural disaster (p<.001 for both), regardless of whether it would occur in the next year or next five years. Only 20% (n=57) and 6.7% (n=19) reported that they believe it is likely that a pandemic will occur during the next five years or next year, respectively (Table 3). Perceived risk for a pandemic in the next five years was significantly higher than for one occurring during the next year (p<.001). Risk perceptions related to a natural disaster or a pandemic affecting the employer's company during the next year or five years were significantly lower than perceived importance for preparing the family or the company for such events (p<.001 for all comparisons).

HR professionals whose employer encouraged him/her to have a personal disaster plan were significantly more likely to report high risk perceptions related to a natural disaster occurring in the next year or five years, or a pandemic occurring in the next five years compared to those whose employers have not encouraged them to have a personal plan (Table 3). There were no significant differences between risk perception related to a pandemic occurring in the next five years and whether the employer encourages staff to have a personal disaster plan (Table 3).

Discussion

This study examined the personal preparedness of HR professionals across the U.S., including identifying predictors of better personal preparedness. Similar to previously published personal preparedness studies among healthcare personnel and the general public, this study found that, although most HR professionals report that personal disaster preparedness is important to them and their family, many lack adequate personal disaster plans. About a third of the respondents had half or fewer of the objectives measures of preparedness that were assessed. This very low level of preparedness means that many HR professionals would lack the resources and supplies needed during a disaster. Researchers indicate that it is vital that individuals and families have the capability of being self-sufficient for a few days during a large-scale disaster before outside resources may be brought into the community and distributed [18]. It is also important that citizens understand that regional and national stockpiles of supplies will not be adequate to address all communities' needs and that households that have prepared in advance will likely fare better after a disaster occurs. The U.S's experiences during the 2009 H1N1 pandemic confirmed that federal resources are inadequate to assist all communities [28], and that event was considered mild compared to the potential for a future pandemic or large-scale disaster [5]. Some researchers have even argued that personal preparedness is a form of social justice, because it allows limited resources to be targeted to the least advantaged members of society, such as those with very low incomes and lack of access to healthcare [12].

It is unclear why so many HR professionals are ill prepared for disasters when the majority of them report that personal preparedness is important to them. Contrary to prior research [17], this study found that risk perceptions of a disaster were not associated with better preparedness. This finding is surprising, given that health promotion theories, such as the Health Belief Model, indicate that perception of risk regarding a negative event or outcome is often associated with choosing to engage in healthy behaviors [16,29]. HR professionals in this study had sub-optimal personal preparedness in terms of having adequate supplies stockpiled and developing a personal disaster plan, regardless of the extent to which perceived a natural disaster or pandemic to be a risk in the next five years. Therefore, other influencing factors must exist that help account for the general lack of preparedness found in this study. One hypothesized reason was the cost associated with stockpiling supplies; however, very few HR professionals in this study reported that developing a plan is too expensive and believing that costs were a significant barrier was not a significant predictor of having a personal disaster plan.

The HR professionals in this study reported having a more robust personal plan that addresses natural disasters and traditional terrorism events; their pandemic preparedness plans were far less thorough. Approximately half of the HR professionals had half or fewer of the objective measures of pandemic preparedness. Biological events require different resources compared to those needed during a natural disaster, such personal protective equipment and over-the-counter medications to treat symptoms of infection. In addition, pandemics are prolonged disasters, with each pandemic wave lasting 6 – 12 weeks; this means that individuals need to have more supplies stockpiled to get them through the disaster until community services are back to full capacity. The extent to which individuals have a personal disaster plan specific to preparing for a biological event has never been evaluated for any occupation or group of individuals, including the general public. However, two studies have reported that K-12 schools' and businesses' disaster plans are more robust for addressing natural disasters compared to their preparedness for biological events [3,22]. Therefore, the lack of personal disaster plans related to biological events identified in this study is not surprising; it simply reflects the lower preparedness for biological events that exists among U.S. businesses. The reasons why HR professionals reported having less robust pandemic preparedness plans are unclear. Perhaps HR professionals are unaware of why a personal disaster plan is needed for a biological event, or they may not know what should be included in such a plan. Future research studies should attempt to further delineate influencing factors that affect individuals from developing personal preparedness plans for all types of disasters, including biological events [7]. Once the reason(s) for non-participation in personal disaster planning have been fully identified, interventions can be developed to address these issues.

Two important predictors for personal preparedness identified in this study include being encouraged by an employer to have a plan and having received disaster preparedness training during the past two years. It would be beneficial to employers to encourage HR professionals to have a personal disaster plan because having such a plan increases the likelihood that staffs are able and willing to work during a disaster [30]. HR professionals will be essential during disaster response because they serve as a source for staffing, training, employee benefits, and employee relations; they will be able to identify and obtain back-up staff during disasters if surge capacity is needed or if personnel are unable or unwilling to work. In addition, HR professionals can help increase company resiliency by encouraging new and existing employees to develop and maintain a personal disaster plan.

Researchers indicate that a policy indicating that administrators or HR professionals encourage staff to develop a personal disaster plan should be implemented on a systems basis and that personnel should be told about the policy when hired and annually after that; HR professionals could be the individuals that inform staff about this policy and monitor personnel's compliance [9,12]. Because recent disaster preparedness training was also associated with better disaster preparedness, it would be beneficial for administrators to encourage staff to participate in disaster planning educational programs or providing such training to employees. Educational programs have been shown to increase staff awareness for the need to better personally prepare for a disaster and to result in higher personal preparedness among emergency department personnel [11].

Similar to previously published studies [16,25], this study found that many HR professionals have low risk perceptions related to natural disasters and biological events. Also similar to previous research [25], this study found that risk perceptions related to natural disasters were higher than perceived risk of a pandemic occurring. Historically, pandemics occur much less frequently than natural disasters and terrorism events. However, pandemics are unpredictable and can occur at any time. For example, the 2009 H1N1 pandemic was completely unexpected; epidemiologists had predicted that avian influenza H5N1 might mutate and cause a pandemic, yet H1N1 occurred seemingly out of nowhere and became a pandemic just two weeks after the first case was identified in the U.S. [31] In addition, other biological events, such as bioterrorism or outbreak of an emerging infectious disease, cause the same response challenges as pandemics, and could occur at any time.

One of the primary strengths of this study is that it is the first to measure individuals' personal preparedness for both natural disasters and biological events. Strength is that it is one of only a few studies to identify predictor variables for personal preparedness; most previous studies have only been descriptive in nature. Some limitations must also be acknowledged. This study involved only HR professionals, and thus is not generalizable to the general public as a whole. In addition, only HR professionals who belong to SHRM were invited to participate; therefore, it may not be generalizable to all HR professionals. There is likely some responder bias in this study, as is common with survey research as a whole. Human resource professionals with an interest in personal disaster planning were likely more willing to participate in this survey, leading to possible bias in the results. This study could not directly assess individual characteristics of the non-responders, and this could potentially limit the generalizability of the findings. Lastly, this study may have some bias related to the finding that having no children was associated with better preparedness. Because participants without children were not penalized for not having an emergency childcare plan (i.e., they were given credit for having that component in their plan), this may have introduced some bias. Future research should examine this issue more closely.

Acknowledgement

The authors would like to thank Dipti Subramaniam for assisting in instrument development and psychometric testing.

References

1. Guha-Sapir D, Vos F, Below R., Ponserre S (2012) Annual Disaster Statistical Review: The Numbers and Trends. Brussels: Centre for Research on the Epidemiology of Disasters (CRED).

2. Levac J, Toal-Sullivan D, O'Sullivan TL (2012) Household emergency preparedness: a literature review. J Community Health 37: 725-733.

3. Rebmann T, Elliott MB, Reddick D, D Swick Z (2012) US school/academic institution disaster and pandemic preparedness and seasonal influenza vaccination among school nurses. Am J Infect Control 40: 584-589.

4. Missouri Department of Health and Human Services (2013).

5. Rebmann T, Wang J, Reddick D, Swick Z, Minden-Birkenmaier C (2013) Healthcare versus non-healthcare businesses' experiences during the 2009 H1N1 pandemic: Financial impact, vaccination policies, and control measures implemented. Am J Infect Control 41: e49-54.

6. American Red Cross (2013) Prepare your home and family.

7. Centers for Disease Control and Prevention. Pandemic Flu Planning Checklist for Individuals and Families. 2007.

8. Centers for Disease Control and Prevention (2013) Emergency preparedness and you.

9. Qureshi K, Gershon RR, Sherman MF, Straub T, Gebbie E, et al. (2005) Health care workers' ability and willingness to report to duty during catastrophic disasters. J Urban Health 82: 378-388.

10. Amaratunga CA, O'Sullivan TL, Phillips KP, Lemyre L, O'Connor E, et al. (2007) Ready, aye ready? Support mechanisms for healthcare workers in emergency planning: a critical gap analysis of three hospital emergency plans. Am J Disaster Med 2: 195-210.

11. Bartley BH, Stella JB, Walsh LD (2006) What a disaster?! Assessing utility of simulated disaster exercise and educational process for improving hospital preparedness. Prehosp Disaster Med 21: 249-255.

12. Kass NE, Otto J, O'Brien D, Minson M 2008) M. Ethics and severe pandemic influenza: Maintaining essential functions through a fair and considered response. Biosecur Bioterror 6: 227-236.

13. Fowkes V, Ablah E, Oberle M, Sandrock C, Fleming P (2010) Emergency preparedness education and training for health professionals: a blueprint for future action. Biosecur Bioterror 8: 79-83.

14. Blessman J, Skupski J, Jamil M, Jamil H, Bassett D, et al. (2007) Barriers to at-home-preparedness in public health employees: implications for disaster preparedness training. J Occup Environ Med 49: 318-326.

15. Rebmann T, Wilson R, LaPointe S, Russell B, Moroz D (2009) Hospital infectious disease emergency preparedness: a 2007 survey of infection control professionals. Am J Infect Control 37: 1-8.

16. Rebmann T, Mohr LB (2008) Missouri nurses' bioterrorism preparedness. Biosecur Bioterror 6: 243-251.

17. Eisenman DP, Wold C, Fielding J, Long A, Setodji C, et al. (2006) Differences in individual-level terrorism preparedness in Los Angeles County. Am J Prev Med 30: 1-6.

18. Ablah E, Konda K, Kelley CL (2009) Factors predicting individual emergency preparedness: a multi-state analysis of 2006 BRFSS data. Biosecur Bioterror 7: 317-330.

19. Eisenman DP, Zhou Q, Ong M, Asch S, Glik D, et al. (2009) Variations in disaster preparedness by mental health, perceived general health, and disability status. Disaster Med Public Health Prep 3: 33-41.

20. Smith DL, Notaro SJ (2009) Personal emergency preparedness for people with disabilities from the 2006-2007 Behavioral Risk Factor Surveillance System. Disabil Health J 2: 86-94.

21. Uscher-Pines L, Hausman AJ, Powell S, DeMara P, Heake G, et al. (2009) Disaster preparedness of households with special needs in southeastern Pennsylvania. Am J Prev Med 37: 227-230.

22. Rebmann T, Wang J, Swick Z, Reddick D, delRosario JL Jr (2013) Business continuity and pandemic preparedness: US health care versus non-health care agencies. Am J Infect Control 41: e27-33.

23. Federal Emergency Management Agency (2009) Are You Ready? Emergency Planning and Checklist.

24. Shadel BN, Rebmann T, Clements B, Chen JJ, Evans RG (2003) Infection control practitioners' perceptions and educational needs regarding bioterrorism: results from a national needs assessment survey. Am J Infect Control. 31: 129-134.

25. Shadel BN, Chen JJ, Newkirk RW, Lawrence SJ, Clements B, et al. (2004) Bioterrorism risk perceptions and educational needs of public health professionals before and after September 11, 2001: a national needs assessment survey. J Public Health Manag Pract 10: 282-289.

26. Rebmann T, Mohr LB (2010) Bioterrorism knowledge and educational participation of nurses in Missouri. J Contin Educ Nurs 41: 67-76.

27. Lynn MR (1986) Determination and quantification of content validity. Nurs Res 35: 382-385.

28. Rebmann T, Wagner W (2009) Infection preventionists' experience during the first months of the 2009 novel H1N1 influenza A pandemic. Am J Infect Control 37: e5-5e16.

29. Janz NK, Champion, VL, Strecher VJ (2008) The Health Belief Model. In: Glanz K, Rimer, B. K., & Viswanath, K, ed. Health behavior and health education: Theory, research, and practice. 4th ed. San Francisco: Jossey-Bass; 2008: 45-66.

30. Goodhue CJ, Burke RV, Ferrer RR, Chokshi NK, Dorey F, et al. (2012) Willingness to respond in a disaster: a pediatric nurse practitioner national survey. J Pediatr Health Care 26: e7-20.

31. Centers for Disease Control and Prevention (CDC) (2009) Swine influenza A (H1N1) infection in two children--Southern California, March-April 2009. MMWR Morb Mortal Wkly Rep 58: 400-402.

18

Predictors of Length of Stay in an Acute Psychiatric Hospital

Muaid H Ithman, Ganesh Gopalakrishna,Niels C Beck, Jairam Das and Gregory Petroski

University of Missouri-Columbia, Columbia, Missouri, USA

Abstract

Length of stay (LOS) in acute psychiatric hospitals has been heightened in recent years with the current economic climate and a growing realization that health care costs need to be contained. This study was designed to identify predictors of LOS which are available at the time of admission. Charts of 391 admissions to an acute psychiatric hospital were reviewed on the basis of a pre-constructed checklist. Regression modeling with the natural logarithm of LOS as the dependent variable was used to identify a multivariate model for LOS. Age, marital status, involuntary admission and diagnosis of an affective disorder or a psychotic disorder were shown to be independent variables that predicted length of stay. These variables in a multivariate model accounted for approximately 19% of the variance in LOS.

Keywords: Length of stay; Acute psychiatric hospital; Chart review; Predictors

Introduction

Length of stay (LOS) in acute psychiatric hospitals has long been a focus of attention and this has been heightened in recent years with the current economic climate and a growing realization that health care costs need to be contained. Length of stay (LOS) has a strong positive relationship with the cost of hospitalization; thus, LOS has become an important marker for hospital administrators, third party payers, patients and also community health providers.

Longer hospital stays do not necessarily mean better mental health care, improved social adjustment or diminished psychopathology [1,2]. The locus of provision of psychiatric care has shifted from institutions to community mental health in USA and many other countries [3-6]. Length of stay in hospitals has drastically dropped in the USA [7].

Many patients are currently on managed healthcare plans and third payers prefer to keep inpatient stays to the minimum. The need of the health care provider to comply with the third party payers, in order to get complete reimbursements and prevent patients from paying out of pocket has put pressure on healthcare professionals to expedite discharges from inpatient facilities and provide optimum care at the same time.

Results from previous studies indicated that some factors which are useful for estimating LOS are available at the time of admission, and these variables might be systematically assessed and incorporated into clinical decision-making. For instance, studies from the past have consistently shown that substance abuse has been associated with shorter length of stay and higher readmission rates [8-10].

Information regarding factors which tend to prolong length of stay has been equivocal across the studies in the past. Some of the demographic variables suggested are: age, fluency in English, gender, marital status, legal status, type of admission, place of residence and employment status [9]. Treatment variables include: number of prior hospitalizations, psychotic features, receiving ECT and need for restraints for violent behavior [10]. Diagnostic variables implicated are: a primary diagnosis of a psychotic or mood disorder, psychiatric symptom severity, co-morbid medical conditions, outpatient treatment, activities of daily living (ADL) functioning at admission, required court proceedings to continue hospitalization [11] or use of involuntary medications. A study conducted in Japan found that strong positive correlations with LOS were inpatient capacity and proportion of involuntary admissions [12]. Higher Brief Psychiatric Rating Scale

(BPRS), positive symptom scores [11] or even subscales of BPRS have consistently been associated with longer length of stay [13].

Although the knowledge generated by such investigations can be useful in identifying significant correlation between single variables and LOS, such findings are of limited applicability when making real-world predictions on a case-by-case basis. At the time of admission, patients possess multiple demographic and diagnostic characteristics, some of which may be positively, and others negatively correlated with LOS. Thus, methods are needed which will somehow combine these multiple influences and arrive at a composite prediction.

Blais et al. conducted a retrospective study of 80 discharged patients to explore the association of 25 demographic, illness and treatment variables from preadmission screening with LOS. Multivariate analysis revealed that 10 variables independently accounted for 62% of the variance in LOS. When the equation obtained from the multivariate regression analysis was applied to the prospective sample, predictive power of the variables shrank to 17% and fewer individual variables were significantly associated with LOS [11].

As Blais et al. [11] point out, although the multivariate methodological approach employed in their study had a number of important advantages over prior work in the area, the study still suffered as a result of relatively small sample size and consequent unfavorable subject to variable ratio, which probably contributed to the degree of shrinkage on cross-validation. The purpose of the present study was to identify predictors of length of stay in an acute psychiatric hospital based on a large sample size of chart review.

Methods

Subjects for this study consisted of every third patient discharged from three adult inpatient units at a publically funded University affiliated acute care psychiatric hospital located in Central Missouri

Corresponding author: Ganesh Gopalakrishna, Assistant Professor, University of Missouri-Columbia, Columbia, Missouri, USA, E-mail: gopalakrishnag@health.missouri.edu

Independent Variable	Parameter Estimate	Significance	Multiplicative Effect (ME)	95% Confidence Interval for ME	
Intercept	1.919	<0.001	6.81	5.68	8.17
Age	0.007	0.006	1.01	1.00	1.01
Married	-0.212	0.029	0.81	0.67	0.98
Involuntary Admission	0.211	0.008	1.24	1.06	1.45
Guardian	0.814	<0.001	2.26	1.53	3.33
Affective disorder	0.196	0.0178	1.22	1.03	1.43
Psychotic disorder	0.558	<0.001	1.75	1.42	2.14

Table 1: Collection of samples from different people.

from January 2006 to September 2009. The patients had to be more than 18 years of age for inclusion.

Data collection

The chart review was reviewed and approved by the ethics committee at the University of Missouri-Columbia. Two psychiatry residents familiar with the medical record used a checklist assessing 14 variables, to abstract data that were utilized for the study. The checklist contained items relating to such topics as diagnosis, prior hospitalizations, admission status (voluntary, involuntary, voluntary by guardian), prior living circumstances (e.g. homeless, supported community living, residential care facility, emergency room, jail or another hospital), as well as demographic variables and diagnostic variables.

Statistical analysis

Univariate analyses were performed to examine the association between LOS and individual diagnosis-related items, demographics, and admission characteristics. Because the distribution of LOS (in days) was highly skewed, nonparametric methods were used, including Spearman's Rank correlation coefficient and the Wilcoxon Rank Sum Test for group comparisons. Regression methods were used to derive a multivariate model of factors associated with LOS. Linear regression methods were used to develop a multivariate description of LOS. Standard linear regression methods derive from the assumption of a normally distributed outcome with constant variance. An examination of regression residuals indicated that neither assumption was satisfied but that regression with the natural logarithm of the LOS as the dependent variable stabilized the variance and normalized the error distribution.

The regression analysis was carried out in several steps. The first step was to fit a model using all diagnosis-related items with sufficient samples size and then remove non-significant (p>0.05) predictors from the model. In this way we identified the most important diagnostic factors before conditioning on demographics. The second step was to add demographics and admission status to the diagnostic model and then exclude what was not statistically significant. Preliminary analysis revealed very low incidence of some diagnoses. Cognitive Affective disorder, Antisocial personality disorder, Anxiety, Borderline Personality Disorder, Mental Retardation, Other personality disorders, Psychotic disorders, & Substance abuse were excluded from the regression analysis as each represented fewer than 10 cases. This was an exploratory study so there was no formal rule used to set the minimum sample size, just a pragmatic decision that 6 was too few and 17 was enough to show an effect. The median overall LOS was 9 days, with an Interquartile range (IQR) of 10 days (25th=6 days, 75th=16).

Results

In all, 391 patients were selected for inclusion in the study during

the time frame in which charts were sampled. Twenty-five charts had multiple missing data values and hence had to be excluded from the analysis. Fifty-six percent of the patients were male, and the average age was 37 years; 90% were Caucasian, 8% were African-American, and 40% were never married; 44% had completed High School or a GED, and 23% had completed college. These demographic variables were closely representative of the general population of the catchment area for this hospital. Diagnostically, 82% suffered from symptoms of a psychotic disorder, 66% carried diagnoses involving substance abuse disorders, and 62% had been hospitalized involuntarily. In terms of length of stay, the average was 14.6 days (SD=18.9).

The sample median LOS was 9 days with a range of 1 to 189 days. Statistically significant predictors of LOS were age, marital status, involuntary admission and a diagnosis of an affective or a diagnosis of a psychotic disorder. These variables in a multivariate model accounted for approximately 19% of the variance. Substance abuse was also shown to be a predictor for a shorter length of stay but was ultimately excluded from the final model based on lack of significance (p=0.083). Regression results for the final log linear model are given in Table 1. Because the model is multiplicative on the LOS scale, the multiplicative effect (ME) and associated 95% confidence interval for each factor is included. Age was mean-centered and the other predictors are coded as 1 for present and 0 for absent. Thus the model-based estimate of LOS is about 7 days for the hypothetical reference individual who is of average age (37 years), unmarried, voluntarily admitted without guardian involvement, and without affective disorder or psychotic diagnoses. LOS increases/decreases by about 1% per year difference from age 37, is about 20% shorter for the married patient, increases by about 24% with an involuntary admission and can be expected to be 26% longer when a guardian is involved. Relative to all other admission diagnoses, affective and psychotic disorders increase expected LOS by 22 and 75% respectively.

Discussion

As expected, utilization of a larger patient sample and a more statistically sound subject/predictor variable ratio resulted in considerable shrinkage in the percent of variance accounted for in LOS. Recall that in contrast to the current finding that about 20% of the variance was accounted for, Blais et al. [11] reported that 62% was accounted for in the analysis of their original sample.

Relative to past research finding in this area, there was significant positive correlation between length of stay and a diagnosis of affective disorder, psychotic disorder or mental retardation. The correlation has been found to be stronger with a diagnosis with psychotic disorders, suggesting that patients with psychotic disorder tend to stay longer in hospitals. This again is consistent with many other studies in the past [8,14,15].

We also found that substance abuse disorders were negatively correlated with the length of stay in our hospital, consistent with the previous studies [8,10]. It is also notable that, though substance abuse disorder was marginally significant in univariate analysis, this variable was not included in the multivariate regression, as these disorders apparently co-vary with other variables, which are included in the multivariate model. Considering the demographic variables, male gender and non-single marital status was associated with a longer length of stay in our hospital. Increased social support in the form of marriage may facilitate discharge. Also, the patient status being involuntary or admitted by a guardian predicted a longer length of stay compared to patients who were admitted voluntarily which is consistent with previous studies [11].

Some of the variables were found to be predictive in previous studies have been excluded from our study, as they do not apply to our hospital. Since we do not use ECT very often in the hospital, this variable was not included, as it would introduce outliers in the data set. Also we do not use BPRS scales at admission, so this variable was unavailable.

Future research in this area needs to focus on variables which might account for the remaining variance in LOS, as the results of the current study indicate that 80% of the variance remains unaccounted for. Although it is doubtful that anything approaching perfect prediction can be achieved, one major source of missing variance may lie in classes of variables that are dynamic in nature [16].

Dynamic variables, in contrast with static variables such as gender and diagnosis, are characterized by their changeable and often situational nature. One class of dynamic variables almost certainly associated with LOS pertains to assessments of psychiatric symptomatology, with particular reference to those symptoms indicative of a patient's propensity for harm to self or others; this variable certainly plays a major role in the admission process, and subsequent to admission, it is almost axiomatic that fluctuations in a patient's assessed likelihood for harm to self or others plays a major role in the decision to ultimately discharge the patient.

When viewed from this perspective, harm to self/others is a variable which takes the form of a trajectory that is monitored by the staff of inpatient units over the hospital course. The heuristic value of this variable class is limited in the sense that a full trajectory of scores would provide only a few hours of lead time to engage in discharge planning, but it is likely that the trajectory of harm to self/others assessments during the first few days of hospitalization may predict LOS, since the maintenance of a high level of risk is almost certainly correlated with continued stay. On the other hand, patients with low levels of self/other harm potential on the day of admission may be relatively likely to be discharged early. In any case, multivariate statistical approaches such as those utilized by the present study and Blais et al. [11] have a distinct advantage under such circumstances, since multivariate predictive equations can accommodate multiple variables and sum both positively correlated and negatively correlated variables into a predictive equation which weighs each in a manner reflective of its predictive power, arriving at a LOS prediction which represents a composite estimate.

Limitations of the study

The current study is a retrospective chart review which implies that only the variables which were recorded and accessible in these records were studied. The multivariate regression model accounts for approximately 18% the variance in LOS. There may be other variables, predicting the length of stay among patients, which could be more apparent in a prospective study. The findings of the study, although consistent with previous studies in other hospitals, may not be generalizable to other hospitals. Testing the model on a prospective sample is needed for further validation.

Conclusions

The retrospective chart review performed as part of this study was able to identify a number of demographic and diagnosis-related variables which were correlated with the length of stay in an acute psychiatric hospital. Gender, employment status, marital status, admission type and diagnosis were correlated with the length of stay in our hospital. Using a multivariate regression model, a male patient who was unemployed, admitted involuntarily or by a guardian, with a diagnosis of an affective or psychotic disorder was likely to have the longest length of stay. However, even when these variables were used in a multivariate equation, they were only able to predict about 20% or one-fifth of the total variance in LOS. A substantial portion of the remaining 80% needs to be accounted for if heuristically meaningful predictions can be generated. We suggest that much of this variance lies in dynamic assessments of psychiatric symptoms, most notably those reflecting changes in the likelihood of harm to self/others.

Implications for Behavioral Health

Length of stay (LOS) in acute psychiatric hospitals has long been a focus of attention, heightened in recent years with the current economic climate and a growing realization that health care costs need to be contained. LOS has a strong positive relationship with the cost of each hospitalization. Longer LOS also puts the hospital at potential financial risk as they must provide adequate documentation for necessity of care. This study was designed to identify predictors of LOS which are available at the time of admission. Identification of predictors for LOS may help early recognition of such key factors as early as the admission and greater emphasis can be focused on such patients to aid in early discharge. This will facilitate efficient allocation of resources to optimize care in behavioral health.

References

1. Johnstone P, Zolese G (1999) Systematic Review of the Effectiveness of Planned Short Hospital Stays for Mental Health. British Medical Journal 318: 1387-1390.

2. Mattes JA (1982) The Optimal Length of Hospitalization for Psychiatric Patients: A Review of the Literature. Hospital and Community Psychiatry 33: 824-828.

3. Gigantesco A, de Girolamo G, Santone G, Rosella M, Angelo P, et al. (2009) Long-stay in Short-stay Inpatient Facilities: Risk Factors and Barriers to Discharge. BMC Public Health 9: 306.

4. Levinson D, Lerner Y, Lichtenberg P (2003) Reduction in Inpatient Length of Stay and Changes in Mental Health Care in Israel Over Four Decades: A National Case Register Study. Israel Journal of Psychiatry and Related Sciences 40: 240-247.

5. Goldberg D (1999) The Future Pattern of Psychiatric Provision in England. European Archives of Psychiatry and Clinical Neuroscience 249: 123-127.

6. Stefansson CG, Hansson L (2001) Mental Health Care Reform in Sweden. Acta Psychiatrica Scandinavica 104: 82-88.

7. Mardis R, Brownson K (2003) Length of Stay at an All-time Low. The Health Care Manager 22: 122-127.

8. Huntley DA, Cho DW, Christman J, Csernansky JG (1998) Predicting Length of Stay in an Acute Psychiatric Hospital. Psychiatric Services 49: 1049-1053.

9. Herr BE, Abraham HD, Anderson W (1991) Length of Stay in a General Hospital Psychiatric Unit. General Hospital Psychiatry 13: 68-70.

10. Compton MT, Craw J, Rudisch BE (2006) Determinants of Inpatient Psychiatric Length of Stay in an Urban County Hospital. Psychiatric Quarterly 77: 173-188.

11. Blais MA, Matthews J, Lipkis-Orlando R, Lechner E, Jacobo M, et al. (2003) Predicting Length of Stay on an Acute Care Medical Psychiatric Inpatient Service. Administration and Policy in Mental Health 31: 15-29.

12. Imai H, Hosomi J, Nakao, H, Tsukino H, Katoh T, et al. (2005) Characteristics of Psychiatric Hospitals Associated with Length of Stay in Japan. Health Policy 74: 115-121.

13. Hopko ER, Lachar D, Bailley SE, Varner RV (2001) Assessing Predictive Factors for Extended Hospitalization at Acute Psychiatric Admission. Psychiatric Services 52: 1367-1373.

14. Oiesvold T, Saarento O, Sytema S, Christiansen L, Göstas G, et al. (1999) The Nordic Comparative Study on Sectorized Psychiatry-Length of In-patient Stay. Acta Psychiatrica Scandinavica 100: 220-228.

15. Pertile R, Donisi V, Grigoletti L, Angelozzi A, Zamengo G, et al. (2010) DRGs and Other Patient-, Service- and Area-Level Factors Influencing Length of Stay in Acute Psychiatric Wards: The Veneto Region Experience. Social Psychiatry and Psychiatric Epidemiology 46: 651-660.

16. Choca JP, Peterson CA, Shanley, LA, Henry R, Elie M (1988) Problems in Using Statistical Models to Predict Psychiatric Length of Stay: An Illustration. Hospital and Community Psychiatry 39: 195-197.

19

Prevalence of Obesity, Overweight and Eating Disorders in a School-Based Population in Southern Brazil

Ricardo Rodrigo Rech[1]*and Ricardo Halpern

Federal University of Health Sciences of Porto Alegre, Brazil. University of Caxias do Sul, Brazil.

Abstract

The health of school-age children and adolescents has been the focus of much attention, since at this stage of life students experience biological, social, emotional and cognitive changes. The aim of this study was to determine the prevalence rates of obesity, overweight and symptoms of eating disorders (ED) among the sixth-grade students of the municipal schools in Caxias do Sul in 2011. A school-based, cross-sectional study evaluated 1230 students (86.80% of the total). A self-report questionnaire and anthropometric measures of weight and height were used in the assessment. The prevalence rates of obesity, overweight and ED symptoms were 7.30%, 22.80% and 33.10%, respectively. The students dissatisfied with their body image were four times more likely (PR=4.01; CI 95%= 2.71–5.93) to have excess weight and nine times more likely (PR=9.30; CI 95%=6.29–13.78) to have symptoms for ED. The prevalence rates of ED symptoms, obesity and overweight of the evaluated students are high and warrant the attention of the community as a whole.

Keywords: Obesity, Eating disorders, Body image, Cross-sectional studies.

Introduction

The health of school-age children and adolescents has been the focus of much attention, since at this stage of life students experience biological, social, emotional and cognitive changes [1]. This is a time when exposure to environment-related risk factors such as inadequate diet and sedentary behavior begins and may persist throughout adulthood [2]. Furthermore, these factors are associated with most chronic non-communicable diseases, such as cardiovascular disease, diabetes and cancer, which are the leading causes of adult death in Brazil [2,3].

The nutritional status of children and adolescents has undergone a shift termed "nutrition transition", which corresponds to increases in the prevalence of obesity and overweight and a reduction in the prevalence of malnutrition [4]. In Brazil, the studies addressing these issues report different prevalence rates and varying associated factors (eating habits, sedentary behavior, level of physical activity, socioeconomic status) depending on the location where the research was conducted and the evaluation methodology applied [5-7]. Other factors that have been associated with overweight are dissatisfaction with the body image and bullying [7].

Depending on the evaluation instrument and the population under study, the prevalence of ED symptoms may vary. In six towns in the interior of Minas Gerais, Vilela et al. [8] found 13.30% of students with possible ED; in Finland[9], a study found 2.60% prevalence for anorexia nervosa, 0.40% for bulimia nervosa and 8.50% for subclinical eating disorders. As with nutritional status, dissatisfaction with the body image is seen as a factor strongly associated to ED [10].

Different prevalence rates were noted for the outcomes in question depending on the study location, a fact that highlights the importance of conducting prevalence studies in the various Brazilian regions by virtue of the cultural, climatic and geographical particularities of each location [5-8,10]. The overall objective of the present study was to determine the prevalence rates of obesity, overweight and ED symptoms among sixth-grade students of the municipal schools in Caxias do Sul, RS, and the possible associations of those outcomes with mother's schooling, economic classification, dissatisfaction with the body image, bullying and lifestyle (physical activity, sedentary behavior and diet).

Methods

The present study is a school-based, cross-sectional, epidemiologic study that represents the first phase of a larger project denominated "Obesity, body image dissatisfaction and symptoms of eating disorders in a student cohort in the *Serra Gaucha*".

A population of 4300 sixth-grade students was found (age range, 11-14 years). To determine sample size, a prevalence of 50% (as the outcomes showed different prevalence rates), a 95% confidence interval (CI) and a 3% error were assumed; thus, it would be necessary to evaluate a minimum of 855 children. In order to secure greater control over the confounding factors, a design effect of 1.40 was calculated, which required the evaluation of 1197 students. The statistical software Epi-Info 6.0 was used to calculate the sample size.

The cluster sampling method was used, by which each school was regarded as a cluster. The randomized selection for the final sample included only the schools that had sixth grade classes. All the schools fulfilling this requirement were included in the selection and had the same chance of study participation according to the number of sixth-graders enrolled in the school on the selection date. All the students of the school who fulfilled the inclusion criteria were invited to participate in the study. Twenty-two schools were randomly selected to complete the minimum number of students to be evaluated (total n= 1417).

The following inclusion criteria were established: age between 11-14 years, no disabilities or any complication preventing the practice of physical activity, informed consent signed by the students' parents or legal guardians, and voluntary participation.

*Corresponding author: Professor Ricardo Rodrigo Rech, Federal University of Health Sciences of Porto Alegre, Brazil, E-mail: ricardo.rech@gmail.com

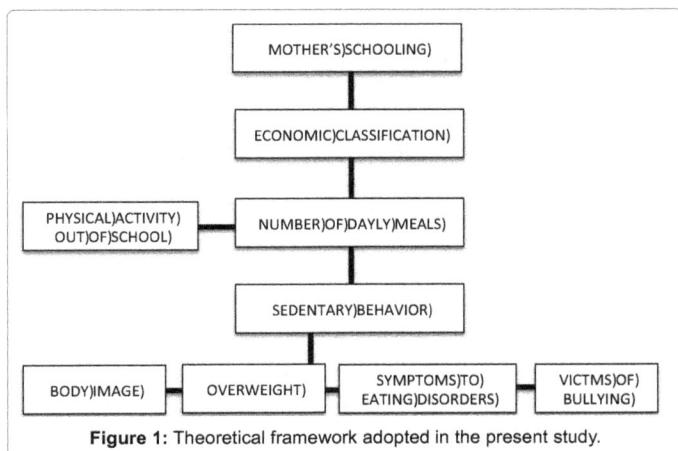

Figure 1: Theoretical framework adopted in the present study.

A self-report questionnaire was used in the assessment of the following variables: economic classification, gender, age, lifestyle habits, Eating Attitudes Test (EAT-26), body image dissatisfaction and bullying. To evaluate the students' eating habits, the number of daily meals was assessed, with the students marking which meals they usually had in a day (response choices: breakfast, morning snack, lunch, afternoon snack, dinner, supper; if others, specify). The students were also questioned as to physical activity out of school (yes or no) and sedentary behavior (number of hours per day involved in activities such as watching television, playing video games and using the computer).

The information concerning the economic classification was organized in accordance with that proposed by Barros and Victora [11], which takes into account 13 variables to constitute the National Wealth Score (Indicador Econômico Nacional, IEN). The students were classified into three categories: low, intermediate and high class.

The EAT-26, an instrument translated and validated for the Brazilian adolescent population by Bighetti [12], was used to screen for symptoms of ED. The EAT-26 evaluates the risks of developing behavior and attitudes typical of patients with anorexia nervosa. This instrument consists of 26 questions with six response choices for each. The established cut-off was 21 points or higher for EAT+ (presence of ED symptoms).

Dissatisfaction with the body image was investigated using the Body Shape Questionnaire (BSQ), which measures the extent of concerns with the body shape and self-depreciation motivated by physical appearance and feelings of being out of shape. The BSQ has been validated for adolescents in its Brazilian version by Conti, Cordás and Latorre [13] and comprises 34 questions with six possible responses.

To characterize victims of bullying, the Kidscape questionnaire was administered [14]. This questionnaire, in the adapted version for the present study, contains 14 questions that identify victims and aggressors. The definition of the outcome victim of bullying was based on the question that elicits the number of times the respondent was subjected to some form of intimidation; bullying is characterized if the fact occurred more than once in the previous month.

In addition to the self-report questionnaire, measurements of total body mass and height were taken. The measurement of total body mass was performed using a Plenna° portable digital scale with accuracy of 0.1 kg. Height was measured with a wall-mounted stadio meter and a set square. The nutritional status of the students was defined using the body mass index (BMI) cut-off points by gender and age

developed by Conde and Monteiro [15]. The children were classified as underweight, healthy weight, overweight and obese. For the bivariate and multivariate analyses, the underweight and healthy weight children were grouped together to compose the "no overweight" variable; the same was done with the overweight and obese children to establish the variable "overweight".

The entire assessment team (15 evaluators) was trained so the evaluations could be standardized; a handbook was prepared and distributed among them for the assessments. A pilot study was undertaken with 15 children of a school that was out of the final study sample, in which the logistic aspects of the project were ascertained, such as questionnaire language verification and standardization of the anthropometric measurements performed by the evaluators. The assessments were conducted in March and April 2011.

Following the collection of the data, these were entered twice in a database formatted in EPIDATA version 3.1. After verifying the consistency of the data, these were exported to the IBM-SPSS software version 19° for analysis. Initially, a descriptive analysis was performed, followed by bivariate (Pearson's chi square test) and multivariate analysis (logistic regression) between the independent variables and outcomes. A significance level of 20% was adopted as a statistical criterion to maintain a variable in the regression model, and also based on the plausibility of the association. The prevalence ratio (PR) and 95% confidence interval (CI) were presented for all associations. The theoretical framework adopted in the present study is outlined in Figure 1. The mother's schooling variable is on the first hierarchical level, followed by socio-economic status on the second level. The number of daily meals was included on the third level and sedentary habits on the fourth.

Regarding the ethical proceedings, informed consent forms were given to all the children in the study sample. In addition to parental consent, the students who composed the sample agreed to participate in the study on a voluntary basis. The research project was approved by the UFCSPA Research Ethics Committee with Opinion 1312/11 and registry no. 741/11.

Results

In total, 1417 children were randomly selected for the study (ages between 11-14 years), and 1230 composed the final sample (86.80% of the total). One child was excluded for not agreeing with the inclusion criteria, 16 refused to participate, and 170 failed to return a signed informed consent. The sample was equally distributed between genders with 606 girls and 624 (50.70%) boys. The assessment comprised 562 (45.70%) students aged 12 years; 452 (36.70%) aged 11 years; 159 (12.90%) aged 13, and 57 (4.60%) students 14 years. The mean age of the evaluated students was 11.85 years (SD=0.82).

In the overall sample, the means for the anthropometric variables weight, height and BMI were, respectively, 44.89 kg (SD=12.72), 1.50 m (SD=0.08) and 19.58 kg/m^2 (SD=3.75). The means for number of daily meals and number of hours sitting by the television, video game and computer were 3.72 (SD=1.24) and 2.21 (SD=1.16), respectively. Eighteen percent of the students were found to be dissatisfied with their body image (24.80% girls and 11.50% boys). The other characteristics of the study participants are shown in Table 1.

The prevalence of obesity, overweight and ED symptoms were 7.30%, 22.80% and 33.10%. Eleven (0.90%) underweight students were also found.

	n	%
Mother's schooling		
Elementary education	701	62,0
High school or higher	430	38,0
Economic classification		
Low	52	4,8
Intermediate	528	48,7
High	505	46,5
Number of daily meals		
Until 3	481	39,2
4 or mor	745	60,8
Sedentary behavior (TV, videogame, computer)		
Until 3 per day	785	64,6
Mor of 3 per day	430	35,4
Physical activity out of school		
Yes	578	47,8
No	631	52,2
Victims of bullying		
No	1104	89,8
Yes	126	10,2

TV= television

Table 1: Characteristics of the study participants (Caxias do Sul, 2011 – n=1230).

For the bivariate and multivariate analyses, the theoretical framework variables were grouped into dichotomous variables. Tables 2 and 3 display the results of the bivariate and multivariate analyses.

The variables mother's schooling, economic classification, physical activity out of school, sedentary habits, bullying, gender and age showed no statistically significant association with overweight ($p>0.05$) in the bivariate and multivariate analyses.

The number of daily meals equal to or greater than, four was found to be a protective factor for weight excess. The students who reported that eating habit were 42% less likely (PR=0.58; CI=0.43-0.78) to be overweight compared to those who ingested up to three meals per day.

The students who felt dissatisfied with their body image were four times more likely (PR=4.01; CI= 2.71-5.93) to be overweight compared with students satisfied with their body image (Table 2).

The variables mother's schooling, economic classification, sedentary habits and age showed no statistically significant association with ED symptoms ($p>0.05$).

The students who had excess weight were 56% more likely to have symptoms of ED compared with those who had no overweight/obesity (PR=1.56; CI=1.12-2.16).

The number of daily meals was significantly associated with the symptoms of ED only in the bivariate analysis, as the students who reported four or more meals per day were 25% less likely (PR=0.75; CI=0.59-0.96) to have ED symptoms relative to the students who had up to three meals per day.

The level of physical activity was associated with ED symptoms. The students who reported no physical activity out of school were 46% less

likely (PR=0.54; CI=0.40-0.74) to show ED symptoms than those who exercised out of school hours. Among the students who reported out-of-school physical activity, 50.40% responded "I think about burning up calories when I exercise" (question 12 of the EAT-26).

The students who declared body image dissatisfaction were nine times more likely (PR=9.30; CI=6.29-13.78) to have symptoms of ED compared with the satisfied students. Being a victim of bullying was associated with ED symptoms only in the bivariate analysis, where the victims were 78% more likely (PR=1.78; CI= 1.23-2.58) to have those symptoms than non-victims of bullying. In the bivariate analysis, the students who were not satisfied with their body image were more than twice as likely to be victims of bullying (PR=2.46; CI=1.64- 3.69).

The boys were 40% less likely (PR=0.60; CI=0.45-0.82) to show ED symptoms than the girls (Table 3).

	Crude PR (bivariate)	CI de 95%	Adjusted PR (multivariate)	CI de 95%
Mother's schooling (1º level)				
Elementary education	1,00		1,00	
High school or higher	1,11	0,86 – 1,45	1,25	0,91 – 1,71
Economic classification (2º level)				
Low and intermadiate	1,00		1,00	
High	1,18	0,91 – 1,54	1,09	0,80 – 1,49
Number of daily meals (3º level)				
Until 3	1,00		1,00	
4 or mor	0,59*	0,46 – 0,76	0,58*	0,43 – 0,78
Physical activity out of school				
Yes	1,00		1,00	
No	1,07	0,83 – 1,38	1,001	0,74 – 1,36
Sedentary behavior (4º level)				
Until 3 per day	1,00		1,00	
Mor of 3 per day	0,93	0,71 – 1,20	1,03	0,76 – 1,40
Body Image (5º level)				
Satisfied	1,00		1,00	
Dissatisfied	5,67*	4,15 – 7,75	4,01*	2,71 – 5,93
Victims of bullying				
No	1,00		1,00	
Yes	1,18	0,79 – 1,76	1,07	0,65 – 1,75
Sex (6º level)				
Female	1,00		1,00	
Male	0,87	0,68 – 1,12	1,31	0,96 – 1,78
Age				
11 years	1,00		1,00	
12, 13 and 14 years	0,90	0,70 – 1,16	0,66	0, 44 – 1,002

CI = Confidence Interval; PR = Prevalence Ratio; *=p<0,05;

Table 2: Bivariate and multivariate analyzes between overweight and dependents variables.

	Crude PR (bivariate)	CI de 95%	Adjusted PR (multivariate)	CI de 95%
Mother's schooling (1° level)				
Elementary education	1,00		1,00	
High school or higher	0,80	0,62 – 1,04	0,86	0,62 – 1,18
Economic classification (2° level)				
Low and intermadiate	1,00		1,00	
High	0,94	0,73 – 1,21	0,94	0,69 – 1,28
Number of daily meals (3° level)				
Until 3	1,00		1,00	
4 or mor	0,75*	0,59 – 0,96	0,99	0,73 – 1,33
Physical activity out of school				
Yes	1,00		1,00	
No	0,72*	0,57 – 0,92	0,54*	0,40 – 0,74
Sedentary behavior (4° level)				
Until 3 per day	1,00		1,00	
Mor of 3 per day	0,81	0,63 – 1,04	0,91	0,67 – 1,24
Overweight (5° level)				
No Overweight	1,00		1,00	
Overweight	2,52	1,95 – 3,26	1,56*	1,12 – 2,16
Body Image				
Satisfied	1,00		1,00	
Dissatisfied	11,31*	8,00 – 16,01	9,30*	6,29 – 13,78
Victims of bullying				
No	1,00		1,00	
Yes	1,78*	1,23 – 2,58	1,26	0,77 – 2,07
Sex (6° level)				
Female	1,00		1,00	
Male	0,56*	0,44 – 0,71	0,60*	0,45 – 0,82
Age				
11 years	1,00		1,00	
12, 13 and 14 years	1,09	0,80 – 1,49	0,96	0,65 – 1,42

CI = Confidence Interval; PR = Prevalence Ratio; *=p<0,05;

Table 3: Bivariate and multivariate analyzes between symptoms for eating disorders and independents variables.

Discussion

The present study found 30.10% of overweight students, a higher rate compared with the study carried out in Denmark [7], in which the children and adolescents had 1.10% obesity and 8.60% overweight. Comparing the results of the current study with other Brazilian studies, they are higher than those found in the cities of Florianópolis, which showed 21.90% of overweight students, Maceió [16], with 13.80% of overweight students, and Sorocaba [17], where 22.10% of the students were overweight or obese.

The present study also yielded higher values than those found in previous Caxias do Sul studies. In 2007[5], 27.90% prevalence

was found for overweight, and in 2010 [18], the prevalence rates for overweight and obesity were 15.10% (half the prevalence noted in the present study). These high prevalence rates can be explained in part by the diet that the Caxias do Sul pre-schoolers have been receiving, especially at home. The children have been consuming fewer adequate foods and more of those with added sugar and chocolate—a behavior that can be regarded as a risk for overweight and obesity, since these habits will be the major determinants of their food intake later in life [18,19].

Regarding ED symptoms, the students evaluated in the current study showed superior values to those found in a study conducted by Vilela et al.[8] (2004) and in public and private schools in the region of Castilla and León in Spain, where a prevalence of 7.80% was reported [20].

The group of students dissatisfied with their body image was four times more likely to be overweight (PR=4.01) and nine times more likely to have symptoms of ED (PR=9.30) relative to the satisfied students. Alves et al.[21], when evaluating 1148 girls in Florianópolis, also found strong associations between symptoms of ED and body image dissatisfaction (OR=14.39), and between excess weight and dissatisfaction with body image (OR=2.07). Other studies developed in Minas Gerais[8] and in several regions of China [22], also showed associations between overweight, ED symptoms and body image dissatisfaction. Eating disorders are characterized by patterns of disordered eating behavior, pathological body weight control and body image distortions [23]. Obese children feel rejected, unhappy with their bodies; they suffer with this situation and would like to change because they are pressured by their social milieu [24].

Another result that could be related to those discussed above: the overweight students were 56% more likely to have symptoms of ED compared with those who were at a healthy weight/underweight (PR=1.56). These are similar results to those found in the cities of São Paulo [25] and Florianópolis [21] as well as in the study conducted in Spain [20], where the children and adolescents with overweight or obesity showed greater likelihood of ED symptoms.

Another trend noted in the present study was the greater prevalence of symptoms of ED in girls, as the boys were 40% less likely (PR=0.60) to have ED symptoms compared with the girls. Perhaps this trend is related to body image, since girls typically exhibit the highest prevalence rates of dissatisfaction and seek methods to alter their body shape, in order to emulate the standards of beauty imposed by society and disseminated by the media [26].

The level of physical activity was associated with ED symptoms. The students who reported no out-of-school physical activity were 46% less likely (PR=0.54) to have ED symptoms. Cross-checking the variable physical activity with the EAT-26 question inquiring whether the child thought about burning calories when he/she exercised, it is possible to note that most children who responded always, very often and sometimes were those who had out-of-school activities, and perhaps this is a compensatory practice for weight control. Exercising with the purpose of losing weight and burning up calories is typical of individuals with ED symptoms [27], since regular and systematic exercise is one of the ways by which body weight control can be achieved [28].

The number of daily meals equal to, or greater than, four was a protective factor for symptoms of ED (PR=0.75; CI=0.59-0.96) and for overweight (PR=0.58; CI=0.43-0.78). A study conducted in Florianopolis with 2826 students also showed a negative correlation between number of daily meals and obesity/overweight [3], as did another study conducted in Caxias do Sul [5], where eating four meals or more in a day was found to be a protective factor for overweight. Dividing the amount of daily food in a greater number of meals per day is a nutritional recommendation that can assist in weight control [29]; epidemiologic studies on the theme have been showing this inverse relationship between number of meals and overweight [3,5].

The present study found 10.20% of victims of bullying. Different results were obtained in a study involving more than 60,000 students of public and private schools in the 26 Brazilian State capitals and the Federal District [30], which found 5.40% of bullying victims. Being a victim of bullying was not associated with overweight; however, in the bivariate analysis, the victims of bullying were 78% more likely (PR=1.78) to show ED symptoms than those who were not bullying victims. Brixval et al.[7], (in Denmark) found an association between bullying and overweight, and posited that body image can account for the association between overweight/obesity and vulnerability to bullying. Given that dissatisfaction with body image and symptoms of ED were strongly associated, this association between being a victim of bullying and ED symptoms observed in the present study could be explained by the relationship between victimization and discontent with body image, since dissatisfied students were more than twice as likely to be the targets of bullying (PR=2.46). Obese children, as a consequence of their body image, are rated as less capable and more indolent; due to this stigma, they are eventually left out of school environment situations [24].

The variables physical activity out of school and sedentary habits were not significantly associated with overweight, as found in the Recife [6] and Sorocaba [17] studies. However, these results counter the findings of another study conducted in Caxias do Sul [5]. It seems that the associations between overweight, physical activity and sedentary habits have not yet been well established in epidemiologic studies—possibly because of the use of indirect measures (such as questionnaires) [6] and not direct measures of health-related physical fitness (such as running track testing) [5].

The variables mother's schooling and socioeconomic status showed no statistically significant association with ED symptoms or with overweight. Other studies [3,16] found this association between better living conditions and overweight, and it may be that obesity and overweight issues are reaching the more underprivileged populations as well [5].

One limitation of the present study was the memory bias that may have occurred in the questions pertaining to eating habits and sedentary behavior. Also, reverse causality may have occurred due to the cross-sectional design of the study.

Because a representative sample of the target population was studied and the number of losses was low, the data of the present study can be extrapolated for the target population within the same age group. Considering the study limitations, it can be said that the prevalence rates of ED symptoms, obesity and overweight of the evaluated students are high.

Body image dissatisfaction was found to be strongly associated with overweight and symptoms of ED. Overweight was also associated with the number of daily meals. Symptoms of ED were associated with overweight, number of daily meals, physical activity, victims of bullying and the female gender.

The results of the present study serve as a warning sign to the study population and the community as a whole. Health promotion programs addressing these topics can be advanced by the town's school community. Further analyses of these students (by the longitudinal study) will more clearly establish the cause-and-effect relationships between the associated variables.

Contributions

Rech RR participated in the making of the project, field work, data analysis, drafting and approval of the final version of the manuscript. Halpern R participated in the making of the project, field work, data analysis, drafting and approval of the final version of the manuscript.

References

1. Legnani E, Legnani RF, Lopes AS, Campos W, Krinski K, et al. (2009) Risk behaviors related to health in adolescents from the tri-border region. RBAFS14:28-37.

2. Malta DC, Sardinha LM, Mendes I, Barreto SM, Giatti L, et al. (2010) Prevalence of risk health behavior among adolescents: results from the 2009 National Adolescent School-based Health Survey (PeNSE). Cien Saude Colet 15 Suppl 2: 3009-3019.

3. Bernardo Cde O, Vasconcelos Fde A (2012) Association of parents' nutritional status, and sociodemographic and dietary factors with overweight/obesity in schoolchildren 7 to 14 years old. Cad Saude Publica 28: 291-304.

4. Wang Y, Monteiro C, Popkin BM (2002) Trends of obesity and underweight in older children and adolescents in the United States, Brazil, China, and Russia. Am J Clin Nutr 75: 971-977.

5. Costanzi CB, Halpern R, Rech RR, Bergmann ML, Alli LR, et al. (2009) Associated factors in high blood pressure among schoolchildren in a middle size city, southern Brazil. J Pediatr (Rio J) 85: 335-340.

6. Alves JG, Siqueira PP, Figueiroa JN (2009) Overweight and physical inactivity in children living in favelas in the metropolitan region of Recife, Brazil. J Pediatr (Rio J) 85: 67-71.

7. Brixval CS, Rayce SL, Rasmussen M, Holstein BE, Due P (2012) Overweight, body image and bullying--an epidemiological study of 11- to 15-years olds. Eur J Public Health 22: 126-130.

8. Vilela JE, Lamounier JA, Dellaretti Filho MA, Barros Neto JR, Horta GM (2004) [Eating disorders in school children]. J Pediatr (Rio J) 80: 49-54.

9. Isomaa R, Isomaa AL, Marttunen M, Kaltiala-Heino R, Björkqvist K (2009) The prevalence, incidence and development of eating disorders in Finnish adolescents: a two-step 3-year follow-up study. Eur Eat Disord Rev 17: 199-207.

10. Yager Z, O'Dea J (2009) Body image, dieting and disordered eating and activity practices among teacher trainees: implications for school-based health education and obesity prevention programs. Health Educ Res 24: 472-482.

11. Barros AJ, Victora CG (2005) A nationwide wealth score based on the 2000 Brazilian demographic census. Rev Saude Publica 39: 523-529.

12. Bighetti F (2003) Tradução e validação do Eating Attitudes Test (EAT-26) em adolescentes do sexo feminino na cidade de Ribeirão Preto - SP [tese de mestrado]. Ribeirão Preto (SP): EERP/USP.

13. Conti MA, Cordás TA, Latorre MR (2009) A study of the validity and reliability of the Brazilian version of the Body Shape Questionnaire (BSQ) among adolescents. Rev Bras Saude Mater Infantil 9:331-8.

14. Kidscape [homepage on the Internet]. Kidscape: preventing bullying, protectin children [cited 2011 Apr 4]. Available from: http://www.kidscape.org.uk

15. Conde WL, Monteiro CA (2006) Body mass index cutoff points for evaluation of nutritional status in Brazilian children and adolescents. J Pediatr (Rio J) 82: 266-272.

16. Mendonça MR, Silva MA, Rivera IR, Moura AA (2010) Prevalence of overweight and obesity in children and adolescents from the city of Maceió (AL). Rev Assoc Med Bras 56: 192-196.

17. Mazaro IA, Zanolli Mde L, Antonio MÂ, Morcillo AM, Zambon MP (2011) Obesity and cardiovascular risk factors in school children from Sorocaba, SP. Rev Assoc Med Bras 57: 674-680.

18. Hoffmann M, Silva AC, Siviero J (2010) Prevalence of hypertension and interrelations with overweight, obesity, food intake and physical activity in students of municipal schools of Caxias do Sul. Pediatria (São Paulo) 32:163-72.

19. Bernardi JR, Cezaro CD, Fisberg RM, Fisberg M, Vitolo MR (2010) Estimation of energy and macronutrient intake at home and in the kindergarten programs in preschool children. J Pediatr (Rio J) 86: 59-64.

20. Vega Alonso AT, Rasillo Rodríguez MA, Lozano Alonso JE, Rodríguez Carretero G, Martín MF (2005) Eating disorders. Prevalence and risk profile among secondary school students. Soc Psychiatry Psychiatr Epidemiol 40: 980-987.

21. Alves E, Vasconcelos Fde A, Calvo MC, Neves Jd (2008) [Prevalence of symptoms of anorexia nervosa and dissatisfaction with body image among female adolescents in Florianópolis, Santa Catarina State, Brazil]. Cad Saude Publica 24: 503-512.

22. Chen H, Jackson T (2008) Prevalence and sociodemographic correlates of eating disorder endorsements among adolescents and young adults from China. Eur Eat Disord Rev 16: 375-385.

23. Saikali CJ, Soubhia CS, Scalfaro BM, Cordas TA (2004) Imagem corporal nos transtornos alimentares. Rev Psiquiatr Clin 31:164-166.

24. Feldmann LR, Mattos AP, Halpern R, Rech RR, Bonne CC et al. (2009) Implicações psicossociais da obesidade infantil em escolares de 7 a 12 anos de uma cidade serrana do sul do Brasil. RBONE 3:255-233.

25. Dunker KL, Fernandes CP, Carreira Filho D (2009) Socioeconomic influence on eating disorders risk behaviors in adolescents. J Bras Psiquiatr;58:156-161.

26. Del Duca GF, Garcia LM, Sousa TF, Oliveira ES, Nahas MV (2010) Body weight dissatisfaction and associated factors among adolescents. Rev Paul Pediatr 28:340-346.

27. Cancela Carral JM, Ayán Pérez C (2011) Prevalence and relationship between physical activity and abnormal eating attitudes in Spanish women university students in Health and Education Sciences. Rev Esp Salud Publica 85: 499-505.

28. Alves JG, Galé CR, Souza E, Batty GD (2008) Effect of physical exercise on bodyweight in overweight children: a randomized controlled trial in a Brazilian slum. Cad Saude Publica 24 Suppl 2: S353-359.

29. Toassa EC, Leal GVS, Wen CL, Philippi ST (2010) Recreational activities in the nutritional guidance of adolescents in the Young Doctor Project. Nutrire: Rev Soc Bras Alim Nutr 35: 17-27.

30. Malta DC, Silva MA, Mello FC, Monteiro RA, Sardinha LM, et al. (2010) [Bullying in Brazilian schools: results from the National School-based Health Survey (PeNSE), Cien Saude Colet 15 Suppl 2: 3065-3076.

20

Prostate Cancer Survivorship

Sanchia S Goonewardene[1]*, Persad R[2], Nanton V[3], Young A[3] and Makar A[4]

[1]*Guys Hospital, Kings College London, UK*
[2]*Bristol Southmead, UK*
[3]*University of Warwick, UK*
[4]*Worcestershire Acute Hospitals, Worcestershire, UK*

Abstract

Background: Due to advances in cancer diagnosis and treatment, the number of prostate cancer survivors are increasing. Yet, with this expanding cohort of patients, very little has been done to develop services.

Objective: A systematic review was conducted to explore prostate cancer survivorship issues. This analysis will inform development of interventions.

Design/setting: A systematic review was conducted using the following databases from 2000 to Decembers 2013: CINAHL and MEDLINE (NHS Evidence), Cochrane, AMed, BNI, EMBASE, Health Business Elite, HMIC, PschINFO. The papers were retrieved and a quality assessment was conducted using a new tool for survivorship care standards.

Participants/Interventions/ Outcome measurements/ results: 76 papers met the criteria for inclusion. These specified papers must be on primary research, related to prostate cancer AND Survivorship OR any one of the categories of nutrition, exercise therapy, psychology, treatment outcomes.

Discussion: The literature is reviewed and the way forward for survivorship discussed. We also identify possible themes for research.

Patient summary: Based on these results, we develop a prostate cancer survivorship care assessment tool and identify areas of practice that can be targeting for further research.

Keywords: Prostate cancer; Survivorship; Patient care; Community based follow-up

Introduction

Over 2 million people in England have a diagnosis of cancer (National Cancer Survivorship Initiative, 2008). Of this, over 250,000 have been diagnosed with prostate cancer [1]. And 130,000 people per year die [2]. The Department of Health is spending £750 million on improving earlier diagnosis and prevention of cancer. During the next decade, a rapid increase in the number of new cancer diagnoses as well as a growing number of cancer survivors are predicted [3].

Hospital clinics are often overbooked with follow-up patients, with little time available for each patient. Yet few studies or guidelines address the broader, multifaceted aspects of cancer survivorship including self-responsibility and patient empowerment [4].

The Quality, Innovation, Productivity and Prevention (QIPP) transformational programme has been set up by the Department of Health to improve the quality of care the NHS delivers while making up to £20billion of efficiency savings by 2014-15. One component involves risk profiling of patients, supported by community based teams and developing shared care/ decision making. As a result any programme which is set up must do the same. This reflects on the cancer survivorship programme, as the basis of this programme, is risk stratification, according to likelihood of recurrence.

Cancer Survivorship

A cancer survivor is any person who has received a diagnosis of cancer from diagnosis until the end of life. Survivorship is defined by Macmillan Cancer Support, a leading UK cancer care and support charity, as someone who has completed initial cancer management with no evidence of apparent disease. According to the National Cancer Institute, cancer survivorship encompasses the "physical, psychosocial, and economic issues of cancer from diagnosis until the end of life." (National Cancer Institute).

Prostate cancer survivors require further investigation as there are concerns current follow-up methods are unsuitable [5]. Due to the growing population of survivors of prostate cancer and the period of austerity for the NHS, patients are not getting the holistic care required during the survivorship phase. Concerns regarding permanent physical, psychosocial, and economic effects of cancer treatment were highlighted by the US Institute of Medicine Report [6]. This defined landmarks for survivorship care: monitoring for recurrence, metastases or side effects and coordination between secondary and primary care.

The unmet needs of cancer survivors, the rising numbers, and pressures to utilise resources efficiently [7] are a significant burden on the health system. These issues have been raised by the National Cancer Survivorship Initiative (NCSI) [8] which highlighted key shifts in attitude towards care.

The current method of follow-up involved focusing on cancer as an acute disease, with monitoring for recurrence, and no focus on the physical, social, emotional or psychological impact of being a Cancer Survivor. However, there is some debate as to the efficacy of this [7].

*Corresponding author: Sanchia S Goonewardene, MBChB BmedSc (Hons) PGCGC Dip, SSC MRCS (Ed) MRCS (Eng) Guys Hospital, Kings College London, UK, E-mail: sanchi7727@gmail.com

Prostate Cancer recurrence can be followed up via PSA, without the actual need to come to clinic. Together with an older population, we have to start formulating pathways to get around this issue in an increasingly financially stricken NHS.

Current Systematic Reviews

Current systematic reviews on prostate cancer survivorship cover a range of topics.

These include symptoms include physical limitations, cognitive limitations, depression/anxiety, sleep problems, fatigue, pain, and sexual dysfunction [9]. This demonstrated cancer survivors can experience symptoms for more than 10 years following treatment. This also highlighted a need for evaluated and managed to optimize long-term outcomes. Another review has highlighted patient requirement for an active part in their healthcare during the survivorship phase [10]. The challenge is in integrating lifestyle support into standardised models of aftercare. EAU guidelines [11] do highlight the need for PSA follow-up in this cohort of patients.

Exercise was found to produce many beneficial effects in the cancer population including improvements in physical function, quality of life, body weight, fatigue levels, and psychological. This improved quality of life; decreased levels of anxiety, fatigue, and depression; and increased levels of functional capacity. Another review indicates exercise interventions are safe, resulting in improvements in physical fitness, QoL, fatigue, and psychosocial outcomes. Positive effects of exercise interventions are more pronounced with moderate- or vigorous exercise. Physical activity guidelines for cancer survivors suggest that physical activity should be an integral and continuous part of care for all cancer survivors [12]. This highlighted future studies should focus on identifying clinical, personal, physical, psychosocial, and intervention. More insight into the working mechanisms of exercise interventions on health outcomes in cancer survivors is needed to improve the efficacy and efficiency of interventions. The challenge, therefore, is in integrating lifestyle support into standardised models of aftercare for cancer survivors [10]. In addition, there is one Cochrane review on this topic, highlighting the importance of interventions to promote exercise including programme goals, prompting practise and self-monitoring and encouraging participants to attempt to generalise behaviours learned in supervised exercise environments. In this case, exercise prescriptions should be designed around individuals.

Diet and wellbeing is also important region for intervention in the survivorship cohort [13]. Exercise and diet interventions can be used to improve health and wellbeing of cancer survivors to develop maximally effective interventions as specified in that review.

Reviews also examined communication between families. Couples, regardless of gender, who are survivors of prostate cancer face a number of challenges and opportunities that impact their health, QOL, communication, and overall relationship satisfaction [14]. In addition, reviews have also highlighted self-management as a method of providing health-care solutions to ameliorate men's functional and emotional problems [15]. However, at the same time satisfied patients, patients with fulfilled information needs, and patients who experience less information barriers, in general have a better HRQoL and lower levels of depression and anxiety [16]. Other reviews have highlighted quality of life tools are lacking [17]. The role of the Nurse practitioner/ specialist nurse also has a strong impact on cancer survivorship care by serving in various roles and settings throughout the cancer trajectory to improve patient outcomes [18]. Reviews have also been conducted

into prostate cancer support-groups: pen-ended, psychoeducational groups with large meetings, expert speakers, and structured, efficient organizations appear most beneficial [19].

Method

A systematic review was conducted. The search strategy (Figure 1) aimed to identify all references related to prostate cancer, survivorship, specific categories and treatment outcomes. (Prostate cancer or prostate neoplasms) and (survivorship or survivor) or (support care or diet therapy or exercise or communication) and (post therapy OR post treatment). Our selection criteria specified papers must be related to Prostate Cancer and Survivorship. The following databases were screened from 1984 to December 2013: CINAHL and MEDLINE (NHS Evidence), Cochrane, AMed, BNI, EMBASE, Health Business Elite, HMIC, PschINFO. In addition, searches using Medical Subject Headings (MeSH) and keywords were conducted using Cochrane databases. Primary research only was included in the the systematic review. Two UK-based experts were consulted in Survivorship care to identify additional studies.

Eligibility

Studies were eligible for inclusion if they reported primary research focusing on prostate cancer survivorship related to nutrition, psychology, physical therapy, treatment outcomes and communication and treatment outcomes. Papers were included if published after 1984 and had to be in English. Studies that did not conform with this were excluded (Figure 1).

Selection criteria

Abstracts were independently screened for eligibility by two reviewers and disagreements resolved through discussion or third opinion. Agreement level was calculated using Cohen's Kappa to test the intercoder reliability of this screening process. The PRISMA flow diagram demonstrates the results of the screening and selection process [ref]. According to criteria 76 papers were identified.

Data Extraction and Quality Assessment of Studies

Data extraction was piloted by SSG and amended in consultation

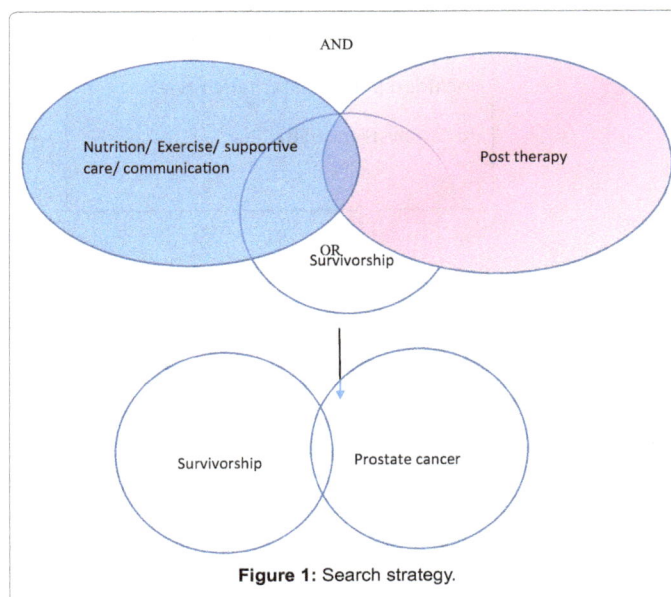

Figure 1: Search strategy.

with the research team. Data extraction included authors, year and country of publication, study aims, setting, intervention aims, number of participants, study methods, intervention components and delivery methods, comparison groups and outcome measures, notes and follow-up questions for the authors. Included studies were quality assessed using for experimental studies, (Popay). for the action research and qualitative studies and the Critical Appraisal Skills Programme for retrospective studies. Individual quality assessment tools enabled us to focus on the specific study designs appropriately.

Results

Flow chart (adapted from Moher PRISMA) of studies related to Prostate cancer survivorship, holistic care, quality of life and follow-up is shown in Figure 2. The searches identified 2495 papers (Figure 2). However, only 76 mapped to search terms. 599 were excluded due to not being applicable to the topic. 1761 were duplicates. Of the 76 papers left, relevant abstracts were identified and the full paper obtained, all of which were in English. There was considerable heterogeneity (numbers/ method, expand) among the included studies therefore a narrative synthesis of the evidence was undertaken. Studies demonstrated a number of problems associated with prostate cancer survivorship care, they did not propose solutions to resolve the issues. What was also demonstrated was significant fracturing of prostate

cancer survivorship care, which was cost inefficient and not properly addressing survivors' needs (Table 1).

UK Studies

Out of 76 papers, there were only 9 UK studies, indicating how far behind in prostate cancer survivorship care we are. However, the ones that were present in this systematic review highlight a number of requirements within survivorship care.

Faithfull [15] examined 22 participants as part of a quasi-experimental: feasibility study with 7 weeks of group and individual sessions. Outcomes were analysed via questionnaire based on urinary symptoms were measured before the intervention and again after 4 months of follow-up through International Prostate Symptom Scores This was conducted by researchers, This pilot study provides data suggesting that a narrowly targeted, cognitive and behavioural self-management intervention can improve LUTS in men who have had radiotherapy treatment for prostate cancer (Moher 'B' quality). This emphasises the importance of contact with secondary care in the survivorship phase [18]. Conducted a descriptive controlled analysis with over 18000 survivors vs controls, examining analysis of consultation rates/ 6 years. Prostate cancer requires 3x more consultations than controls. (Moher 'B' quality). This again emphasises the same point.

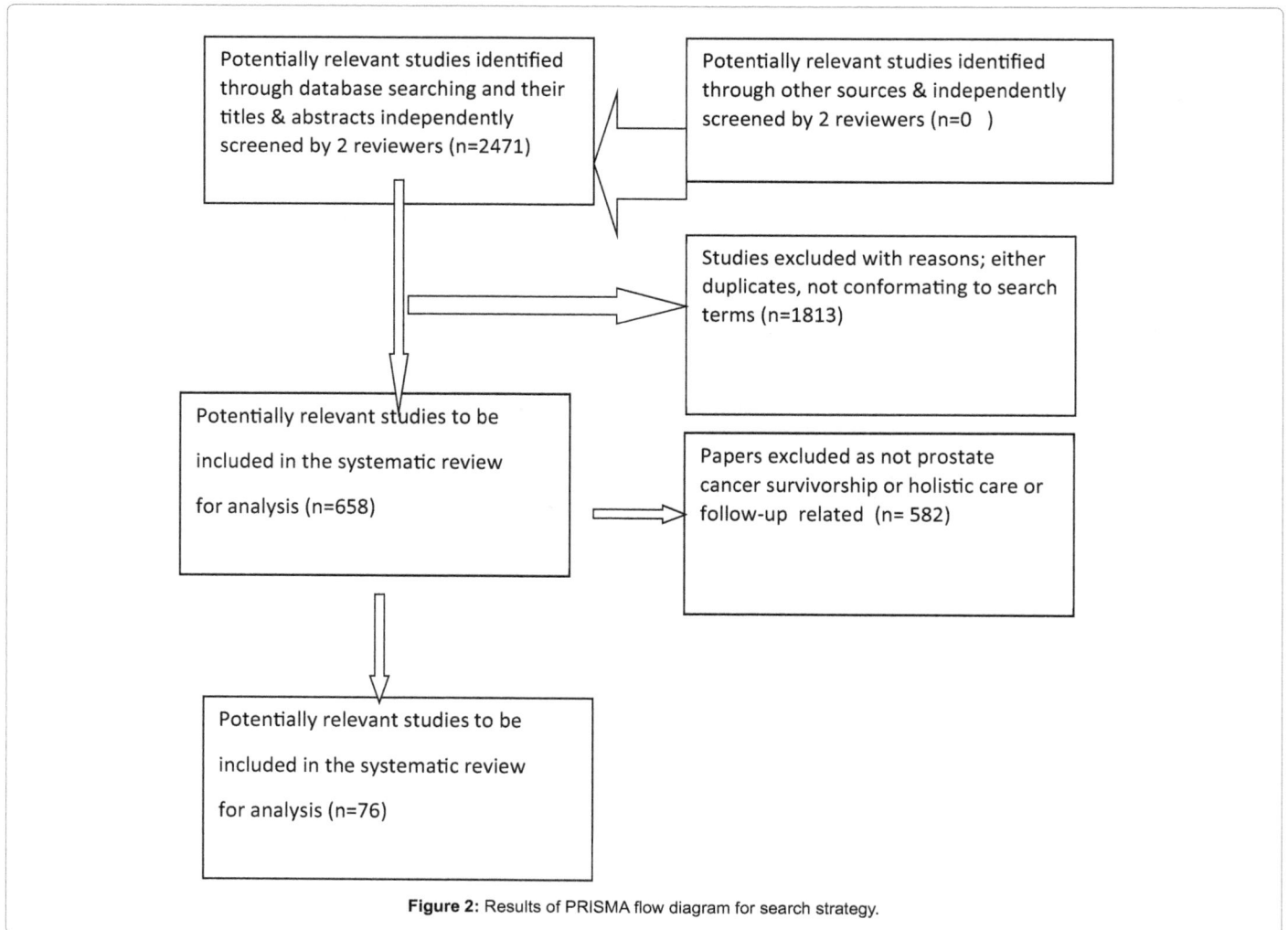

Figure 2: Results of PRISMA flow diagram for search strategy.

Type of study design	Papers
Randomised controlled trials	(Demark-Wahnefried, W) [36], (Synder DC) [13]. (Miller) [25], (Synder DC) [13].
Randomised trial:	Perkins H., 2009
Cross-sectional studies:	(Kent et al.) [32]. (Mols et al.) [16]. (Skolarus et al.) [39], (Del-Giudice et al.) [38]. (Miller et al.) [25]. (Schaefer et al.) [28]. (Taskilaa et al.) [27]. (Lindbohn et al.) [27]
Cross sectional case control	(Miller et al.) [25]
Control- cross over study	(Demark-Wahnefried et al.) [36]
Case- control study	(Mols et al.) [16]. (Synder et al.) [13]. (Skolarus et al.) [39].
Cohort Study	(Sheriff et al.) [37].
Quasi Experimental study	(Faithfull et al.) [15].
Experimental	Badger et al. [29].
Feasibility study	(Campbell et al.) [24], (Skolarus et al.) [39].
Descriptive study	(Skolarus et al.) [39], (Takisila et al.) [27].
Longitudinal study	(Taylor-Ford et al.) [31], (Skolarus et al.) [39]
Qualitative studies	(Grunfield et al.) [39] (Faithfull et al.) [15]
Descriptive controlled study	(Synder et al.) [34], (Del Giudice et al.) [38], (Grov) [30]

Table 1: Characteristics of studies.

Country	Study
USA	Synder et al. [34] Segrin et al. [29], Campbell et al. [24] DEimling et al. [28] Badger et al. [29] Grov et al. [30] Platek et al., Demark-Wahnefried et al. [36] Kent et al. [32] Synder et al. [13]. Sheriff et al. [37]. Skolarus et al. [39]. Synder et al. [13]. Badger et al. [29]. Miller et al. [25], Miller et al. [25]
UK	Faithfull et al. [15] Goonewardene SS [21] Goonewardene SS [22]
Norway	Grov et al. [30] Takisila et al. [27] Linbohn [27]
Netherlands	Mols et al. [16]
Finland	Takiskila et al. [27]
Australia	Zucca et al. [26], Lynch et al. [35]
Sweden	Taylor-Ford et al. [31]
Canada	Del Giudice et al. [38]

Table 2: Country of origin.

Ashley [20]. Conducted a feasibility study with 886 prostate cancer survivors, over 15 months. Questionnaire based analysis focused on generic, cancer-specific and cancer diagnosis-specific outcome measures. This was conducted by researchers who demonstrated a computer based system, with the potential to provide an affordable UK-scalable technical platform to facilitate and support longitudinal cohort research, and improve understanding of cancer survivors (Moher 'B' quality).

Elliott J, conducted a cross-sectional study with 780 prostate cancer survivors, using a National Health interview survey used to measure outcomes, in terms of health needs. This demonstrated Cancer survivors have ongoing health needs that are not currently being addressed (Moher 'A' quality study).

Harrington [9]. Conducted a cross sectional questionnaire survey on discharge status, provision of time/ information prior to discharge, feelings at discharge and satisfaction with how discharge was managed. They demonstrated discharge of patients from hospital -requires additional time, support and information, again emphasising the extra support needed for this cohort.

Goonewardene [21] 178 Qualitative 1 year Improvement

A quality Goonewardene [21] 178 Quantifiable improvement Qualitative

A quality Goonewardene [22] 500 patients, 20 GPS Cross sectional qualitative study Questionnaire based, GP views on Survivorship programme, to give further support to GPS to manage A quality (Table 2).

The systematic review required narrative analysis. Study designs varied and were conducted by a range of members from the multidisciplinary team including specialist nurses, doctors and in addition, researchers. Number of participants: 258139 patients and 330 primary care physicians.

These papers within this systematic review examine the following topics:

- Cognitive interventions: (Segrin et al.) [23], (Campbell, et al.) [24], (Badger et al.) [23].

- Cancer-related symptoms: (Cherrier), (Van Dis), (Badger et al.) [23], (Miller et al.) [25]

- Work (Zucca et al.) [26], (Gilbert et al.) [25].

- Familial impact (Taskilaa et al.) [27]

- Psychological distress (DEimling et al.) [28]. physical and mental health, Depression and anxiety, psychological QOL in PCSs (Badger et al.) [29] Psychometric analysis

- Patient satisfaction (Grov et al.) [30].

- Cognitive and behavioural self-management for symptoms (Faithfull et al.)[15], problem-focused and support-seeking strategies

- Body image (Taylor-Ford et al.) [31].

- Unmet information needs (Kent et al.) [32].

- Physical activity (Livingston et al.) (LaStayo, et al.) [33] (Blanchard et al.) (Synder et al.) [34] (Lynch et al.) [35].

- Lifestyle interventions (Synder, Demark- Wahnefried et al.) [36] (Sheriff et al.) [37].

- Ongoing health needs (Elliott et al.) [1] healthcare input (Mols et al.) [16] increased primary health care use (Heins) [16], (Rodgers et al.), (Khan et al.), (SAbatino et al.), (Del Giudice et al.) [38] GP input (Goonewardene et al.) [22].

- Comorbid conditions (Aarts et al.), (Skolarus et al.) [39] (Khan et al.), (Lafata et al.).

- Discharge of patients from hospital (Harrison et al.).

- Survivorship Issues (Baker et al.).

- Fragmented prostate cancer survivorship care and cost (Skolarus et al.) [39].

- Multi-speciality working (Weaver et al.).

- Suboptimal health behaviors (Mosher et al.).

- Patient expectations (Nesse et al.)

- Survivorship care (Goonewardene et al.) [21].

- Impact of cancer (Foley et al.).

- Qol (Mols et al.), (Van Dis et al.), (Blanchard et al.), (Lemasters et al.).

- Patients empowerment (Litwin et al.).

- Return to normal health (Schag et al.).

- Survivorship measures (AVIS et al.).

- Sexual HRQOL, Sexual counselling (Miller et al.) [25].

- Cancer survivorship research (Carmen).

Risk of Bias

13 studies were of 'C' quality, 27 were of 'A' quality, 36were of 'B' quality using the criteria of Moher. All studies described withdrawal and dropout rates, including follow-up methodologies, and presented the interventions' outcome results. Blinding was not applicable in any trial. The flow of participants was represented in a consort style diagram in 20 studies. Allocation concealments of participants were not appropriate and the methods used for each study were. Greater than 80% of participants did provide follow-up data of interest, and outcomes were clearly defined. Only 3 studies had sample size calculated. An adequate summary of results for each outcome was provided, including for non-significant results. Sample results were explicitly defined, as was the method of recruitment and intervention.

Development and Types of Interventions, Components and Delivering of Interventions

All studies were complex interventions composed of components acting independently and/ or interdependently. Interventions were as follows, below.

- 6 weeks of telephone based cognitive therapy, coping skills training vs. normal care, Campbell, L.C [24].

- 7 weeks of group and individual sessions. Outcomes analysed via questionnaire based on Urinary symptoms were measured before the intervention and again after 4 months of follow-up through International Prostate Symptom Scores (IPSS), Faithfull [15].

- Telephone counselling and personalised work book, Kent E.E [32].

- Thrice weekly exercise stepping, Outcomes, muscles measurements and mechanical force, Synder [36].

- Physical acivity measured via accelerometer data and waist circumference over 1 week, Lynch [35].

- Telephone analysis: The 7-Day Physical Activity Recall and the Diet History Questionnaire, quality of life; risk for depression; social support; comorbidity; perceived health; self-efficacy for exercising, Demark-Wahnefried [36].

- National Health interview survey used to measure outcomes, Elliott [1].

- Intervention: work book and telephone counselling over 12 month s Assessment over telephone with dietary recall, Synder [36].

- Personalised mail intervention, telephone surveys to assess dietary habits at 1 and 2 years, (Christy et al.).

- Intervention: workbook and unit materials, telephone survey, Demark-Wahenfried [36].

- Point analysis, phone interview, on educational materials and, (Nesse et al.).

- Goonewardene [21].

- Randomised to received tailored vs none tailored diet and exercise intervention. Analysis on Qol via physical activity recall, Ottenbacher.

One study used a telephone delivered quality of life instrument questionnaire [39]. One used focus groups to explore patient experience and benefit of exercise therapy [18]. Mail survey was also used to gain physicians' opinions of routine follow-up. Only study used financial incentives [38]. Study periods varied from cross sectional to three days to analysis over years [39]. All studies had no follow up beyond the specified study period. There were a range of settings used for studies including secondary care, primary care [38] both primary and secondary care university research.

Outcomes measures ranges from sexual and urinary tract functioning to QoL experiences, short and long term preventative outcomes associated with prostate cancer and examination of primary care physicians views on survivorship [38].

Discussion of papers

Impact on Community based Survivorship Care

This systematic review clearly highlights the large areas of Survivorship Care that are currently being unaddressed (Figure 3).

What patients want

Survivors report few cancer-related symptoms and high QoL [26]. However some had deteriorated work abilities due to cancer with more problems post therapy [27]. Telephone based interventions are a feasible approach that can successfully enhance coping [24].

Psychological impairment

Many have psychological distress due to cancer and its treatment. These are strongest predictors of depression and can persist with symptom control [28]. Tailored interventions are appropriate and should be considered in these cases. Further research is however required [29].

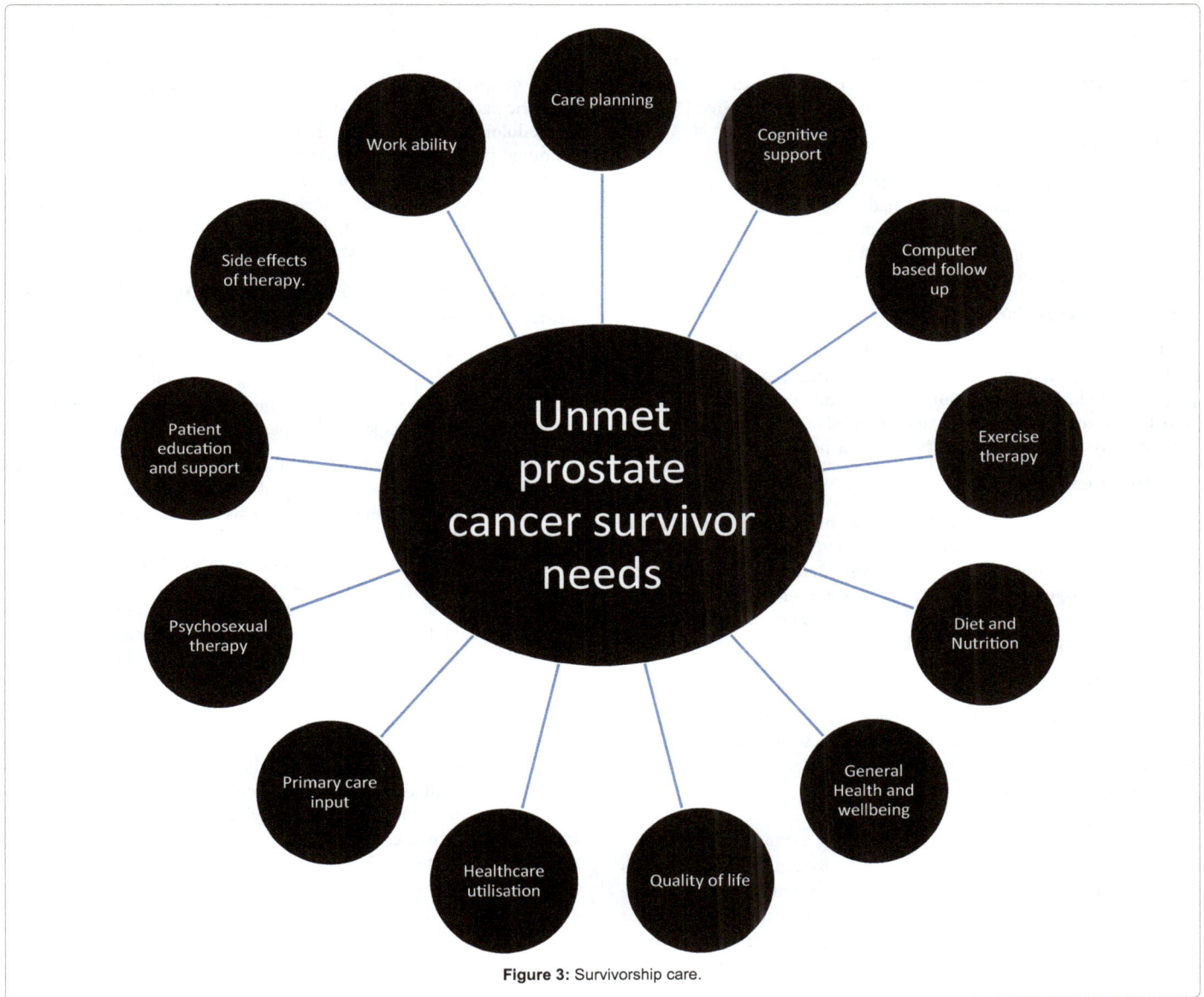

Figure 3: Survivorship care.

Healthcare utilisation

Survivors demonstrate a higher rate of decreased self-rated health, more physical impairment and thyroid diseases, daily use of medication and psychotropics and higher level of anxiety [30]. Increased primary health care use is the result, more significant in younger patients. There is a high prevalence of suboptimal health behaviors among older, long-term survivors with appropriate information and support in place, PCPs reported being willing to assume responsibility for the follow-up care of adult cancer survivors [38]. Cardiovascular disease risk factors are common, yet not discussed with relevant healthcare teams. This highlights more inter-speciality working is required. Due to the increased demands, changes in health care, more efficiency, are required to manage increasing demand [16]. The number of physician visits, particularly primary care input, are important factors associated with successful survivorship care [34]. With appropriate information and support in place, multispeciality working together with primary care can manage this cohort.

Cormorbid conditions and side effects of treatment

Suvivors suffer sexual, urinary, and bowel dysfunction. Another issues which together with erectile dysfunction, could be addressed by adequate Survivorship care. [25].

Social support

This is increasingly important to the prostate cancer survivor and there carer. As a result any programme which is set up, must also be made accessible to the carer/ relative of the survivors [23]. Direct associations are present between perceived support and the use of problem-focused and support-seeking strategies, whereas inverse associations emerged with self-blame, wishful thinking, and avoidance [40]. Healthcare professionals must aim to promote the former.

Exercise therapy

Exercise interventions have been shown to improve health related quality of life. There are also clear long term health benefits of participating in physical activity programs. Older cancer survivors represent a vulnerable population who we must target and for alteration of health behaviours. This can be a hard-to-reach population [34]. Increasing moderate-to-vigorous activity may assist this population with weight management, however more research is required [35].

Health related Qol

Most long-term survivors retrospectively report that cancer either positively influenced their lives or had little long-term impact [41]. Those who express Resentment report that pain, physical deformities, and social isolation significantly reduced their long-term HRQL. This is significant, as it highlights a cohort we need to target.

Lifestyle interventions

Home-based diet and exercise interventions hold promise in improving lifestyle behaviors. However, further research is required [36] even in older survivors [36]. That diet and other lifestyle practices were important predictors of patient QOL [37]. As a cohort, we need to focus on physical, functional and social well-being. [1].

Post treatment care

Despite high levels of satisfaction, discharge of cancer survivors from hospital follow-up could be improved with the provision of additional time, information and support. Better structuring of the final hospital appointment or a review appointment in primary care at this time could help to ensure that discharge from hospital follow-up is managed optimally for cancer survivors. [29].

Psychosexual

Only 43% of men said their partners had encouraged them to find help. This highlights an area of survivorship care which is not properly addressed. This must be corrected to improve sexual rehabilitation in this cohort post therapy.

Cost effectiveness

None of the studies address cost effectiveness of interventions directly, however one [39] does. This study examined that telephone follow-up is a feasible strategy for or assessing prostate cancer survivor QOL and could provide a low cost, sustainable, and systematic approach to measuring patient-centred outcomes, conducting comparative effectiveness research, and monitoring the quality of prostate cancer care [39].

Statement of main findings

Our review found a small number of papers of similar research design. All studies reported positive survivorship outcomes or gave further evidence for a way forward. This demonstrates how well adapted the interventions were structured, coupled with the fact that key points were investigated leading to good care. The studies were of moderate quality in relation to the characteristics of their particular design.

Prostate cancer survivors were the focus of these interventions research in all studies. This is a very sizable group, not just in the UK but through the world.

Strengths and limitations

The search criteria of this review included prostate cancer and survivorship. Interventions of any research design (from a wide range of sources including experts) were assessed and included using the novel survivorship care assessment tool to ensure the inclusion of all relevant interventions previously undertaken in the area. Therefore, this design was robust because previous systematic reviews have limited their search to specific survivorship topics, not looking at survivorship as a holistic package of care. The included studies were assessed for both methodological quality and strength of survivorship care. The review is limited by the different methodological studies. It was a relatively heterogeneous population, indicating the conclusions published are valid. In addition, as only published studies were included, some relevant ongoing studies may have been excluded. The definitions of 'Survivor' have been signposted in this review.

Findings in Relation to Other Survivorship Studies and Trends, Literature

Concerns regarding permanent physical, psychosocial, and economic effects of cancer treatment were highlighted by the US Institute of Medicine Report [6]. These include impact on life for example, financial, occupational or performance concerns.

The Institute of Medicine produced a report on the focus of survivorship care plans including the chronic effects of cancer, monitoring for and preventing late effects e.g. malignancies, and promoting healthy lifestyles. There is a lack of evidence in this field, with regard to patient follow up and whether it should be led by primary or secondary care, and also a lack of follow up into a patients' wellbeing and quality of life. Survivorship care plans are recommended as an important tool to facilitate communication and allocation of responsibility as part of this. Self -management is part of this, with patient driven assessment of outcomes (National Cancer Intelligence Network) [5].

A survey conducted by Macmillan of 1001 survivors demonstrated current services were falling short of their needs [42]. 94% said they would expect a full assessment of their on-going needs; 92% said they would expect to discuss potential side effects of treatment; 89% would expect a personalised care plan to support them after therapy. There is also a suggestion that 70% of patients living with and beyond cancer could self-manage their symptoms.

The unmet needs of cancer survivors, the rising numbers, and pressures to utilise resources efficiently [7] are a significant burden on the health system. These issues have been raised by the National Cancer Survivorship Initiative (NCSI) (Giarelli) [8].Which highlighted key shifts in attitude towards care. The focus is now more on recovery and return to work. This includes personalised approach to individual risk assessment and patient self-management.

This is supported by research conducted by the Picker Institute, an independent nonprofit organization dedicated to advancing the principles of patient-centered care. Their research demonstrated 43% of respondents would have liked more information and advice, 75% did not hae or did not know if they had, a care plan. 75% reported not knowing who to contact for advice outside of office hours. Further results from mapping exercises conducted by NCIS include psychological, physical and occupational problems, with a lack of information [7].

The patient consensus meeting concluded patients are not averse to new approaches to follow-up care and support. However they need to have access to good quality information and rapid access to specialist treatment -should they need it.

An important pre-requisite for survivorship care, is a good insight into the patients' needs and preferences. Providing cancer patients with information about their disease and treatment helps them to make decisions about treatment. In addition they are able to overcome fear, develop realistic expectations, manage side effects and comply with treatment. Individualised information sessions have been associated with lower anxiety, better psychological well-being and higher treatment satisfaction [43]. Continuity and coordination of care is difficult, with many patients unclear about who is responsible for their ongoing survivorship care [38]. However, to date, there has been little consensus on the value and organisation of follow-up.

One area which is infrequently addressed is that of sexual dysfunction. This affects many prostate cancer survivors. The incidence of varies between 20% and 88%. Changes in body image, pain, and loss of desire, long-term physical and psychological side effects from cancer treatments can affect sexual functioning.

Other Follow-ups Programmes

There is a lack of evidence in this field, with regard to patient follow up and whether it should be led by primary or secondary care, and also a lack of follow up into a patients' wellbeing and quality of life. The current method of follow-up involved focusing on cancer as an acute disease, with monitoring for recurrence, and no focus on the physical, social, emotional or psychological impact of being a Cancer Survivor. However, there is some debate as to the efficacy of this [7].

The associated clinical improvement section ran pilot models of improved care and support for survivors [7]. As a result of this, five key phases to survivorship care were identified: care via primary treatment from diagnosis, enable as rapid and full a recovery as possible, ensure recovery is sustained, manage side effects of treatment, monitor for recurrence or disease progression.

This has been taken one step further by the Queensland government, who have developed a framework allowing patients to make and participate in decisions, build and sustain partnerships, possess the capacity to manage the impact of their health in functioning, emotions and interpersonal relationships and monitor and manage symptoms and signs of recurrence.

Interventions based on rehabilitation and self-management requires further research is required.

Conclusion and Recommendations for Future

This systematic review has defined landmarks for survivorship care: monitoring for recurrence, metastases or side effects and coordination between secondary and primary care. This has also demonstrated a requirement for further holistic support for patients in the survivorship cohort, which is not being addressed. In addition patients with psychological, emotional, social and financial concerns as well as sexual health concerns were also highlighted as not having their problems addressed leading to poorer quality of life. Since writing this systematic review, based on SSGs recommendation, Prostate Cancer Survivorship and Supportive Care has been added as a section to the EAU congress. This is the way forward.

References

1. Maddams J, Brewster D, Gavin A, Steward J, Elliott J, et al. (2009) 101: 541-547.

2. Improving Outcomes in Cancer (2011) Department of Health Publication.

3. Ganz PA (2009) Survivorship adult cancer survivors.Prim Care 36: 721-41.

4. Centers for Disease Control and Prevention. Cancer survivorship—United States (2004) MMWR Surveill Summ 53: 526-529.

5. National Cancer Intelligence Network UK (2008) Lifetime prevalence for all cancers and colorectal, lung, breast and prostate cancers.

6. Hewitt M, Greenfield W (2006) From Cancer Patient to Cancer Survivor. In: Stovall E (eds.) The National Academies Press, Washington.

7. National Cancer Survivorship Initiative (2008).

8. Giarelli E (2004) A model of survivorship in cancer genetic care. Semin Oncol Nurs 20: 196-202.

9. Harrington C, Hansen J, Moskowitz MT, Feuerstein BL, Michael L (2010) It's not over when it's over: Long-term symptoms in cancer survivors: A systematic review. International Journal of Psychiatry in Medicine 40: 163-181.

10. DaviesBedford Hospital, BatehupSupport L, Addenbrooke's Programme (2011) The role of diet and physical activity in breast, colorectal and prostate cancer survivorship. a review of the literature British Journal of Cancer 105: 52-73.

11. Mottet N, Bellmunt J, Bolla M, Joniau S, Mason M, et al. (2011) EAU guidelines on prostate cancer. Part II: Treatment of advanced, relapsing, and castration-resistant prostate cancer. Eur Urol 59: 572-583.

12. Buffart LM, Galvão DA, Brug J, Chinapaw MJM, Newton RU (2014) Evidence-based physical activity guidelines for cancer survivors: Current guidelines, knowledge gaps and future research directions Cancer Treatment Reviews 40: 327-340.

13. Snyder DC, Morey Miriam C, Sloane R, Stull V, Cohen HJ, et al. (2009) Reach out to Enhance Wellness in Older Cancer Survivors (RENEW).design, methods and recruitment challenges of a home-based exercise and diet intervention to improve physical function among long-term survivors of breast, prostate, and colorectal cancer. Psycho-Oncology 18: 405-411.

14. Michael E, Galbraith, Regina Fink, Wilkins Gayle G, Couples Surviving Prostate Cancer. Challenges In Their Lives And Relationships Seminars in Oncology Nursing 27: 300-308.

15. Jane Cockle-Hearne, Sara Faithfull (2010) Self-management for men surviving prostate cancer. a review of behavioural and psychosocial interventions to understand what strategies can work,for whom and in what circumstances Psycho-Oncology 19: 909-922.

16. Husson O, Mols F, Van de Poll-Franse LV (2011) The relation between information provision and healthrelated quality of life, anxiety and depression among cancer survivors: a systematic review Annals of Oncology 22: 761-772.

17. Barbara Muzzatti , Antonietta Annunziata M (2013) Assessing quality of life in long-term cancer survivors: a review of available tools Supportive care in cancer 21: 3142-3152.

18. Martin E, Bulsara C, Naumann F, Magrani Do Rosario P, Smith C, et al.(2014) What men and women want: The experiences of men and women in a group exercise counselling cancer recovery programme. Journal of Science and Medicine in Sport 14: 117-118.

19. Lyn Thaxton, Emshoff James G, Omar Guessous MA (2005) Prostate Cancer Support Groups.Journal of Psychosocial Oncology 23: 25-40.

20. Jacobs LA, Vaughn DJ, Cotton D, Taichman D, Williams S (2013) In the clinic care of the adult cancer survivor. Annals of Internal Medicine 158: 6-16.

21. Goonewardene SS, Symons M, McCormack G, Makar A (2012) The Worcestershire Prostate Cancer Survivorship Programme:a new concept for long term support and follow-up. Journal of American College of Surgeons 215: 143.

22. Goonewardene SS, Young A, Symons M, Sullivan A, McCormack, et al. (2013) The prostate cancer survivorship program: A new concept for holistic long-term support and follow-up. Journal of Clinical Oncology 30 (5 SUPPL. 1).

23. Chris Segrin, Terry A (2010) Badger Psychological Distress in Different Social Network Members of Breast and Prostate Cancer Survivors. Researchin Nursing & Health 33: 450-464

24. Campbell Lisa C, Keefe Francis J, Cindy Scipio BA, McKee Daphne C, et al. (2007) Facilitating Research Participation and Improving Quality of Life for African American Prostate Cancer Survivors and Their Intimate Partners A Pilot Study of Telephone-Based Coping Skills Training CANCER Supplement 109: 2.

25. Gilbert SM, Miller DC, Hollenbeck BK, Montie JE, Wei JT (2008) Cancer

survivorship.Challenges and changing paradigms. Journal of Urology 179: 431-438.

26. Zucca Alison C, Allison W (2012) Quality of Life and Physical Symptom Clusters in Long-Term Cancer Survivors Across Cancer Types Journal of Pain and Symptom Management 43: 720-732.

27. Taina Taskilaa, Rami Martikainenb, Pa¨ivi Hietanenc, Marja-Liisa Lindbohma (2007) Comparative study of work ability between cancer survivors and their referents.European journal of cancer 43: 914-920.

28. Deimlinga Gary T, Boaz Kahanab, Bowmanc Karen F, Schaefer Michael L (2002) Cancer Survivorship And Psychological Distress In Later Life Psycho-Oncology 11: 479-494.

29. Badger Terry A, Chris Segrin, Figueredo Aurelio J, Joanne Harrington, Kate Sheppard, et al. (2013) Who benefits from a psychosocial counselling versus educational intervention to improve psychological quality of life in prostate cancer survivors.Psychology & Health 28: 336-354.

30. Grov Ellen K, Fossål Sophie D, Dahl Alv A Morbidity, life style and psychosocial situation in cancer survivors aged 60-69 years: results from The Nord-Trøndelag Health Study (The HUNT-II Study)

31. Megan Taylor-Ford, Meyerowitz Beth E, D'Orazio Lina M, Christie Kysa M, et al. (2013) Body image predicts quality of life in men with prostate cancer. Psycho-Oncology 22: 756-761.

32. Kent Erin E, Neeraj K, Arora C, Julia H, Rowland B, et al. (2012) Health information needs and health-related quality of life in a diverse population of long-term cancer survivors. Patient Education and Counseling 89: 345-352.

33. LaStayo Paul C, Marcus V, Dibble Lee E, Smith Sheldon B, Beck Susan L, et al. (2009) Psycho-Oncology 18: 429-439.

34. Snyder CF, Frick KD, Herbert RJ, Blackford AL, Neville BA, et al. (2011) Preventive care in prostate cancer patients: following diagnosis and for five-year survivors. Journal of Cancer Survivorship 5: 283-91.

35. Lynch BM, Dunstan DW, Winkler E, Healy GN, Eakin E, et al. (2011) Objectively assessed physical activity, sedentary time and waist circumference among prostate cancer survivors: findings from the National Health and Nutrition Examination Survey. European Journal of Cancer Care 20: 514-519.

36. Demark-Wahnefried W, Morey Miriam C, Clipp Elizabeth C, Pieper Carl F, Snyder DC, et al. (2003) Leading the Way in Exercise and Diet: intervening to improve function among older breast and prostate cancer survivors.Controlled Clinical Trials 24: 206-223.

37. Sheriff Sara K, Shohara Ryo A, Dumican Sarah B, Small Eric J, Carroll Peter R, et al. (2005) Lifestyle Correlates of Health Perception and Treatment Satisfaction in a Clinical Cohort of Men with Prostate Cancer. Clinical Prostate Cancer 3: 239-245.

38. Del Giudice ME, Grunfield E, Harvey B J, Piliotis E, Verma S (2009) Primary Care Physicians views of routine follow-up of cancer survivors 20: 3338-3345.

39. Skolarus TA, Holmes-Rovner M, Hawley ST, Dunn RL, Barr KL, et al. (2012) Monitoring quality of life among prostate cancer survivors: The feasibility of automated telephone assessment. Urology 80: 1021-1026.

40. Ptacek JT, Pierce Gregory R, Ptacek John J (2002) The Social Context of Coping with Prostate Cancer, Journal of Psychosocial Oncology 20: 61-80.

41. Saad F, Finelli A, Dranitsaris G, Goldenberg L, Bagnell S (2006) Canadian surgical wait times (SWAT) initiative. Can J Urol 13: 16-24.

42. Productivity and Prevention National Cancer Institute (2012) The Quality, Innovation NCCS Charter.

43. Hummel S, Simpson EL, Hemingway P, Stevenson MD, Rees A (2010) Intensity-modulated radiotherapy for the treatment of prostate cancer: a systematic review and economic evaluation. Health Technol Assess 14: 1-108.

21

Quality of Life among Persons Aged 60-84 Years in Europe: The Role of Psychological Abuse and Socio-Demographic, Social and Health Factors

Joaquim JF Soares[1]*, Örjan Sundin[2], Eija Viitasara[1], Maria Gabriella Melchiorre[3], Mindaugas Stankunas[4,5], Jutta Lindert[6], Francisco Torres-Gonzales[7], Henrique Barros[8] and Elisabeth Ioannidi-Kapolou[9]

[1]Department of Public Health Sciences, Mid Sweden University, Sundsvall, Sweden
[2]Department of Psychology, Mid Sweden University, Östersund, Sweden
[3]Italian National Institute of Health and Science on Aging, INRCA, Ancona, Italy
[4]Department of Health Management, Lithuanian University of Health Sciences, Kaunas, Lithuania
[5]School of Public Health, Griffith University, Gold Coast Campus, Queensland, Australia
[6]Department of Public Health Science, Protestant University of Applied Sciences, Ludwigsburg, Germany
[7]Network of Biomedical Research on Mental Health Centers, University of Granada, Spain
[8]Department of Hygiene and Epidemiology, University of Porto, Medical School, Porto, Portugal
[9]Department of Sociology, National School of Public Health, Athens, Greece

Abstract

Background: Elder abuse and its effects are a serious public health issue. However, little is known about the relation between psychological abuse, other factors (e.g. social support) and quality of life (QoL) by domain. This study addressed differences in QoL by domain between psychologically abused and non-abused. While considering other factors such as social support.

Methods: The respondents were 4,467 (2,559 women) randomly selected persons aged 60-84 years living in 7 European cities. The mean response across countries was 45.2%. The cross-sectional data were analyzed with bivariate/multivariate methods.

Results: Abused respondents contrasted to non-abused scored lower in QoL (autonomy, 67.42 ± 21.26 vs. 72.39 ± 19.58; intimacy, 55.31 ± 31.15 vs. 67.21 ± 28.55; past/present/future activities, 62.79 ± 19.62 vs. 68.05 ± 18.09; social participation, 65.03 ± 19.84 vs. 68.21 ± 19.77). Regressions showed that abuse was negatively associated with autonomy, intimacy and past/present/future activities, and positively with the social participation. All QoL dimensions were negatively associated with country and depressive/anxiety symptoms, and positively with social support. Further, variables such as age, sex and somatic symptoms were negatively associated with some of the QoL dimensions and others such as family structure, education, health care use and drinking positively. The regression model "explained" 32.8% of the variation in autonomy, 45.6% in intimacy, 44.8% in past/present/future activities and 41.5% in social participation.

Conclusions: Abuse was linked to lower QoL in most domains, but other factors such as depressive symptoms also carried a negative impact. Social support and to some extent family structure had a "protective" effect on QoL. Abuse, health indicators (e.g. depressive symptoms) and social support should be considered in addressing the QoL of older persons. However, QoL was influenced by many factors, which could not be firmly disentangled due to the cross-sectional approach, calling for longitudinal research to address causality.

Keywords: Older persons; Psychological abuse; QoL; Demographics/socio-economics; Mental health; Social support; Europe

Background

Elder abuse is acknowledged as a public health problem and generates increasing concern specially as current projections indicate that persons aged 60-plus will increase from 760 million 2011 to 2 billion by 2050 [1-3]. Prevalence rates of elder abuse vary contingent on various factors such as operational definition of abuse and type of sample. For instance, a review of 49 studies reported a mean elder abuse rate of 13%, and rates in the general population varied between 3.2-27.5% and over 6% had been abused during the last month [4]. Recent studies in the USA, Israel and Europe with general population/community samples observed abuse rates ranging between 0.6-27.1% depending on the type [5-7]. Among selected samples such as older persons living in a residence home, abuse rates up to 55% depending on the type have been reported [4]. Elder abuse, not least physical, co-exists with detrimental effects such as depression, premature death and reduced social support [5,8-16]. Psychological abuse, e.g. being excluded and repeatedly ignored, seems to be the most commonly reported by elders, with prevalence rates up to 52% [4,5,7]. In a recent WHO report [3], it was estimated that 29 million of persons aged 60 years and over are psychologically abused each year in Europe. Psychological abuse often co-occurs with other abuse categories, e.g. financial [5,17,18] and has been associated with poor health, e.g. trauma [5,19-22]. Further, psychological abuse may be more damaging for older persons than other abuse types [5,23].

Various factors such as poor mental health and lack of social support have been connected with decreased quality of life (QoL) among older

*Corresponding author: Joaquim JF Soares, Institution for Health Sciences, Department of Public Health Sciences, Mid Sweden University, Holmgatan 10, Humlegården, Hus M, 851 70 Sundsvall, Sweden,
E-mail: joaquim.soares@miun.se

persons [e.g. 24-34] and abuse may also be an important contributor to it. Yet, the linkage between abuse, perceived QoL and other factors such as depressive symptoms among older persons has not attracted great attention. To our knowledge, only two studies have investigated this issue [35,36]. Although both reported a relation between abuse/neglect and decreased QoL, they differed substantially. For instance, the operational definition of abuse/neglect and what is meant with QoL is unclear in one of the studies [35]. In the other study [36], there is an unusual operational definition of for instance psychological abuse, e.g. an act of psychological abuse was considered only if it occurred 10 or more times, suggesting under estimation of abuse.

A further examination of the influence of abuse (particularly psychological), while considering other factors such as depressive symptoms upon perceived QoL by domain among older adults from the general population may be useful in several ways. First, by addressing some of the limitations of available studies as described above, we may provide a more accurate description of the relationship between abuse, other factors such as depressive symptoms and QoL among older persons. Second, as far as we know, there are no studies about the relationship between psychological abuse, other factors such as depressive symptoms and QoL with general population samples of older adults. Third, abused older persons in many countries such as Spain, Portugal and Lithuania are not being systematically and consistently assisted, although the importance of prevention has been stressed [1,2]. Therefore, by exploring the relationship between psychological abuse, other factors such as depressive symptoms and QoL among older persons from different countries (e.g. Spain, Portugal, Lithuania), we may provide reliable data on their experiences that could support policy makers and health planers/providers in the development of effective interventions for targeting abuse and improving QoL. Finally, limited attention has been paid to the identification of correlates of QoL (subjective) among older adults, particularly regarding the role of psychological abuse. Considering factors such as depressive symptoms may help to better understand the actual contribution of psychological abuse towards "explaining" the variation in QoL, not least as psychological abuse may be the most commonly reported form of abuse by older persons and more damaging that other abuse forms. Thus, our main aims were to: (i) Compare the subjective experience of QoL by domain (autonomy, fear of death/dying, intimacy, past/present/future activities, sensory-abilities, social participation) between psychologically abused and non-abused persons aged 60-84 years; and (ii) Scrutinize, among all respondents, the association between psychological abuse, other factors such as depressive symptoms and QoL by domain.

Methods

Respondents

The respondents were randomly selected women/men from the general population living in 7 European cities (Stuttgart; Athens; Ancona; Kaunas; Porto; Granada; Stockholm) that took part in the survey "Elder abuse: A multinational prevalence survey, ABUEL" during January-July 2009. Inclusion criteria were age 60-84 years, no cognitive problems (e.g. dementia) [1] or sensory impairments (e.g. blindness), national citizens or documented migrants, living within the community (own/rented houses) or homes for elderly and proficiency in the native languages.

The sample size was estimated on based on municipal census (number of women/men aged 60-84 years) in each city and expected abuse prevalence ranges. Departing from an abuse prevalence of

13%, with a precision of 2.6 percent derived from a recent review [4], a sample size of 633 persons in each city was necessary. Overall, the sample consisted of 4,467 respondents (2,559 women, 57.3%) and mean response across countries was 45.2%. Details regarding for instance the target population, sampling procedures, completion rates, refusal rates and differences between countries are reported in a separate ABUEL method paper by Lindert et al. [37]. Data on demographics/socio-economics are shown in Lindert et al. [37] and Macassa et al. [7].

Definition of quality of life

The definition of QoL proposed by the WHOQOL group was used in this study: "An individuals' perceptions of their position in life in the context of the culture and value systems in which they live, and in relation to their goals, expectations, standards and concerns. It is a broad ranging concept affected in a complex way by the persons' physical health, psychological state, level of independence, social relationships and their relationship to salient features of their environment" [38-40].

Measures

Quality of Life (QoL) was assessed with the WHOQOL-OLD [38]. It contains 24 items graded 1-5 (e.g. not at all-extremely), but after transformation scores range from 0-100 [41]. The items can be summed into a total QoL and divided into 6 domains with four items in each, i.e. autonomy (e.g. freedom to make own decisions); fear of death/dying (e.g. scared of dying); intimacy (e.g. feel a sense of companionship in life); past/present/future activities (e.g. satisfied with achievements); sensory-abilities (e.g. loss of sensory abilities affecting participation in activities); and social participation (e.g. have enough to do each day). High scores correspond to high QoL. Cronbach α (standardized items) for QoL across the included countries was 0.92.

Abuse was assessed with 52 items based on the Conflict Tactic Scales 2 [42] and the UK survey of abuse/neglect of older people [36]. The items were arranged in 5 abuse sub-scales, i.e. psychological, physical, sexual, injury and financial. Additionally, neglect was assessed with 13 items (e.g. routine housework) and data were collected on other factors such as the perpetrators age and sex. The abuse acts may have occurred (how often) once, twice, 3-5, 6-10, 11-20 or >20 times during the past year (chronicity), did not occurred the past year, but before or never occurred. In this study, only the responses regarding psychological abuse (11 items, e.g. threatened to hit or throw something at you) during the past year were analysed. If respondents answered that abuse had not occurred during the past year, they were considered as no abuse cases (no). If respondents answered that they had been abused during the past year independently of chronicity, they were considered as abuse cases (yes). Cronbach α (standardized items) for psychological abuse across the includedcountries was 0.85.

Somatic symptoms were assessed with the short version of the Giessen Complaint List [43]. It contains 24 items graded 0-4 (not affected-very affected). The items can be summed into a total somatic symptoms and arranged in 4 domains with 6 items in each: exhaustion (e.g. tiredness); gastrointestinal (e.g. nausea); musculoskeletal (e.g. pains in joints or limbs); and heart distress (e.g. heavy, rapid or irregular heart-throbbing). The total score for all items is 96 and 24 for each symptom domain. The higher the scores, the more one is affected. Cronbach α (standardized items) for somatic symptoms across the included countries was 0.92.

Depressive and anxiety symptoms were assessed with Hospital Anxiety and Depression Scale [44]. It contains 14 items graded 0-3 (e.g. not at all-most of the time), of which 7 pertain to depression (e.g. I feel as if I am slowed down) and 7 to anxiety (e.g. I get sudden feelings of panic). The total score for depression and anxiety is 21 each. No cases correspond to a score of 0-7, possibly cases to 8-10 and probable cases to 11-21. High scores correspond to high depression and anxiety levels. Cronbach α (standardized items) for anxiety across the included countries was 0.81 and for depression 0.80.

Health care use was assessed as the number of contacts with health care staff (e.g. physician) and health care services (e.g. primary care). We also assessed the number of diseases (e.g. cardiovascular), which the respondents suffered from presently. The items were derived from the Stockholm County Council health survey [45].

Social support was assessed with the Multidimensional Scale of Perceived Social Support [46]. It contains 12 items graded 1-7 (very strongly disagree-very strongly agree). The items can be summed into a total social support and divided into 3 domains with 4 items in each: support from family (e.g. my family really tries to help me); significant others (e.g. there is a special person who is around when I am in need); and friends (e.g. I can talk about my problems with my friends). The total score ranges from 12-84, 4-28 for each domain. High scores correspond to high social support. Cronbach α (standardized items) for social support across the included countries was 0.92.

Life-style variables were assessed as alcohol and cigarette use, and body mass index (BMI). Alcohol was assessed with items derived from The Alcohol Use Disorders Identification Test [47]. First, the respondents were asked if they presently used alcohol (do you drink alcohol? yes/no). If they answered yes, 3 items derived from Audit were applied: (1) how often do you have a drink containing alcohol? (once a month or less, 2-4 times a month, 2-3 times a week, 4 or more times a week); (2) how many drinks containing alcohol do you have on a typical day when you are drinking? (1 or 2, 3 or 4, 5 or 6, 7, 8, or 9, 10 or more); (3) how often do you have six or more drinks on one occasion? (Never, less than monthly, monthly, weekly, daily or almost daily). Finally, we asked respondents about their past use of alcohol (if you do not drink alcohol now, have you ever been drinking alcohol? yes/no). Smoking was assessed in a similar way. This study focused on use of alcohol and cigarettes in a yes/no format. A BMI, based on self-reported height and weight, was calculated for each respondent with the formula kg/m^2 (Mean/SD, 26.68/4.19; CI95% 26.55-26.80).

Demographic/socio-economic and household variables were assessed, i.e. country, age, sex, marital status, ethnic background, education, profession, financial support, financial strain, housing, living situation, household size and if still on work. Financial strain (worries with how to make ends meet) was measured with one item (no/sometimes/often/always format). A participant was defined as having "financial strain" if she/he chose any response other than no. Four items (e.g. place of birth) assessed whether the respondents were migrants or native inhabitants. These factors were tailored for each country, but similar in content.

Design/Procedure

The design was cross-sectional. The recruitment of respondents and data gathering were conducted during January-July 2009. The data were collected via face-to-face interviews or a combination of interviews and self-response[1]. The scales (if not available) were translated into each country´s language, back-translated and culturally adapted. Only GBB, the Multidimensional Scale of Perceived Social Support and health questions were applied the above mentioned procedure based on previously defined protocol for some of the countries. A similar strategy was applied for other materials such as information letters. Interviewers in each city (n=5-20) received training in various issues (e.g. ethical behavior). The respondents were carefully informed about the research in writing/verbally, and signed a consent form. Great emphasis was put on confidentiality, anonymity and the respondent´s rights[1]. Ethical permission was received in each participating country. For further details on design/procedure see Lindert et al. [37].

Statistical analyses

Differences in QoL by domain between psychologically abused and non-abused respondents were analyzed with ANOVAs. A significant level of P<0.05 was accepted for bivariate and multivariate analyses. Differences between psychologically abused and non-abused respondents in various areas such as demographics/socio-economics are shown elsewhere [7,37]. Additionally, we conducted collinearity statistics on the regressions, with VIF´s for autonomy ranging from 1.085 to 8.552; for past/present/future activities from 1.067 to 7.079; for social participation from 1.066 to 9.596; and for intimacy from 1.066 to 8.943. The VIF´s were below accepted levels, up to 10 (detailed data not shown here). Furthermore, Pearson correlation analyses showed positive correlation coefficients ranging from 0.000 to 0.501 and negative from -0.001 to -0.584. The overwhelming majority of negative/positive correlations were below 0.20.

Further, 4 multiple linear regressions were computed to scrutinize the associations between the dependent variables (autonomy, intimacy, past/present/future activities, and social participation) and other covariates (independent variables) among all respondents[2]. The independent variables were selected based on statistical inference, i.e. factors such as socio-economics that differentiated abused/non-abused respondents in previous analyses [7,37] and the literature on QoL. The independent variables were psychological abuse, country, age, sex, marital status, migrant background, living situation, housing, education, profession, financial support, still work, financial strain, alcohol and cigarette use, household size, BMI, health care use, diseases number, anxiety, depression, somatic symptoms and social support. Associations between the variables were expressed as unstandardized Betas/Std.Error, standardized Betas, CI95% and R^2.

Results

QoL and psychological abuse

As shown in table 1, psychologically abused respondents contrasted to non-abused scored lower in autonomy, intimacy, past/present/future activities and social participation, indicating that they experienced their QoL in these areas as lower. There were no differences regarding fear of death/dying and sensory abilities (Table 1).

Correlates of QoL by domain

As shown in table 2, autonomy was positively associated with all education levels (low, secondary, university), alcohol use and social support. Being from any other country than Germany, aged 80-84 years, financially strained and financially supported by social/sickness benefits/other pension benefits (e.g. sick pension), and experiencing anxiety, depressive andsomatic symptoms and abuse was negatively associated with autonomy. The model "explained" 32.8% of the variation in autonomy.

Past/present/future activities were positively associated with social support. Being from any other country than Germany, financially strained and financially supported by social/sickness benefits/other pension benefits (e.g. sick pension), and experiencing anxiety, depressive and somatic symptoms and abuse was negatively associated with past/present/future activities. The model "explained" 44.8% of the variation in activities (Table 2).

As shown in table 3, social participation was positively associated with still on work, alcohol use, social support and abuse. Being from any other country than Germany, aged 80-84 years, man and financially supported by social/sickness benefits/other pension benefits (e.g. sick pension), smoking, and experiencing anxiety, depressive and somatic symptoms were negatively associated with social participation. The model "explained" 41.5% of the variation in social participation.

Intimacy was positively associated with being married/cohabitant, financially strained and financially supported by spouse/partner income, living with spouse/partner, spouse/partner/other[3], other persons[4] and in large households, using health care frequently and social support. Being from any other country than Germany, and experiencing anxiety and depressive symptoms and abuse were negatively associated with intimacy. The model "explained" 45.6% of the variation in intimacy (Table 3).

Variables	Abused n	Not –abused n	Anova
Autonomy[b]	873	3505	($F_{(1,4376)}$=43.66, $p<0.0001$)
Mean ± SD	67.42 ± 21.26	72.39 ± 19.58	
Fear of death/dying[b]	871	3475	($F_{(1,4344)}$=1.38, $p=0.2408$)
Mean ± SD	60.92 ± 26.75	62.17± 28.47	
Intimacy[b]	870	3521	($F_{(1,4389)}$=116.84, $p<0.0001$)
Mean ± SD	55.31 ± 31.15	67.21 ± 28.55	
Past/present/future activities[b]	876	3534	($F_{(1,4408)}$=57.24, $p<0.0001$)
Mean ± SD	62.79 ± 19.62	68.05 ± 18.09	
Sensory-abilities[b]	880	3547	($F_{(1,4425)}$=0.12, $p=0.9121$)
Mean ± SD	73.42 ± 24.54	73.31 ± 26.66	
Social participation[b]	874	3537	($F_{(1,4409)}$=8.54, $p=0.0035$)
Mean ± SD	65.03 ± 19.84	68.21 ± 19.77	

[a]=WHOQOL-OLD=World Health Organization Quality of Life-Old; [b]=sub-scales, 0-100 each one.

Table 1: Means/SD of quality of life[a] by psychological abuse.

Discussion

QoL and psychological abuse

Psychologically abuse was related to lower scores in autonomy, intimacy, past/present/future activities and social participation. There were no differences between abused and non-abused respondents in fear of death/dying and sensory abilities, which may have been more affected by the ageing process than abuse. Subsequent regressions confirmed that abuse was negatively associated with autonomy, intimacy and past/present/future activities, and positively with social participation.

Psychological abuse consists of acts such as being undermined and belittled over one´s activities, excluded and repeatedly ignored and prevented from seeing others. This seems contrary to QoL goals and expectations such as freedom to make own decisions (autonomy), being able to have personal and intimate relationships (intimacy), satisfaction with achievements in life (past/present/future activities) and opportunity to participate in community activities (social participation).

An explanation could be that the abuse led to feelings of worthlessness, powerlessness, hopelessness, unhappiness and insecurity. Over time these feelings may have resulted, for instance, in experiences of not being able to make own decisions, a sense that companionship with a partner or other close person was not shared to the extent desired and doubts over achievements. Elder abuse has been previously associated with poor self-esteem and unhappiness [48-50], and psychological abuse may be more damaging than other forms of abuse [5,23]. The negative effects of abuse could have been strengthened as the main perpetrators were spouses/partners (37.1%) and significant other, e.g. offspring (34.1%). Older persons often rely on spouses/partners and/or significant other for assistance with daily activities, provide affection, care for their health, and may be the main source of personal care and well-being [51,52]. Being abused by near one´s may have highly stressful for the older persons, for instance, in terms of effects on intimacy. It is also possible, in view of the respondents situation in other areas such as mental health problems and financial strain that for example the spouses/partners and/or significant other felt highly exasperated, dissatisfied and burdened by the situation, resulting in abuse and subsequently in the respondents experience of decreased QoL. Findings indicate that dependency on others due to physical/cognitive problems may increase abuse "risk" [53]. On the other hand, the respondents may have expressed frustration and discontentment with their QoL (e.g. poor intimacy), which led to abuse.

Abuse was positively linked to social participation (e.g. increased satisfaction with the opportunity to participate in community activities). This finding seems odd considering that abuse involved, among other acts, being prevented from seeing others. It is possible that although prevented to see others, the respondents nevertheless took part in community activities and valued them highly. Social participation could have functioned as a way to cope with the strains of abuse as the older persons may have been able to express their experiences and received support. Social support has been shown to attenuate the experience of abuse [7,54].

Abuse has been associated with decreased QoL [35,36], but as indicated previously these studies have several limitations (e.g.

[3-5]Daughter.

Independent variables	Autonomy Past/present/future activities					
	β(SE)[l]	β[m]	CI95[n]	β(SE)[l]	β[m]	CI95[n]
Country[b]						
Greece	-5.317(1.253)	-0.096****	-7.773/-2.861	-4.855(1.046)	-0.094****	-6.906/-2.803
Italy	-11.478(1.150)	-0.204****	-13.733/-9.223	-7.259(0.961)	-0.138****	-9.144/-5.374
Lithuania	-3.931(1.180)	-0.075***	-6.246/-1.617	-6.257(0.986)	-0.128****	-8.191/-4.323
Portugal	-5.668(1.110)	-0.106****	-7.845/-3.491	-5.272(0.926)	-0.106****	-7.088/-3.456
Spain	-3.949(1.291)	-0.064**	-6.481/-1.417	-6.100(1.081)	-0.106****	-8.219/-3.980
Sweden	-5.566(1.088)	-0.101****	-7.699/-3.433	-3.979(0.909)	-0.078****	-5.762/-2.196
Germany[c]		1			1	
Age[b]						
65-69	0.448(0.812)	0.010	-1.145/2.041	0.991(0,683)	0.024	-0.349/2.331
70-74	0.252(0.885)	0.005	-1.484/1.988	0.890(0,744)	0.020	-0.568/2.349
75-79	0.601(0.971)	0.011	-1.302/2.504	0.736(0.814)	0.015	-0.861/2.333
80-84	-2.665(1.081)	-0.044*	-4.785/-0.545	-0.023(0.910)	0.001	-1.806/1.761
60-64[c]		1			1	
Sex[b]						
Male	-0.430(0.650)	-0.011	-1.704/0.844	-2.116(0.546)	0.032	-4.431/0.418
Female[c]		1			1	
Migrant background[b]						
Yes	-2.039(1.211)	-0.024	-4.413/0.335	-1.233(1.008)	-0.016	-3.210/0.744
No[c]		1			1	
Marital status[b]						
Married/cohabitant	-2.231(2.058)	-0.054	-6.266/1.804	-0.666(1.717)	-0.017	-4.033/2.700
Divorced/separated	0.322(1.469)	0.004	-2.557/3.202	-2.007(1.235)	-0.030	-4.428/0.415
Widow/er	0.560(1.314=	0.011	-2.016/3.137	0.744(1.103)	0.016	-1.419/2.906
Single[c]		1			1	
Living situation[b]						
Spouse/partner	-3.399(1.922)	-0.087	-7.168/0.370	-1.463(1.599)	-0.040	-4.599/1.672
Spouse/partner/other[e]	-1.932(2.149)	-0.037	-6.144/2.280	-2.866(1.793)	-0.058	-6.382/0.650
Other[f]	-3.928(1.228)	-0.039	-6.150/2.286	-2.178(1.033)	-0.034	-4.432/0.419
Alone[c]		1			1	
Housing[b]						
Rent	-1.707(0.738)	-0.026	-4.419/0.339	-2.907(0.620)	-0.033	-4.431/0.420
Other[g]	-3.563(1.609)	-0.030	-4.543/0.343	-1.827(1.354)	-0.017	-4.482/0.828
Own[c]		1			1	
Household size	-0.543(0.333)	-0.033	-1.196/0.111	0.668(0.280)	0.043*	0.119/1.218
Education[b]						
Low education[h]	4.164(2.028)	0.102*	0.189/8.140	1.483(1.707)	0.039	-1.864/4.830
Middle education[i]	4.958(2.107)	0.124*	0.826/9.089	1.768(1.774)	0.048	-1.710/5.246
High education[j]	6.067(2.241)	0.128**	1.674/10.461	2.505(1.885)	0.057	-1.191/6.201
Cannot read/write[c]		1			1	
Profession[b]						
Blue-collar agricultural/fishery/crafts	1.014(0.948)	0.024	-0.845/2.873	0.219(0.795)	0.006	-1.340/1.778
Low white-collar worker	1.361(0.867)	0.031	-0.339/3.060	-1.138(0.726)	-0.028	-2.561/0.286
Armed forces/similar	1.600(2.588)	0.009	-3.474/6.675	-0.129(2.179)	-0.001	-4.400/4.143
Housewives/husbands	-1.810(1.398)	-0.028	-4.552/0.931	-2.536(1.169)	-0.033	-0.513/3.870
Middle/high white-collar worker[c]		1			1	
Financial support[b]						
Work	1.470(1.327)	0.025	-1.133/4.072	1.679(1.116)	0.031	-0.510/3.867
Social/sickness/other pension benefits	-4.672(1.276)	-0.053****	-7.175/-2.170	-2.776(1.071)	-0.035**	-4.876/-0.675
Spouse/partner income	0.262(1.190)	0.004	-2.070/2.595	0.446(0.999)	0.008	-1.512/2.404
Other income[k]	-1.239(1.829)	-0.010	-4.825/2.347	0.536(1.524)	0.005	-2.452/3.524
Work pension[c]		1			1	
Still wrork[b]						
Yes	-1.170(1.130)	-0.023	-3.386/1.046	0.263(0.951)	0.006	-1.602/2.128
No[c]		1			1	
Financial strain[b]						
Yes	-2.621(0.629)	-0.064****	-3.854/-1.389	-2.620(0.528)	-0.069****	-3.655/-1.586
No[c]		1			1	
Smoking[b]						
Yes	0.676(0.859)	0.011	-1.009/2.361	-1.400(0.725)	-0.025	-2.821/0.021
No[c]		1			1	
Drinking[b]						
Yes	2.847(0.650)	0.069****	1.573/4.121	0.412(0.546	0.011	-0.660/1.483
No[c]		1			1	
BMI[d]	0.111(0.068)	0.023	-0.022/0.245	0.044(0.057)	0.010	-0.068/0.155
Health care use[d]	0.104(0.102)	0.015	-0.096/0.303	0.071(0.086)	0.011	-0.098/0.239
Physical diseases[d]	0.396(0.223)	0.029	-0.041/0.833	-0.126(0.188)	-0.010	-0.494/0.242
Anxiety symptoms[d]	-0.286(-0.286)	-0.058**	-0.466/-0.105	-0.538(0.077)	-0.118****	-0.689/-0.387
Depressive symptoms[d]	-1.470(0.099)	-0.302****	-1.664/-1.276	-1.620(0.083)	-0.357****	-1.782/-1.458
Somatic symptoms[d]	-0.138(0.026)	-0.103****	-0.188/-0.087	-0.061(0.022)	-0.049**	-0.103/-0.018
Social support[d]	0.223(0.021)	0.164****	0.181/0.265	0.311(0.018)	0.247****	0.276/0.347
Psychological abuse[b]						
Yes	-2.482(0.699)	-0.051****	-3.852/-1.113	-1.643(0.586)	-0.036**	-2.792/-0.494
No[c]		1			1	
R²	32.8%			44.8%		

[a]=WHOQOL-OLD, sub-scales; [b]=categorical variables; [c]=comparison variable; [d]=continuous variables; [e]=e.g. daughter; [f]=without spouse/partner, but other e.g. daughter; [g]=e.g. homes for elderly; [h]=primary school/similar; [i]=secondary school/similar; [j]=university/similar; [k]=e.g. own capital; [l]=un-standardised betas and standard error; [m]=standardized betas; [n]=lower/upper bound; VIF´s for autonomy ranged from 1.085-8.552; VIF´s for past/present/future activities range from 1.067-7.079; * p<0.05; **p<0.01; ***p<0.001; ****p<0.0001.

Table 2: Correlates of quality of life by domain (multiple linear regression analyses).

Independent variables	Social participation			Intimacy		
	β(SE)[l]	β[m]	CI95[n]	β(SE)[l]	β[m]	CI95[n]
Country[b]						
Greece	-2.976(1.153)	-0.054**	5.238/-0.715	-9.748(1.681)	-0.117****	-13.044/-6.453
Italy	-5.424(1.061)	-0.096****	-7.504/-3.344	-9.736(1.543)	-0.115****	-12.761/-6.712
Lithuania	-2.795(1.086)	-0.054**	-4.925/-0.665	-32.025(1.585)	-0.407****	-35.133/-28.917
Portugal	-2.722(1.020)	-0.051**	-4.722/-0.723	-8.947(1.497)	-0.109****	-11.882/-6.012
Spain	-3.285(1.190)	-0.054**	-5.617/-0.952	-11.269(1.737)	-0.122****	-14.675/-7.863
Sweden	-5.979(0.999)	-0.109****	-7.938/-4.021	-13.957(1.462)	-0.169****	-16.823/-11.090
Germany[c]		1			1	
Age[b]						
65-69	0.771(0.753)	0.017	-0.705/2.248	-0.150(1.099)	-0.002	-2.305/2.006
70-74	0.739(0.823)	0.016	-0.874/2.352	-2.212(1.196)	-0.031	-4.556/0.132
75-79	0.302(0.898)	0.006	-1.460/2.063	0.697(1.311)	0.009	-1.873/3.267
80-84	-3.357(1.002)	-0.056***	-5.322/-1.391	-1.708(1.465)	-0.019	-4.581/1.165
60-64[c]		1			1	
Sex[b]						
Male	-3.454(0.601)	-0.088****	-4.633/-2.275	1.030(0.878)	0.017	-0.691/2.750
Female[c]		1			1	
Migrant background[b]						
Yes	-2.138(1.116)	-0.025	-4.325/0.049	-0.474(1.641)	-0.004	-3.691/2.743
No[c]		1			1	
Marital status[b]						
Married/cohabitant	-3.601(1.890)	-0.087	-7.308/0.105	7.299(2.772)	0.117***	1.864/12.734
Divorced/separated	-2.527(1.358)	-0.035	-5.189/0.136	1.262(1.998)	0.011	-2.656/5.180
Widow/er	-1.625(1.213)	-0.033	-4.003/0.754	0.209(1.785)	0.003	-3.291/3.709
Single[c]		1			1	
Living situation[b]						
Spouse/partner	-0.414(1.761)	-0.011	-3.868/3.040	10.620(2.582)	0.180****	5.557/15.683
Spouse/partner/other[e]	-1.080(1.975)	-0.020	-4.953/2.793	9.544(2.892)	0.120***	3.874/15.214
Other[f]	-3.118(1.141)	-0.037	-5.191/0.139	4.133(1.682)	0.042**	0.836/7.430
Alone[c]		1			1	
Housing[b]						
Rent	-0.656(0.682)	-0.014	-1.994/0.681	-0.223(0.999)	-0.003	-2.182/1.736
Other[g]	-0.905(1.493)	-0.008	-3.831/2.021	-4.075(2.218)	-0.024	-8.424/0.274
Own[c]		1			1	
Household size	0.090(0.309)	0.005	-0.515/0.696	0.973(0.451)	0.039*	0.089/1.857
Education[b]						
Low Education[h]	0.302(1.881)	0.007	-3.386/3.990	-0.375(2.782)	-0.006	-5.829/5.080
Middle Education[i]	0.242(1.955)	0.006	-3.590/4.075	1.038(2.889)	0.017	-4.625/6.702
High Education[j]	0.504(2.078)	0.011	-3.570/4.579	1.483(3.063)	0.021	-4.523/7.488
Cannot read/write[c]		1			1	
Profession[b]						
Blue-collar/agricultural/fishery/crafts	0.217(0.878)	0.005	-1.504/1.939	-0.549(1.281)	-0.009	-3.062/1.963
Low white-collar worker	-0.224(0.800)	-0.005	-1.794/1.345	-0.716(1.169)	-0.011	-3.007/1.576
Armed forces/similar	2.936(2.427)	0.016	-1.822/7.694	3.700(3.499)	0.013	-3.159/10.560
Housewives/husbands	-1.229(1.293)	-0.019	-3.765/1.306	-0.333(1.877)	-0.003	-4.013/3.347
Middle/high white-collar worker[c]		1			1	
Financial support[b]						
Work	-1.161(1.232)	-0.020	-3.577/1.255	-0.052(1.810)	0.001	-3.600/3.496
Social/sickness/other pension benefits	-5.090(1.179)	-0.058****	-7.401/-2.779	2.297(1.740)	0.017	-1.115/5.708
Spouse/partner income	0.017(1.100)	0.001	-2.140/2.173	3.885(1.612)	0.041*	0.725/7.046
Other income[k]	0.969(1.681)	0.008	-2.326/4.264	1.234(2.461)	0.006	-3.592/6.060
Work pension[c]		1			1	
Still work[b]						
Yes	3.634(1.052)	0.071***	1.571/5.696	2.516(1.547)	0.033	-0.517/5.549
No[c]		1			1	
Financial strain[b]						
Yes	-1.044(0.582)	-0.026	-2.186/0.098	2.760(0.848)	0.045***	1.097/4.423
No[c]		1			1	
Smoking[b]						
Yes	-1.601(0.798)	-0.027*	-3.166/-0.037	-0.758(1.159)	-0.008	-3.030/1.515
No[c]		1			1	
Drinking[b]						
Yes	1.504(0.603)	0.037**	0.321/2.686	0.489(0.881)	0.008	-1.238/2.217
No[c]		1			1	
BMI[d]	-0.101(0.063)	-0.021	-0.224/0.022	-0.102(0.092)	-0.014	-0.282/0.078
Health care use[d]	-0.006(0.094)	-0.001	-0.191/0.179	0.429(0.138)	0.042****	0.159/0.700
Physical diseases[d]	-0.124(0.207)	-0.009	-0.531/0.282	0.431(0.302)	0.021	-0.162/1.024
Anxiety symptoms[d]	-0.217(0.085)	-0.044**	-0.384/-0.050	-0.471(0.124)	-0.064****	-0.714/-0.228
Depressive symptoms[d]	-2.044(0.092)	-0.420****	-2.223/-1.864	-1.358(0.134)	-0.185****	-1.620/-1.096
Somatic symptoms[d]	-0.138(0.024)	-0.104****	-0.185/-0.091	-0.015(0.035)	-0.007	-0.083/0.053
Social support[d]	0.269(0.020)	0.200****	0.230/0.308	0.530(0.029)	0.258****	0.473/0.586
Psychological abuse[b]						
Yes	1.517(0.647)	0.31**	0.249/2.784	-6.861(0.945)	-0.094****	-8.714/-5.007
No[c]		1			1	
R²	41.5%			45.6%		

a=WHOQOL-OLD, sub-scales; b=categorical variables; c=comparison variable; d=continuous variables; e=e.g. daughter; f=without spouse/partner, but other e.g. daughter; g=e.g. homes for elderly; h=primary school/similar; i=secondary school/similar; j=university/similar; k=e.g. own capital; l=un-standardised betas and standard error; m=standardised betas; n=lower/upper bound; VIF´s of social participation ranged from 1.066-9.596; VIF´s of intimacy ranged from 1.066-8.943;* p<0.05; **p<0.01; ***p<0.001; ****p<0.0001.

Table 3: Correlates of quality of life by domain (multiple linear regression analyses).

methodological). In any case, our study may be the first to demonstrate a clear relationship between psychological abuse and decreased QoL, although mainly regarding autonomy, intimacy and past/present/future activities.

QoL and Country

All QoL domains (autonomy, intimacy, past/present/future activities, social participation) were negatively related to being from any other country in contrast to Germany (reference country). This in line with a study across 21 countries (e.g. Germany), i.e. older persons from developing countries scored lower on these domains than those from medium and high-development countries [55]. However, it is hazardous to compare results as only four of our countries were included (Germany, Lithuania, Spain, Sweden) and none of these were developing countries.

Further, other data show that individuals from our countries (except Sweden) contrasted to those from Germany experience less autonomy, with some of the underlying reasons being lower levels of social services and incomes [24-27]. The discrepancy regarding Sweden may pertain to that the financial situation of older persons in this country, particularly the oldest, has deteriorated during the past years (e.g. low incomes) and this could have had a negative effect on their autonomy [56]. Additional findings show that autonomy depends on various factors such as disease, financial resources and social support [26,57-61].

As to intimacy, available findings tend to involves elected groups such as frail older persons and the bulk of studies focus on the sexual expression of intimacy and emphasize its importance for well-being [62-66]. Our findings are unlikely to reflect that the respondents from the other included countries compared to those of Germany differed in their living situation (who lived with the respondent) and were more often singles, divorced/separated or widowers in view that there were no major differences in total percentages. It is possible for instance that the respondents from the other included countries compared to those from Germany experienced a less "tolerant" environment to give/receive intimacy, and therefore the lower scores, but this issue was not directly addressed.

Regarding past/present/future activities, it is likely that the expression of achievement values among older persons depends on factors such as life satisfaction, self-esteem and individual/societal economic development. In line with this, data indicate that older persons in most of the included countries experienced a lower life satisfaction contrasted to those from Germany [24,27] due to various reasons such as economic difficulties. Poverty levels among older persons in Germany are lower than in most of our included countries [67,68]. Self-esteem declines in older age [69,70], but the decline may have been less evident among respondents in Germany. Thus, the respondents satisfaction with opportunities in life and how satisfied they were with what they achieved in life may have been influenced by the above mentioned factors.

As to social participation, it is likely that poverty levels [67,68] were an obstacle for participation in social activities, at least in some countries such as Portugal, and data show indeed that low income levels are associated with decreased QoL [24,27]. Decreased social participation could also be an indirect measure of loneliness. Older persons from Southern European countries feel lonelier than those from Germany pertaining to factors such as economic deprivation, although our results concerning Sweden and Lithuania seem at odds [71,72]. Poverty, loneliness or both could thus be an obstacle for social participation and therefore the dissatisfaction.

QoL, Demographics/socio-Economics and Life-Style

Age 80-84 years was negatively associated with autonomy and social participation. This at odds with results from Norway, i.e. no differences in these domains between persons aged below 75 years and those aged 75 years and over [73]. Sample differences, for instance, may explain the discrepancy. In general, older cohorts compared to younger have worse health, depend more on others, are more isolated and have lower incomes, and these factors negatively affect their well-being and QoL [67,68,74-82]. Thus, such circumstances may have hindered our respondents to do the things they like to do and to take part in activities as desired.

Male gender was negatively associated with social participation. Thisis in line with a Norwegian study among older adults, i.e. men scored lower on social participation than women [73]. Our findings seem to reflect that older men contrasted to older women have less extensive social ties and participate less in social activities [83,84].

Being married/cohabitant, living with spouse/partner/other[5] and in large households were positively associated with intimacy. This indicates that spouses/partners and significant other are vital for the well-being of older persons as for instance givers of affection. Family and significant other also provide companionship and support when health declines and the older person need help. Our findings seem to bean indirect indicator that some of our respondents lived in harmonious relationships. For example, harmonious marriages positively affect for instance the psychological well-being of individuals, including older persons [85-91]. Living in large households suggests that the older persons had multi-levels of support and opportunities to receive/give love, and indeed living in extended families and/or receiving inter generational support has been shown to provide benefits for older persons, particularly in relation to health [92,93] although the quality of the relationships in the family may be more important than the number of persons in it [94]. Thus, living in large households may also be beneficial for intimacy.

All types of education compared to no education were positively associated with autonomy. Contrary to our findings, a recent Brazilian study with older adults reported no major impact of education on autonomy [95]. Our findings seem also at odds with data showing that individuals, including older persons, with high educational attainment experience greater QoL than those with lower educational attainment. However, we confirmed that individuals with the highest educational attainment report greater QoL than those without any educational attainment and the opposite [96-98]. Differences, for instance, in the definition of educational levels may account for the discrepancy between our findings and those of others.

Financial support based on social/sickness benefits/other pension benefits was negatively associated with autonomy, past/present/future activities and social participation. Being supported by benefits (e.g. social) indicates financial difficulties and thus in contrast to higher social groups those who are on benefits may be less happy and in control of their situation [99]. Further, there is a link between income and health which affects QOL, showing that within countries, poorer health is associated with lower income [100,101]. Low income levels seem also to lead to decreased QoL [24,27]. On the other hand, the above mentioned association could reflect that people with poor health, which affects QOL, are more likely to be on special types of benefits (e.g. social) usually a sign of economic problems [102-104]. Thus, disease, financial problems or both may have hindered respondents to make own decisions freely and to participate in activities to the extent desired, and thus experienced that there wasn´t much to look forward to.

Financial strain was negatively associated with autonomy, intimacy and past/present/future activities, illustrating further the importance of finances for the older person´s well-being. Income levels decline in older age and there is a close relationship between poverty rates and older ages [67,68]. The rates of poverty among older persons are greater than in the population as a whole in some Southern/Eastern European countries, but also in Nordic countries incertain aspects such as low net real assets, and during the past years the financial situation in Europe has deteriorated with increases in living costs and cuts or stagnation of benefits/services [56,67,68,105-107]. These circumstances are likely to have led to the experience of financial strain, and, consequently to decreased QOL in various domains. Financial strain may have hindered the respondents to make own decisions about different aspects of their lives and to participate in activities. Financial strain may have also led to disagreements between respondents and those close to them, which would be an obstacle to give and receive love. Studies have shown indeed an association between financial strain/problems/income inequality, poor mental/physical health and decreased QOL among different groups, including older persons [108-112].

An additional finding on the importance of economy in QoL was the positive association between still working and social participation. Employment tends to provide the status, self-esteem and financial resources, which facilitates social relationships, social connections or participation in social activities, and thus the high scores in social participation. However, data on the relation between still working (paid work) and social participation are however ambiguous, with findings indicating that work impacts positively on social participation [113] and others not [114].

Being financially supported by the spouses/partners income was positively associated with intimacy. Financial dependency on a spouse/partner concerning one´s living situation is indicative of little decision latitude for the dependent person and greater influence in how the resources are spent and who spends them for the financial contributor [115-117]. A longitudinal analysis of dual-earner couples showed that the husband´s financial dependence was linked with lower levels of perceived marital quality among husbands [118], but cross-sectional data found no connection between a husband's economic dependence and his reports of marital satisfaction [119]. Further, recent findings suggest an association between marital dissatisfaction and poorer physical health over time for both men and women, particularly among older persons [120], and being the secondary earner seems to have negative effects on the health of highest-income men [121]. Thus, one could expect financial dependency to be detrimental to intimacy because of marital discord, negative effects on health or both. We found the opposite, i.e. financial dependency was related to increased satisfaction with intimacy. A plausible explanation is that at the age of the respondents issues regarding, for instance, who is the bread winner and who has the final say played little role. The couples were likely to share financial intimacy and this had a positive influence on intimacy.

Alcohol use was positively associated with social participation and autonomy. Slightly over 64% of our respondents used alcohol and 82.7% drank 1-2 drinks a day, indicating that they were moderate drinkers[6]. Of the alcohol users, 68.2% used alcohol in conjunction with social activities, e.g. meeting friends. [7]Moderate alcohol use has been associated with beneficial effects on mortality risk, health and QoL among older persons [122-125]. Thus, the positive relation between alcohol use and social participation may be a reflection of this. As to the relation between autonomy and alcohol use, one could hypothesize that alcohol use gave the respondents a sense that they could make their own decisions.

QoL and health

Not surprisingly, depressive and anxiety symptoms were negatively associated with all QoL domains, and somatic symptoms with autonomy, past/present/future activities and social participation. Depression, anxiety and somatic symptoms have been associated with decreased QoL among various types of elder samples and in different settings/countries [28-32,76], and in a recent study among older persons it was found that psychological well-being predicted QoL [126]. Thus, our findings seem to confirm those of a plethora of studies. The mechanisms underlying the connection between these conditions and decreased QoL are likely to be complex. For example, depressed persons may have reduced interest or pleasure in all activities, or almost all; diminished ability to make own decisions; and are unlikely to engage and/or find satisfaction, or at least seldom, in such events as participation in daily activities and give intimacy. Hence, it may be foreseeable that they report a decreased QoL. On the other hand, a reverse pattern could be possible in some cases. For instance, persistent refusal of intimacy and lack of appreciation over achievements could over time have led to depressive, anxiety or somatic symptoms.

QoL and social support

High scores in social support were positively related to all QoL domains. Social support (e.g. having help from friends)[8] and social engagement has a positive influence on health, QoL and life satisfaction and the opposite regarding low social support/social isolation [33,34,127-130]. Thus, our results seem in accord with previous observations. The mechanisms underlying the connection between social support and the QoL domains were not addressed in our study. Nevertheless, it is possible for example that social support functioned as a "mechanism" buffering the negative effects of stress and enhancing personal coping abilities such as self-esteem and self-efficacy [131], which would positively affect the older persons perception of various components of QoL as receivers and givers.

Limitations

This study has limitations. First, the cross-sectional nature of the data did not allowed to firmly conclude about causality. Second, the respondents may not have been representative for rural samples and other countries in Europe or elsewhere (e.g. USA) as they were recruited in urban centers from only seven specific European countries. Thus, the generalizability of our findings cannot be guaranteed. Third, the non-

---

[6]One drink represents one unit and is equivalent to 10 grams of alcohol.
[7]Details on alcohol use patterns and activities are not shown here.
[8,9]In some cases the studies include also young persons.

use of objective measures to corroborate the respondents' subjective assessments of their situation affects the accuracy. For example, the presence of somatic symptoms (e.g. pain) was not objectively confirmed. On the other hand, the used instrument (GBB) has good psychometric properties and is sensitive to age [e.g. 43]. Fourth, GBB, Multidimensional Scale of Perceived Social Support and health items needed to be translated into some of the included country's languages, back-translated and culturally adapted. Although this was done with great caution and precision, errors could have occurred raising questions about the validity of what was measured. Fifth, the high non-response rate could have led to the "selection" of women/men with characteristics differing from those of women/men in general. For instance, we may have an over-representation of men who were psychologically abused [7]. However, there were no major divergences (age and gender) between responders and non-responders nor did they differ from the population in each participating state [37]. Sixth, the burden of the perpetrators such as spouses/cohabitants and offspring was not assessed and thus we cannot conclude on whether it influenced their abusive behaviors. Seventh, sleep disturbances are common among older persons [132,133] and may lead to deteriorated QoL [134,135], but this issue was not directly addressed here precluding any conclusion about its influence on QoL. In spite of the limitations, the strength of this study lies in its careful methodology, large sample and multi-country approach. It also provides an overview and opportunity to compare older persons from cities in seven European countries with respect to the impact of psychological abuse on QoL by domain considering other factors such as depression and social support.

Conclusions

Several of the QoL domains were negatively affected by psychological abuse, but other factors such as depressive and anxiety symptoms and country of origin also impacted negatively on QoL. Social support, for example, had a positive effect on the QoL dimensions. Interventions to improve the QoL of older persons should consider these factors, not the least the role of psychological abuse, social support and mental health. Overall, our results seem to have shed further light on the experience of QoL in relation to psychological abuse and other factors such as mental health and social support in older persons; may be useful for changing advocacy and policies regarding older person's experience of QoL, but also for changing public perceptions of it; pointed to the importance of psychological abuse, mental health and social support for the experience of QoL; may be useful for the development of interventions to improve QoL, but also for the development of prevention/treatment interventions to deal with psychological abuse and to decrease mental health and social isolation; and may serve as stimulation for further research across cultures and considering the relationship between various types of elder abuse, QoL, mental health and social support. Notwithstanding, our findings reveal that the QoL of older persons is influenced by many factors, which could not be firmly disentangle. More research, in particular longitudinal, is therefore necessary to conclude about causality.

Authors' contributions

Joaquim J.F. Soares has made significant contributions to the conception, design, data collection, analyses and interpretation of data. He was also involved in drafting the manuscript and revising it critically. EV and ÖS were involved in the analyses and interpretation of data, and in drafting the manuscript and revising it. MGM, MS, JL, FT-G, HB and EI-K were involved in the gathering, analyses and interpretation of data, and in drafting the manuscript and revising it.

References

1. United Nations (2010) World population ageing 2009. Department of Economic and Social Affairs, Population Division. New York, United Nations.

2. WHO (2002) The world report on violence and health. World Health Organization, Geneva.

3. WHO (2011) European report on preventing elder maltreatment. World Health Organization, Regional Office for Europe, Copenhagen.

4. Cooper C, Selwood A, Livingston G (2008) The prevalence of elder abuse and neglect: a systematic review. Age Ageing 37: 151-160.

5. Acierno R, Hernandez MA, Amstadter AB, Resnick HS, Steve K, et al. (2010) Prevalence and correlates of emotional, physical, sexual, and financial abuse and potential neglect in the United States: the National Elder Mistreatment Study. Am J Public Health 100: 292-297.

6. Lowenstein A, Eisikovits Z, Band-Winterstein T, Enosh G (2009) Is elder abuse and neglect a social phenomenon? Data from the First National Prevalence Survey in Israel. J Elder Abuse Negl 21: 253-277.

7. Macassa G, Viitasara E, Sundin Ö, Barros H, Gonzales FT, et al (2013) Psychological abuse among older persons in Europe: A cross-sectional study. J Aggress Confl Peace Res 5:16-34.

8. AbathMde B, Leal MC, MeloFilho DA, Marques AP (2010) Physical abuse of older people reported at the Institute of Forensic Medicine in Recife, Pernambuco State, Brazil. Cad SaudePublica 26: 1797-1806.

9. Bonnie R, Wallace R (2003) Risk Factors for Elder Mistreatment. In Elder mistreatment: Abuse, neglect, and exploitation in an aging America. Edited by Bonnie R, Wallace R. Washington, DC: The National Academies Press.

10. Dong X, Simon MA (2008) Is greater social support a protective factor against elder mistreatment? Gerontology 54: 381-388.

11. Dong X, Simon M, Mendes de Leon C, Fulmer T, Beck T, et al. (2009) Elder self-neglect and abuse and mortality risk in a community-dwelling population. JAMA 302: 517-526.

12. Dong XQ, Simon MA, Beck TT, Farran C, McCann JJ, et al. (2011) Elder abuse and mortality: the role of psychological and social wellbeing. Gerontology 57: 549-558.

13. Fulmer T, Paveza G, VandeWeerd C, Fairchild S, Guadagno L, et al. (2005) Dyadic vulnerability and risk profiling for elder neglect. Gerontologist 45: 525-534.

14. Lachs MS, Williams CS, O'Brien S, Pillemer KA, Charlson ME (1998) The mortality of elder mistreatment. JAMA 280: 428-432.

15. Lee M, Kolomer SR (2005) Caregiver burden, dementia, and elder abuse in South Korea. J Elder Abuse Negl 17: 61-74.

16. Shugarman LR, Fries BE, Wolf RS, Morris JN (2003) Identifying older people at risk of abuse during routine screening practices. J Am Geriatr Soc 51: 24-31.

17. Cambridge P, Beadle-Brown J, Milne A, Mansell J, Whelton R (2006) Exploring the incidence, risk factors, nature and monitoring of adultprotection alerts. Canterbury: Tizard Centre.

18. McCallum J, Matiasz S, Graycar A (1990) Abuse of the elderly at home: The range of theproblem. National Centre for Epidemiology and Population Health. Canberra.

19. Abbey L (2009) Elder abuse and neglect: when home is not safe. Clin Geriatr Med 25: 47-60, vi.

20. Kim OS, Yang KM, Kim KH (2005) [Dependency, abuse, and depression by gender in widowed elderly]. Taehan Kanho Hakhoe Chi 35: 336-343.

21. Wolf RS (1997) Elder abuse and neglect: causes and consequences. J Geriatr Psychiatry 30: 153-174.

22. Wu L, Chen H, Hu Y, Xiang H, Yu X, et al. (2012) Prevalence and associated factors of elder mistreatment in a rural community in People's Republic of China: a cross-sectional study. PLoS One 7: e33857.

23. Swagerty DL Jr, Takahashi PY, Evans JM (1999) Elder mistreatment. Am Fam Physician 59: 2804-2808.

24. Anderson R, Mikulic B Vermeylen G, Lyly-Yrjanainen M, Zigante V (2009) Second European quality of life survey: Overview. European foundation for the improvement of living and working conditions.

25. KnesebeckOvd, Wahrendorf M, Hyde M, Siegrist J (2007) Socio-economic position and quality of life among older people in 10 European countries: results of the SHARE study. Ageing Soc 27: 269-284.

26. Walker A (2005) Quality of life in old age in Europe. In Growing older in Europe. Editor: Walker A. Suffolk: Open University Press.

27. Watson D, Pichler F, Wallace C (2010) Second European quality of life survey subjective well-being in Europe. European Foundation for the Improvement of Living and Working Conditions.

28. Baumeister H, Hutter N, Bengel J, Härter M (2011) Quality of life in medically ill persons with comorbid mental disorders: a systematic review and meta-analysis. Psychother Psychosom 80: 275-286.

29. Brenes GA (2007) Anxiety, depression, and quality of life in primary care patients. Prim Care Companion J Clin Psychiatry 9: 437-443.

30. Gallegos-Carrillo K, Mudgal J, Sánchez-García S, Wagner FA, Gallo JJ, et al. (2009) Social networks and health-related quality of life: a population based study among older adults. Salud Publica Mex 51: 6-13.

31. Halvorsrud L, Kalfoss M, Diseth Å, Kirkevold M (2012) Quality of life in older Norwegian adults living at home: a cross-sectional survey. J Res Nurs 17: 12–29.

32. Porensky EK, Dew MA, Karp JF, Skidmore E, Rollman BL, et al. (2009) The burden of late-life generalized anxiety disorder: effects on disability, health-related quality of life, and healthcare utilization. Am J Geriatr Psychiatry 17: 473-482.

33. Hawton A, Green C, Dickens AP, Richards SH, Taylor RS, et al. (2011) The impact of social isolation on the health status and health-related quality of life of older people. Qual Life Res 20: 57-67.

34. Fernandez-Ballesteros R (2002) Social support and quality of life among older people in Spain. J Soc Issues 58: 645-659.

35. Dong X, Simon MA, Gorbien M (2007) Elder abuse and neglect in an urban chinese population. J Elder Abuse Negl 19: 79-96.

36. O´ Keeffe M (2007) UK study of abuse and neglect of older people: Prevalencesurvey report. London: Department of health.

37. Lindert J, Luna J, Torres-Gonzalez F, Barros H, Ioannidi-Kapolou E, et al. (2012) Study design, sampling and assessment methods of the European study 'abuse of the elderly in the European region'. Eur J Public Health 22: 662-666.

38. Power M, Quinn K, Schmidt S (2005) Development of the WHOQOL-old module. Qual Life Res 14: 2197-2214.

39. The WHOQOL Group (1994) Development of the WHOQOL: Rationale and current status. Int J Ment Health 23: 24-56.

40. (1995) The World Health Organization Quality of Life assessment (WHOQOL): position paper from the World Health Organization. Soc Sci Med 41: 1403-1409.

41. Power M, Schmidt S, WHOQOL Group (2006) WHOQOL-OLD manual. World Health Organization.

42. Straus MA, Hamby SL, BoneyMcCoy S, Sugarman DB (1996) The revised Conflict Tactics Scales (CTS2). Development and preliminary psychometric data. J Fam Issues 17: 283-316.

43. Brähler E, Scheer JW (1995) Der gießenerbeschwerdebogen (GBB) (2. Aufl). Bern: Huber.

44. Zigmond AS, Snaith RP (1983) The hospital anxiety and depression scale. Acta Psychiatr Scand 67: 361-370.

45. Folkhälsorapport (2007) Folkhälsan i Stockholmslän 2007 [In Swedish]. Stockholm: Centrum förfolkhälsa, Stockholmslänslandsting.

46. Zimet GD, Dahlem NW, Zimet SG, Farley GK (1988) The multidimensional scale of perceived social support. J Pers Assess 52: 30-41.

47. Babor TF, Higgins-Biddle JC, Saunders JB, Monteiro MG (2001) The Alcohol Use Disorders Identification Test: Guidelines for use in primary care. (2ndedn) Geneva: World Health Organization Department of Mental Health and Substance Dependence.

48. Kleinschmidt KC (1997) Elder abuse: a review. Ann Emerg Med 30: 463-472.

49. Luo Y, Waite LJ (2011) Mistreatment and psychological well-being among older adults: exploring the role of psychosocial resources and deficits. J Gerontol B Psychol Sci Soc Sci 66: 217-229.

50. Podkieks E (1992) National survey on abuse of the elderly in Canada. J Elder Abuse Neg l4: 5-58.

51. Gray A (2009) The social capital of older people. Ageing Soc 29: 5-31.

52. Stroebe W (2000) Moderators of the stress-health relationship. In Social psychology and health. Editor: Stroebe W, Philadelphia, PA: Open University Press.

53. Lachs MS, Williams C, O'Brien S, Hurst L, Horwitz R (1997) Risk factors for reported elder abuse and neglect: a nine-year observational cohort study. Gerontologist 37: 469-474.

54. Melchiorre MG, Chiatti C, Lamura G, Torres-Gonzales F, Stankunas M, et al. (2013) Social support, socio-economic status, health and abuse among older people in seven European countries. PLoS One 8: e54856.

55. Molzahn AE, Kalfoss M, Schick Makaroff K, Skevington SM (2011) Comparing the importance of different aspects of quality of life to older adults across diverse cultures. Age Ageing 40: 192-199.

56. Buber I, Kuhn M, Philipov D, Prskawetz A, Schuster J (2010) The economic situation of older cohorts in Europe. Vienna Institute of Demography of the Austrian Academy of Sciences.

57. Low G, Molzahn AE (2007) Predictors of quality of life in old age: a cross-validation study. Res Nurs Health 30: 141-150.

58. Welford C, Murphy K, Wallace M, Casey D (2010) A concept analysis of autonomy for older people in residential care. J Clin Nurs 19: 1226-1235.

59. Haak M (2006) Participation and independence in old age – Aspects of home and neighbourhood environments. InstitutionenförHälsa, VårdochSamhälle, LundsUniversitet, Sverige.

60. Hwang HL, Lin HS, Tung YL, Wu HC (2006) Correlates of perceived autonomy among elders in a senior citizen home: a cross-sectional survey. Int J Nurs Stud 43: 429-437.

61. Matsui M, Capezuti E (2008) Perceived autonomy and self-care resources among senior center users. Geriatr Nurs 29: 141-147.

62. DeLamater J (2012) Sexual expression in later life: a review and synthesis. J Sex Res 49: 125-141.

63. Frankowski AC, Clark LJ (2009) Sexuality and intimacy in assisted living: Residents' perspectives and experiences. Sex Res Social Policy 6: 25-37.

64. Lindau ST, Gavrilova N (2010) Sex, health, and years of sexually active life gained due to good health: evidence from two US population based cross sectional surveys of ageing. BMJ 340: c810.

65. Rheaume C, Mitty E (2008) Sexuality and intimacy in older adults. Geriatr Nurs 29: 342-349.

66. Robinson JG, Molzahn AE (2007) Sexuality and quality of life. J Gerontol Nurs 33: 19-27.

67. Zaidi A, Makovec M, Fuchs M, Lipszyc B, Lelkes O, et al. (2006) Poverty of elderly people in EU25. Vienna: European Centre for Social Welfare Policy and Research.

68. Zaidi A (2010) Poverty risks for older people in EU countries – An Update. Policy Brief Series, Vienna: European Centre for Social Welfare Policy and Research.

69. Orth U, Trzesniewski KH, Robins RW (2010) Self-esteem development from young adulthood to old age: a cohort-sequential longitudinal study. J Pers Soc Psychol 98: 645-658.

70. Robins RW, Trzesniewski KH (2005) Self-esteem development across the lifespan. Curr Dir Psychol Sci14: 158-162.

71. Fokkema T, De Jong Gierveld J, Dykstra PA (2012) Cross-national differences in older adult loneliness. J Psychol 146: 201-228.

72. Sundström G, Fransson E, Malmberg B, Davey A (2009) Loneliness among older Europeans. Eur J Ageing 6:267-275.

73. Kalfoss M, Halvorsrud L (2009) Important issues to quality of life among norwegian older adults: an exploratory study. Open Nurs J 3: 45-55.

74. Babatsikou F, Zavatsanou A (2010) Epidemiology of hypertension in the elderly. Health Sci J 4: 24-30.

Quality of Life among Persons Aged 60-84 Years in Europe: The Role of Psychological Abuse...

121

75. Blazer DG (2009) Depression in late life: Review and commentary. Focus 7: 118-136.

76. Breivik H, Collett B, Ventafridda V, Cohen R, Gallacher D (2006) Survey of chronic pain in Europe: prevalence, impact on daily life, and treatment. Eur J Pain 10: 287-333.

77. Hawthorne G (2008) Perceived social isolation in a community sample: its prevalence and correlates with aspects of peoples' lives. Soc Psychiatry Psychiatr Epidemiol 43: 140-150.

78. Jemal A, Bray F, Center MM, Ferlay J, Ward E, et al. (2011) Global cancer statistics. CA Cancer J Clin 61: 69-90.

79. Lenze EJ, Wetherell JL (2011) A lifespan view of anxiety disorders. Dialogues ClinNeurosci 13: 381-399.

80. Shaw JE, Sicree RA, Zimmet PZ (2010) Global estimates of the prevalence of diabetes for 2010 and 2030. Diabetes Res Clin Pract 87: 4-14.

81. Iliffe S, Kharicha K, Harari D, Swift C, Gillmann G, et al. (2007) Health risk appraisal in older people 2: the implications for clinicians and commissioners of social isolation risk in older people. Br J Gen Pract 57: 277-282.

82. Lloyd-Jones D, Adams R, Carnethon M, De Simone G, Ferguson TB, et al. (2009) Heart disease and stroke statistics--2009 update: a report from the American Heart Association Statistics Committee and Stroke Statistics Subcommittee. Circulation 119: 21-181.

83. James BD, Wilson RS, Barnes LL, Bennett DA (2011) Late-life social activity and cognitive decline in old age. J Int Neuropsychol Soc 17: 998-1005.

84. Kendler KS, Myers J, Prescott CA (2005) Sex differences in the relationship between social support and risk for major depression: a longitudinal study of opposite-sex twin pairs. Am J Psychiatry 162: 250-256.

85. Brockmann H, Klein T (2004) Love and death in Germany: The marital biography and its effect on mortality. J Marriage Fam 66: 567-581.

86. Di Tella R, MacCulloch RJ, Oswald AJ (2003)The macroeconomics of Happiness. Rev Econ Stat 85:809-827.

87. Diener E, Gohm C, Suh E, Oishi S (2000) Similarity of the relations between marital status and subjective well-being across cultures. J Cross Cul Psychol 31: 419-436.

88. Koball H, Moiduddin E, Henderson J, Goesling B, Besculides M (2010) What do we know about the link between marriage and health? J Fam Issues 31: 1019-1040.

89. Schoenborn CA (2004) Marital Status and Health: United States, 1999-2002. Adv Data 15: 1-32.

90. Wilson CM, Oswald AJ (2005) How does marriage affect physical and psychological health? A survey of the longitudinal evidence. IZA Discussion Paper No. 1619.

91. Wood RG, Goesling B, Avellar S (2007) The effects of marriage on health: A synthesis of recent research evidence. Princeton, NJ: Mathematica Policy Research.

92. Silverstein M, Gans D (2006) Intergenerational support to aging parents: The role of norms and needs. J Fam Issues 27: 1068-1084.

93. Turagabeci AR, Nakamura K, Kizuki M, Takano T (2007) Family structure and health, how companionship acts as a buffer against ill health. Health Qual Life Outcomes 5: 61.

94. Ryan AK, Willits FK (2007) Family ties, physical health, and psychological well-being. J Aging Health 19: 907-920.

95. Guedes DP, Hatmann AC, Martini FA, Borges MB, Bernardelli R Jr (2012) Quality of life and physical activity in a sample of Brazilian older adults. J Aging Health 24: 212-226.

96. Bowles S, Durlauf S, Hoff K (2006) Poverty traps. Princeton University Press.

97. Lacey EA, Walters SJ (2003) Continuing inequality: gender and social class influences on self perceived health after a heart attack. J Epidemiol Community Health 57: 622-627.

98. Marmot M, Wilkinson R (2006) Social determinants of health, (2ndedn). Oxford: Oxford University Press.

99. Krause NM, Jay GM (1994) What do global self-rated health items measure? Med Care 32: 930-942.

100. Berkman L, Kawachi I (2000) Social epidemiology. New York: Oxford University Press.

101. Wilkinson R, Pickett K (2010) The spirit levelwhy more equal societies almost always do better. London: Penguin Books.

102. Al-Windi A (2005) The relations between symptoms, somatic and psychiatric conditions, life satisfaction and perceived health. A primary care based study. Health Qual Life Outcomes 3: 28.

103. Hoedeman R, Blankenstein AH, Krol B, Koopmans PC, Groothoff JW (2010) The contribution of high levels of somatic symptom severity to sickness absence duration, disability and discharge. J Occup Rehabil 20: 264-273.

104. Ihlebaek C, Eriksen HR, Ursin H (2002) Prevalence of subjective health complaints (SHC) in Norway. Scand J Public Health 30: 20-29.

105. Eurostat (2008) The life of women and men in Europe: A statistical portrait. Luxembourg: Eurostat.

106. Grundy E (2006)Ageing and vulnerable elderly people: European perspectives. Ageing Soc 26: 105–134.

107. Winquist K (2002) Women and men beyond retirement. Statistics in focus, population and social conditions, Luxembourg: Eurostat.

108. Chiao C, Weng LJ, Botticello AL (2012) Economic strain and well-being in late life: findings from an 18-year population-based Longitudinal Study of older Taiwanese adults. J Public Health (Oxf) 34: 217-227.

109. Fryers T, Melzer D, Jenkins R (2003) Social inequalities and the common mental disorders: a systematic review of the evidence. Soc Psychiatry Psychiatr Epidemiol 38: 229-237.

110. Hall SE, Williams JA, Senior JA, Goldswain PR, Criddle RA (2000) Hip fracture outcomes: quality of life and functional status in older adults living in the community. Aust N Z J Med 30: 327-332.

111. Ladin K, Daniels N, Kawachi I (2010) Exploring the relationship between absolute and relative position and late-life depression: evidence from 10 European countries. Gerontologist 50: 48-59.

112. Mikulic B, Sándor E, Leoncikas T (2012) Experiencing the economic crisis in the EU: Changes in living standards, deprivation and trust. European Foundation for the Improvement of Living and Working Conditions.

113. Sampaio PY, Ito E (2013) Activities with higher influence on quality of life in older adults in Japan. Occup Ther Int 20: 1-10.

114. Paskulin L, Vianna L, Molzahn AE (2009) Factors associated with quality of life of Brazilian older adults. Int Nurs Rev 56: 109-115.

115. Blood R, Wolfe D (1960) Husbands and wives: The dynamics of married living. New York: Free Press.

116. Ferree MM (1990) Beyond separate spheres: Feminism and family research. J Marriage Fam 52: 866-884.

117. Pahl J (1990) Household spending, personal spending and the control of money in marriage. Sociology 24: 119-138.

118. Brennan RT, Barnett RC, Gareis KC (2001) When she earns more than he does: A longitudinal study of dual-earner couples. J Marriage Fam 63: 168-182.

119. Pappenheim H, Graves G (2005) Bringing home the bacon: Making marriage work when she makes more money. New York: William Morrow.

120. Umberson D, Williams K, Powers DA, Liu H, Needham B (2006) You make me sick: marital quality and health over the life course. J Health Soc Behav 47: 1-16.

121. Springer KW (2010) Do wives' work hours hurt husbands' health? Reassessing the care work deficit thesis. Soc Sci Res 39: 801-813.

122. Anderson P, Baumberg B (2006) Alcohol in Europe. London: Institute of Alcohol Studies.

123. Holahan CJ, Schutte KK, Brennan PL, Holahan CK, Moos BS, et al. (2010) Late-life alcohol consumption and 20-year mortality. Alcohol Clin Exp Res 34: 1961-1971.

124. Kaplan MS, Huguet N, Feeny D, McFarland BH, Caetano R, et al. (2012) Alcohol use patterns and trajectories of health-related quality of life in middle-aged and older adults: a 14-year population-based study. J Stud Alcohol Drugs 73: 581-590.

125. Paganini-Hill A, Kawas CH, Corrada MM (2007) Type of alcohol consumed, changes in intake over time and mortality: the Leisure World Cohort Study. Age Ageing 36: 203-209.

126. Bowling A, Iliffe S (2011) Psychological approach to successful ageing predicts future quality of life in older adults. Health Qual Life Outcomes 9: 13.

127. de Belvis AG, Avolio M, Spagnolo A, Damiani G, Sicuro L, et al. (2008) Factors associated with health-related quality of life: the role of social relationships among the elderly in an Italian region. Public Health 122: 784-793.

128. George LK (2006) Perceived Quality of Life. In Handbook of aging and the social sciences.(6thedn), Editors: Binstock RH, George LK. San Diego, CA: Elsevier.

129. White AM, Philogene GS, Fine L, Sinha S (2009) Social support and self-reported health status of older adults in the United States. Am J Public Health 99: 1872-1878.

130. Martinez-Martin P, Prieto-Flores M, Forjaz MJ, Fernandez-Mayorales G, Rojo-Perez F, et al. (2012) Components and determinants of quality of life in community-dwelling older adults. Eur J Ageing 9: 255-263.

131. Cohen S, Wills TA (1985) Stress, social support, and the buffering hypothesis. Psychol Bull 98: 310-357.

132. Gureje O, Kola L, Ademola A, Olley BO (2009) Profile, comorbidity and impact of insomnia in the Ibadan study of ageing. Int J Geriatr Psychiatry 24: 686-693.

133. LeBlanc M, Mérette C, Savard J, Ivers H, Baillargeon L, et al. (2009) Incidence and risk factors of insomnia in a population-based sample. Sleep 32: 1027-1037.

134. Faubel R, Lopez-Garcia E, Guallar-Castillón P, Balboa-Castillo T, Gutiérrez-Fisac JL, et al. (2009) Sleep duration and health-related quality of life among older adults: a population-based cohort in Spain. Sleep 32: 1059-1068.

135. Lo CM, Lee PH (2012) Prevalence and impacts of poor sleep on quality of life and associated factors of good sleepers in a sample of older Chinese adults. Health Qual Life Outcomes 10: 72.

22

Speech-Language Disorders in Children with Hearing Loss Connected with Otitis Media with Effusion

Broz Frajtag Jasenka*

Department for Otolaryngology, University Clinical Hospital Center, Croatia

Abstract

Introduction: Otitis media with effusion is accompanied with conductive hearing loss. The aim of the study is to find out effect of long term or recurrent conductive hearing loss on speech descrimination.

Method: Tonal audiometry timpanometry, speech audiometry (free sound field, head phone for left and right ear respectively) performed in 18 girls (mean age 8 years) and 27 boys (mean age 7 year). All of the children undergo speech/language screening tests.

Results: Results of speech recognition showed no ear side effect in girls and right ear advantage in boys. Girls showed earlier in age central auditory processing disorder. Boys showed lower scores in words discrimination while hearing throught the head-phones on left ear. Poorer speech recognition at boys is accompanied with motorical immaturty, undeveloped articulation, poor vocabulary, lack of syntax in sentences, substitution of R and L, unable to focus on school tusk.

Conclusion: Children with conductive hearing loss associated to otitis media with effusion are pronounced auditory processing disorder and speech/language discrimination disturbance. Associative thinking and solving of abstract problems are more affected in females than males.

Keywords: Conductive hearing loss; Speech discrimination; Effusion; Otitis

Introduction

Communication disorders are the most frequent health problem world-wide. Hearing loss is the most common birth defect and needs emergency audiologic intervention otherwise sequels have implications not only on speech and language and cognition development delay, but also social adaptation, academic skills, behavior, motoric skills, learning problems, communication in noise background is difficult. Central auditory processing disorder results from hearing developmental disorder because of long term central auditory processing disorder and lack of processing in some frequencies, especially speech frequencies. Most common symptom is difficulty of speech discrimination in the back-ground noise and balance in space, even when hearing level is normal. Hearing loss, during development, leads to central deficit that persists even after the restoration of peripheral function [1]. Although these effects are particularly severe following long period of auditory deprivation, even the temporary elevation of thresholds can disrupt auditory processing, the most frequent birth defect in humans. It can be difficult to recognize and often goes undetected until the child is older. Such children should be tested for hearing impairment as soon after birth as possible.

Otitis media with effusion is accompanied with conductive hearing loss. The aim of the study is to find out effect of long term or recurrent conductive hearing loss on speech descrimination. OME associated with conductive hearing loss is the most frequent disease in childhood with incidence of 80% until 3 years of age fluid in the middle ear and edema of the mucosa present in the otitis media with effusion disrupts transmission of the acoustic sound from the outside through the middle ear to the cochlea.

Aims of Performed Study

Aims of performed study is to investigate influence of long term peripheral hearing loss on primary auditory cortical function, receptive and expression language; possible gender, age and ear side influence and accordingly possible further sequels on cognition and behavior.

Method

To find out capability of speech discrimination and central auditory processing we performed retrospective research study in group children suffer from hearing loss associated with otitis media with effusion. For testing of negative effect of fluid in the middle ear and possible effect to central auditory processing, receptive and expressive language, changing of behavior in the presence of the sound and cognition we carried out our research study based on results of audiologic testing and speech-pathologic testing (Speech Audiometry-We scored expressive speech and defiend if exist diferences between left ear, right ear and free field, *Clinical Evaluation of Language fundamentals*-evaluaties understanding and use of language including word meaning (semantics), word and sentence structure (sintax) and retrieval of spoken language (auditory memory) of children, *Picture Vocabulary test*-picture naming, test which measures a childs naming (expressive vocabulary skills) of our patients who are in audiologic follow-up and permanent speech and language rehabilitation program.

Tonal audiometry timpanometry, speech audiometry (free sound field, head phone for left and right ear respectively) performed in 18

***Corresponding author:** Broz Frajtag Jasenka, Professor, Department for Otolaryngology, University Clinical Hospital Center, Zagreb, Rebro, Kišpatićeva 12, Croatia, E-mail: brozfrajtag@gmail.com

girls (mean age 8 years) and 27 boys (mean age 7 year). Results were analyzed statistically with SPSS 7 program for Word.

Results

Preliminary results of our study showed that characteristics of conductive hearing loss associated with otitis media with effusion according to gender, age and ear side have different damage of speech understanding and different level of developmental development of cognition and fine motor development of hand. Secondary effects and disorders which came out as results of unrecognized conductive hearing loss associated with otitis media with effusion are clinically more complicated for treatment and rehabilitation and can last even for 2 years after peripheral hearing loss which have been restored. Incidence of boys (60%) in this random study was higher than in girls (40%) (Figure 1).

Boys were older than girls for mean age of 2-5 years. Girls displayed central auditory processing disorders continuously from earlier age than boys. Frequency increases and reaches peak around 5 years of age, decreases from age of 6 years to the older ages but maintained equalized and permanent up to adolescence [2]. Boys started to display central auditory processing disorders at 7 years of age and maintains permanent but not equalized frequency with relapsed that matched with relapses of the otitis media (Table 1). Tonal audiometry showed in male and female groups a higher level of hearing loss for lower frequencies (500 Hz, 1000 Hz) than for high frequencies (2000 Hz, 4000 Hz) ($p=0.008$) (Table 2).

Frequency of 1000 Hz has the highest level of hearing loss in both genders. Females displayed on both ears for 4000 Hz higher level of hearing loss than males do average hearing threshold for speech frequencies in tested groups of ears do not excides 27 dB for left and 26 dB for right ears (Figures 2 and 3). Females shows for both ear side higher average of hearing loss at speech frequencies than males ($p=0.0052$). Speech audiometry shows no significant difference in females between speech discrimination threshold in free sound field and each ear separately when tested by the help of earphones ($p=0.891$). There was also no ear side advantage (Table 2). Females, if compared with males, have a higher level of speech discrimination threshold in free sound field and for right ($p=0.016$) and left ear separately, when tested by the help of earphones. In males, right ears when tested by the help of earphones, showed better speech discrimination threshold than their left ears and threshold in free sound filed. Right ears in males showed advantage when reaching 100% in speech discrimination test if compared with left ears of males ($p=0.016$) and both side of ears in females ($p=0.012$, $p=0.008$).

Girls showed earlier in age central auditory processing disorder. Boys showed lower scores in words discrimination while hearing throught the head-phones on left ear. Poorer speech recognition at boys is accompanied with motorical immaturty, undeveloped articulation, poor vocabulary, lack of syntax in sentences, substitution of "R and L", unable to focus on school tusk. Handzic and all showed ear side related differences of hearing loss in OME children with orofacial clefts and out of malformations. Previous studies indicated that CHL (conductive hearing loss) profoundly affects short term synaptic depression and spike adaptation, increases synaptic latencies and evoked postsynaptic potentials were longer and more variable [3]. Females have advantage in process of hearing, it was not described if there exist gender differences in sensitivity for hearing loss in case of prolonged presence of conductive hearing loss to the central auditory processing. Impact of milder forms of conductive hearing loss on the auditory cortex is still

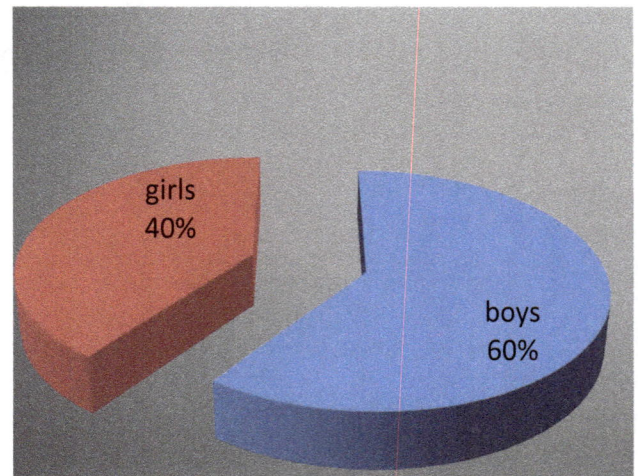

Figure 1: Sex distribution.

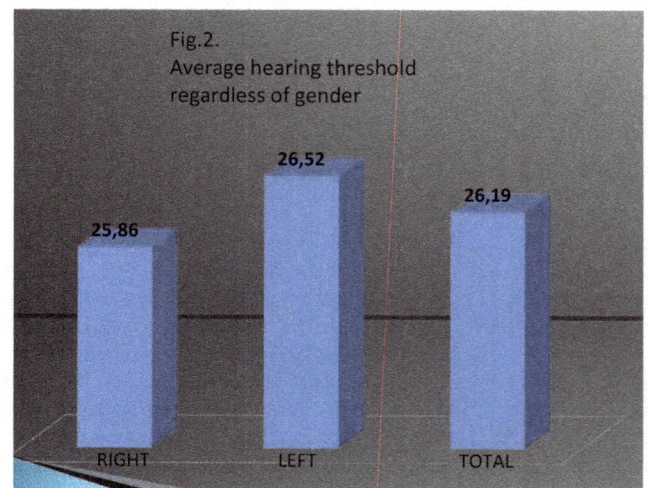

Figure 2: Average hearing threshold regardless of gender.

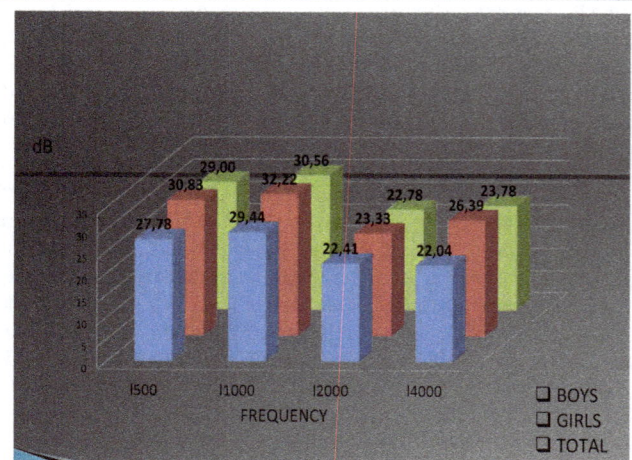

Figure 3: Average hearing threshold–left ear.

Age/Year	3	4	5	6	7	8	9	10	11	12	13	14	Min	Max	Average	N
Boys	0	0	0	7	4	2	3	2	1	1	2	1	6	14	8.52	23
Girls	1	3	5	2	0	2	0	1	0	1	1	0	3	13	6.44	16
Total	1	3	5	9	4	4	3	3	1	2	3	1	3	14	7.69	39

Table 1: Distribution of boys and girls longitudinally according to aging.

Gender	Speech audiometry Free sound field 10 words list Speech discrimination threshold dB	Speech audiometry Free sound field 10 words list 100% words discrimination threshold dB	Speech audiometry Headphones right ear 10 words list Speech discrimination threshold dB	Speech audiometry Headphones left ear 10 words list Speech discrimination threshold dB	One-way ANOVA p-level	Speech audiometry right ear 10 words list 100% words discrimination dB	Speech audiometry left ear 10 words list 100% words discrimination dB	One-way ANOVA p-level
Male	17.04	42.96	12.41	15.74	0.169	36.11	42.78	0.016
SD	8.80	10.94	8.13	9.38	-	9.94	9.74	-
Female	20.83	44.72	20.00	20.56	0.891	45.56	46.67	0.799
SD	9.12	11.18	12.25	11.87	-	14.13	11.76	-
One-way ANOVA p-level	0.169	0.603	0.016	0.137	-	0.012	0.234	-
Total	28.11	29.44	22.67	29.00	0.029	23.22	30.56	0.008
SD	12.85	15.75	12.14	11.71	-	16.38	13.02	-

Table 2: Speech audiometry testing-results for free sound field and headphones for each ear separately, thresholds and 100% discrimination.

undefined. Children with otitis media with effusin they have difficulties in pronunciation dyslalila. Damage in pronunciation become in profile of omission, supstitution and distortion, almoust always mistake in frikatives and afrikates, poor vocabular of children in social less environment, disorders in perception and behavior (hyperactivity) (Figure 4).

Conclusion

Children with conductive hearing loss associated to otitis media with effusion are pronounced auditory processing disorder and speech/language discrimination disturbance. Associative thinking and solving of abstract problems are more affected in females than males. Prevention of hearing loss and secondary effects with irreversible sequels is one of the most important goals because of its high incidence in early childhood and orofacial malformations. Preschool and school preventive testing would be performed and children with disorders or disbalances would be included in program creating to their needs. Males at age of 8.5 years and females at age 6.5 years do not show lateralization of the peripheral hearing loss for the average hearing loss on speech frequencies

In both gender lower frequencies of 500 Hz and 1000 Hz displayed higher level of hearing loss, male shows improvement of hearing level on 2000 Hz and 4000 Hz, females showed higher level of hearing loss at 2000 Hz and 4000 Hz than males with no improvement with aging.

In female's development of receptive and expressive language started from the early childhood, earlier than in males became developmental priority, reaches peak at the age of 5 years when dominate cognitive disorder and after that frequency keeps continuing through the adolescence. Males displayed later than females disorders of receptive and expressive language as results of central auditory processing disorder which starts and reach peaks at the age of 6 years, then frequency keeps continuing through the adolescence with tendency of relapsing at the ages which matches with ages when hearing loss associated with OME relapses. In males at earlier age dominant symptoms of central auditory disorder are behavioral problems and spatial disorientation, males displayed later than females receptive and expressive language

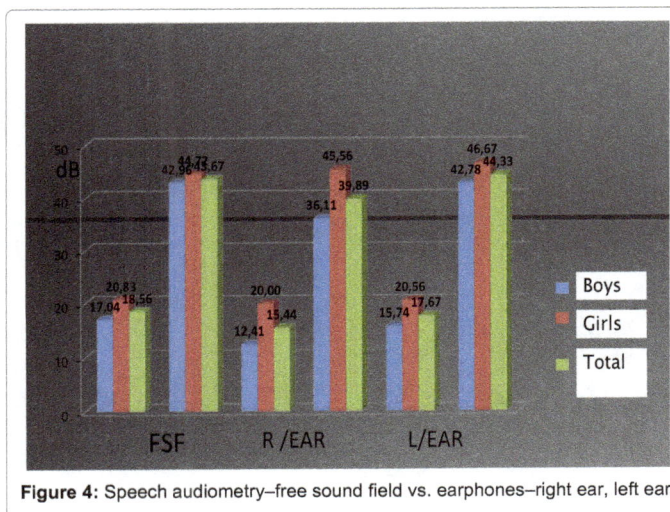

Figure 4: Speech audiometry–free sound field vs. earphones–right ear, left ear.

disturbance which are mostly overlooked until preschool age when verbal skills, syntax of sentences and articulation started to be important. Females display diffuse central auditory processing damage, both intra-hemisphere and inter-hemisphere auditory processing damage which influence to the quality of solving math and spoken language skills in the school and displayed no laterality. Males display central auditory processing disorder laterality with domination of left intra-hemispheric processing damage and females displayed no laterality. Central processing disorder in females mostly affect cognition while in boys affect more behavior than cognition.

Summary

Males and females show central auditory processing and left hemispheric processing differences in quality according to the advantage of the right ear in the males and no ear advantage in the females. Aging have negative effects in girls if exist speech-language disorders. Girls have more problems with solving mathematics problems while boys have more problems in classes of spelling and reading of maternal language. Both groups have problems with syntax of sequences and speech articulation particularly fricatives. Some of them have problems in behavior and have delay in learning if compare with counterparts with no hearing problems.

Both groups male and female children, which is also described in literature, have had deficit of attention, motor skills, untidy handwriting, missed information's in school because children are unable to be focus on the problem, misbehavior and low rate of social adaptation. Deficit of attention and hyperkinetic behavior in such children are not entity per se but sign of developmental motor delay. Most of children in early childhood, preschool and school age have communication problems which are not recognized and need urgent audiologic rehabilitation-habilitation to prevent permanent sequel in cognition, behavior, spatial orientation social adaptation and academic skills.

References

1. Handzic J, Radic B, Bagatin T, Savic A, Stambolija V, et al. (2012) Hearing in children with otitis media with effusion-clinical retrospective study. Coll Antropol 36: 1273-1277.

2. Isaacson G (2016) Acute Otitis Media and the Crying Child. Pediatr Infect Dis J.

3. Schilder AG, Chonmaitree T, Cripps AW, Rosenfeld RM, Casselbrant ML, et al. (2016) Otitis media. Nat Rev Dis Primers 2: 16063.

23

Stress and Coping among the Parents of Children with Congenital Heart Disease

Babita Singh* and Pratima Ghimire

National Medical College Nursing Campus, Birgunj, Nepal

Abstract

Introduction: Congenital heart defects are the most common, pervasive and serious chronic illness of all congenital malformations. The birth of a child can be stressful enough for many parents, turn into one of dashed joy and feeling of distress so there may be necessary for parents to obtain enough support from health professionals.

Methods: A descriptive Correlational study was conducted among 142 parents of children with Congenital Heart Disease attending Pediatric Medical Out Patient Department in Shahid Gangalal National Heart Center, Bansbari, Kathmandu. Data were collected using pre-tested structured interview schedule in Nepali version. The obtained data were analyzed by descriptive statistics (frequency, percentage, mean and standard deviation) and inferential statistics (chi-square and Karl Pearson's coefficient of correlation).

Results: The findings of the study revealed that near about three forth (71.8%) of parents had moderately level of stress whereas 28.2% had low level of stress and 79.6% had moderately helpful level of coping and 20.4% had minimally helpful level of coping. There was negative correlation between stress and coping (r=-0.076 and p-value=0.367) of parents. There were no any statistical association between socio-demographic characteristics of parents and stress level. Similarly, there were statistically significant association of level of coping with relationship with child, religion and occupation of parents (p-value 0.004, 0.002 and 0.005) respectively.

Conclusion: The study concluded that with increased level of stress, there is decreased level of coping among the parents. Further, the findings suggest that health personnel must assess parenting stress at each visit to provide appropriate support and anticipatory guidance to families of children with Congenital Heart Disease.

Keywords: Stress; Coping; Parents; Children with congenital heart disease

Introduction

A new baby is the beginning of wonders, hopes and dreams and becoming parents is one of life's greatest blessings. A parent's dream of giving birth to the perfect child but the birth of a child with congenital heart disease challenges those dreams. This forces families to deal with a crisis for which they may be completely unprepared. Discovering one's child has a disability causes major stress, this can disrupt the total family functioning [1].

Congenital heart disease (CHD) is now estimated to be the second most prevalent chronic illness may have effects that pervasive consequence for family life. Recently, focused on resiliency variables, especially support and coping strategy, regulating the impact of stress. In the resiliency model of family stress, adjustment and adaptation, social support is viewed as one of the primary mediators between stress and well-being [2].

India has a large population with a perceived incidence of congenital heart disease in 8 per 1000 live births in children; nearly 180,000 kids are born yearly with this problem. Of these 60,000 to 90,0000 are critical and need early treatment. Nearly 10% of the infant mortality seen is due to congenital heart defects. As the number of centers capable of handling this is very few, a huge number of children are added to this pool each year of Congenital Heart Disease [3].

It can be a great burden for parents to be informed that their child is suffering from heart disease. The whole family might be affected and might undergo a stressful adjustment process, experiencing challenges such as attempting to understand the disease's effects, coping with uncertainty, and seeking reassurance from healthcare providers. Experiences such as somatization, depression, anxiety, distress,

hopelessness, and social isolation can also arise. Mothers might also feel guilt and might wrongly blame themselves or they might feel frustration over not having a healthy baby. Those who have multiple children might additionally experience neglecting the healthy children [4].

Parents of children with heart disease were more likely than the normative population to report excessive parenting stress, especially related to characteristics of the child that make them difficult to parent. These parents expressed difficulty with setting limits or discipline of the child with heart disease. Parenting stress was related to the severity of the child's heart disease, family socioeconomic status, or time since most recent surgery. Clinicians must assess parenting stress at each health care visit to provide appropriate support and anticipatory guidance to families of children with heart disease [5].

The objectives of the present study were to find out the level of stress and coping, to determine the relationship between stress and coping among the parents of children with Congenital Heart Disease and to find out the association of level of stress and level of coping with selected socio demographic variables.

---

*Corresponding author: Babita Singh, National Medical College Nursing Campus, Birgunj, Nepal, E-mail: bobysin71@hotmail.com

Materials and Methods

A descriptive Correlational study was conducted among 142 parents of children with Congenital Heart Disease attending Pediatric Medical Out Patient Department in Shahid Gangalal National Heart Center, (SGNHC) Bansbari, Kathmandu. Non-probability purposive sampling technique was adopted to select 142 parents as a sample for this study. Sample size was calculated at 95% confidence level and 5% confidence interval. The prevalence of children with Congenital Heart Disease (AVSD) being 10.3% [6]. The Inclusion criteria for the sample were Parents of children with the age of 6 months - 15 years having Congenital Heart Disease, who were able to speak and understand Nepali and had stayed at least for 6 months with the child as a primary caregiver. A total of 142 parents were interviewed from dated 31st January 2016 to 27th February 2016 by using pretested structured interview schedule which was developed in consultation with eleven expertise in the related field. Data were collected after getting ethical clearance from Institutional Review Committee (IRC) National Medical College and Teaching Hospital, (NMCTH) Birgunj and IRC of SGNHC, Bansbari, Kathmandu. The collected data were organized and coded and entered in Epi.data 3.1 and export to IBM Statistical Package for Social Science (SPSS 20) version and appropriate statistical tests were performed to draw the inference

Results

The findings of the study revealed that majorities (54.2%) of the parents were father, 43.0% were mother, and the least (2.8%) were primary care-givers. Half of respondents (50%) belonged to the range of 31-40 age groups. Similarly, 58% were male and 41% female. More than half (57%) of them were Hindu, followed by Buddhist (26.8%) and others (0.7%). Likewise, 23% of the respondents were educated up to secondary level, 18.3% were educated up to higher secondary and the least 3.5% were master and above. Near about one forth (22.5%) parents were home-makers and 9.2% were Governmental officers. More than half (54.9 %) were living in Urban whereas 16.2% were living in Semi-urban. Half of the respondents (50.0%) were from nuclear family and 3.5% were from extended family. Similarly, 54.9% had three members in family and 41.5% parents had a monthly family income of NRs. 5000-15,000 monthly.

Regarding the socio-demographic of child, 28.2% belonged to the age group of 3-6 years. More than half (57.7%) were male and 42.3% were female. Among the number of siblings, 51.4% had two siblings. Likewise, the type of disease, 33.1% had Atrial Septal defect and 57% were diagnosed at the age of below 1 year. Similarly, numbers of hospitalization, 50.0% of the children were admitted 1-3 times.

Data presented in Table 1 depicts, area-wise stress among the parents, which shows that parents were having more physical stress with mean percentage score (45.25) followed by family and work stress with mean percentage score (35.8), psychological stress with mean percentage score (35.64) and financial stress with mean percentage score (26.66). Data presented in Table 2 reveals that near about three forth (71.8%) of parents had moderately level of stress whereas 28.2% had low level of stress.

Data presented in Table 3 shows the area-wise coping score among the parents, which shows that parents were having more coping on understanding the health care situation through communication with other parents and consultation with the health care team with mean percent score (41.22) followed by maintaining social support, self-esteem and psychological stability with mean percent score (35.77) and family integration, cooperation and an optimistic definition of the situation with mean percent score (33.41).

Data presented in Table 4 reveals that 79.6% had moderately helpful level of coping and 20.4% had minimally helpful level of coping among Parents of Children with Congenital Heart Disease.

Data presented in Table 5 illustrates that there is negative correlation between Stress and Coping among the parents of Children with Congenital Heart Disease with r=-0.076 and p-value=0.367 which was not statistically significant.

Data presented in Table 6, declaims that there was statistical positive correlation between financial stress and understanding health care situation as well as in family and work stress and total coping with r=0.189* and r=0.212* with p-value 0.024 and 0.011 respectively. Likewise, there were statistical negative correlation between family and work stress and maintaining social support, self-esteem and psychological stability as well as in family and work stress and understanding health care situation with r=-0.210* and r=-0.235** with p-value 0.012 and 0.005 respectively.

The study findings also revealed that there were no any statistical association between socio-demographic characteristics of parents and stress level. Similarly, there were statistically significant association of level of coping with relationship with child, religion and occupation of parents (p-value 0.004, 0.002 and 0.005) respectively.

Discussion

Regarding the socio-demographic characteristics of the parents of children with Congenital Heart Disease attending medical OPD of SGNHC revealed that 54.2% were father, 43.0% were mother and only 2.8% were primary care givers whose aged ranged from 31-40 years. More than half 58% were male and 41% female. Similarly, 57% of them were Hindu, followed by Buddhist (26.8%) and others (0.7%). Likewise, 23% of the parents were educated up to secondary level, 18.3% were educated up to higher secondary and the least 3.5% were master and above. Near about one forth (22.5%) parents were home-makers and 9.2% were Governmental officers. More than half (54.9 %) were living in Urban whereas 16.2% were living in Semi-urban. Half of the respondents (50.0%) were nuclear family and 3.5% were extended family. Similarly, 54.9% had three members in the family.

Regarding the socio-demographic of child information, 28.2% belonged to the age group of 3-6 years. More than half (57.7%) were male and 42.3% were female. Among the number of siblings, 51.4% had two siblings. Likewise, the type of disease, 33.1% had Atrial Septal defect and 57%were diagnosed at the age of below 1 year. Similarly regarding the numbers of hospitalization, 50.0% of the children were admitted 1-3 times.

Sub-scales	Mean Score ± SD	Percentage of mean Score	Range	Maximum Possible Score
Physical stress	9.05 ± 1.55	45.25	4-13	20
Psychological stress	16.04 ± 3.89	35.64	9-31	45
Family and work stress	12.53 ± 3.69	35.8	7-22	35
Financial stress	4.19 ± 1.58	26.66	3-11	15

Table 1: Stress score according to sub-scales among parents of children with congenital heart disease (n=142).

Level of stress	Frequency	Percentage
Moderate stress	102	71.8
Low stress	40	28.2

Table 2: Level of stress score among parents of children with congenital heart disease. n=142.

Area-wise Sub-scale	Mean score ± SD	Percent of mean Score	Range	Maximum possible score
Family Integration, Cooperation and an Optimistic Definition of the Situation	26.73 ± 3.13	33.41	21-40	80
Maintaining Social Support, Self –esteem and Psychological Stability	35.77 ± 3.32	35.77	29-44	100
Understanding the Health Care Situation through Communication with other Parents and Consultation with the Health Care Team	18.55 ± 1.86	41.22	13-24	45

Table 3: Coping score according to sub-scale among parents of children with congenital heart disease. n=142.

Level of Coping	Frequency	Percentage
Minimally helpful	29	20.4
Moderately helpful	113	79.6

Table 4: Level of Coping among parents of children with congenital heart disease. n=142.

Characteristics	Mean score ± SD	Correlation	p-value
Stress	41.83 ± 7.15	-0.076	0.367
Coping	81.07 ± 7.16		

Table 5: Correlation between stress and coping score among the parents of children with congenital heart disease. n=142.

Stress / Coping	Physical stress	Psychological stress	Family and work stress	Financial stress	Total stress
Family Integration, Cooperation and an Optimistic Definition of the Situation	0.057 (0.501)	0.051 (0.548)	-0.122 (0.148)	-0.011 (0.896)	-0.025 (0.764)
Maintaining Social Support, Self –esteem and Psychological Stability	-0.0017 (0.843)	0.028 (0.740)	-0.210* (0.012)	0.143 (0.089)	-0.065 (0.440)
Understanding the Health Care Situation through Communication with other Parents and Consultation with the Health care Team	-0.067 (0.426)	-0.073 (0.390)	-0.235** (0.005)	0.189* (0.024)	-0.134 (0.112)
Total coping	0.000 (0.997)	0.016 (0.846)	0.212* (0.011)	0.111 (0.189)	-0.076 (0.367)

*Statistically Significant at the level of (p=0.05); **Statistically Significant at the level of (p=0.01)

Table 6: Correlation between sub-scales of stress and coping among the parents of children with congenital heart disease. n=142.

Regarding level of stress, result revealed that majority of parents (71.8%) had moderate stress and 28.2% parents had low stress. This finding was supported by the study findings of Katherine, which showed moderate (58.3%), followed by high (25%) and low (16.7%) level of stress in parents of children with Congenital Heart Disease.

Regarding the level of coping, majority (79.6%) had moderately helpful level of coping and 20.4% had minimally helpful level of coping among parents of children with Congenital heart disease. Findings of the study is supported by the study conducted by Sullivan and Kathryn [7], which reported coping strategies related to maintaining family integration and an optimistic definition were significantly associated with spirituality. By being able to recognize factors associated with parental coping the medical and social support community able to better facilitate positive coping mechanisms for parents of children with CHD which was concluded that there was moderately helpful of the coping patterns.

Regarding the correlation between stress and coping, there were negative correlation between stress and coping with r=-0.076 and p-value=0.367. The findings of the study were supported by the study

findings of Katherine Jo Greshik [8-19] which reported negative correlation between stresses and coping.

Conclusion

On the basis of findings, it can be concluded that there was moderate level of stress and moderately helpful of coping pattern among the parents of children with Congenital Heart Disease and negative correlation between stress and coping. There were no association between stress and socio-demographic characteristics of parents and there was only significant association between coping and relation with child, religion and occupation of the parents. So, it is recommended that the health professionals must assess the parenting stress at each follow up to promote appropriate support, guidance and counseling to the parents of children with Congenital Heart Disease.

References

1. Margaret M (2008) A Descriptive Study to Assess the Level of Stress and its Association with the Quality of Life of Parents having Children with Major Congenital Anomalies. Indira Gandhi Institute of Child Health, Bangalore.

2. Tak YR, McCubbin M (2002) Family stress, perceived social support and

coping following the diagnosis of a child's congenital heart disease. Journal of advanced nursing 39: 190-198.

3. Saxena A (2007) Consensus on Timing of Intervention for Common Congenital Heart Disease. Journal of Indian Pediatric 45: 117-126.

4. Bruce E, Lilja C, Sundin K (2014) Mothers' lived experiences of support when living with young children with congenital heart defects. Journal for specialists in pediatric nursing 19: 54-67.

5. Uzark K, Jones K (2003) Parenting Stress and Children with Heart Disease. Journal of Pediatric Health Care 17: 163-168.

6. Kapoor R, Gupta S (2008) Prevalence of Congenital Heart Disease of Kanpur India. Indian Pediatric 45: 309-311.

7. Katherine JG (1999) Stress and Coping of Parents of Pediatric Heart Transplant Patients and Parents of Pediatric Patients with Chronic Heart Disease: A Comparative Study Implications for Health Care Providers, USA.

8. Sullivan L, Kathryn J (2011) Coping Patterns among Parents of Children with Congenital Heart Disease.

9. Jackson AC, Frydenberg E, Liang RP, Higgins RO, Murphy BM (2015) Familial impact and coping with child heart disease: a systematic review. Pediatric cardiology. 36: 695-712.

10. Bahadur KC, Sharma D, Shrestha MP, Gurung S, Rajbhandari S, et al. (2002) Prevalence of Rheumatic and Congenital Heart Disease in School Children of Kathmandu Valley in Nepal. Indian Heart Journal 55: 615-618.

11. Lee S, Yoo J, Yoo Y (2007) Parenting Stress in Mothers of Children with Congenital Heart Disease. Asian Nursing Research 1: 116-124.

12. Marelli AJ, Ionescu-Ittu R, Mackie SS, Guo L, Dendukuri N, et al. (2014) Lifetime Prevalence of Congenital Heart Disease in the General Population from 2000 to 2010. Journal of American Heart Association 130: 749-756.

13. Sadowski SL (2009) Congenital cardiac disease in the newborn infant: past, present, and future. Critical care nursing clinics of North America 21: 37-48.

14. Saied H (2006) Stress, Coping, Social Support and Adjustment among Families of CHD Children in PICU After Heart Surgery. Case Western Reserve University, Ohio.

15. Shah GS, Singh MK, Pandey TR, Kalakheti BK, Bhandari GP (2008) Incidence of congenital heart disease in tertiary care hospital. Kathmandu University Medical Journal 6: 33-36.

16. Soulvie MA, Desai PP, White CP, Sullivan BN (2012) Psychological distress experienced by parents of young children with congenital heart defects: A comprehensive review of literature. Journal of Social Service Research 38: 484-502.

17. Yildiz A, Celebioglu A, Olgun H (2009) Distress levels in Turkish parents of children with congenital heart disease. Australian Journal of Advanced Nursing 26: 39-46.

18. Bajracharya S, Shrestha A (2016) Parental coping mechanisms in children with congenital heart disease at tertiary cardiac centre. Asian Journal of Medical Sciences 7: 75-79.

19. Basnet NB (2006) Congenital Heart Disease in Nepalese Children. Journal of Nepal Medical Association 45: 281-282.

24

Study of Implicit Preferences in Facial Expression Recognition of Urban Internet-Addicted Left-Behind Children in China

Ying Ge[1,2]*, Jinfu Zhang[1] and Yuanyan Hu[2]

[1]Faculty of Psychology, Key Laboratory of Personality and Cognition, Ministry of Education, Southwest University, Beibei, Chongqing, China
[2]Laboratory of Cognition and Mental Health, Chongqing University of Arts and Sciences, Yongchuan, Chongqing, China

Abstract

For the purpose for exploring the differences in implicit preferences in facial expression recognition between urban internet-addicted left-behind children and urban left-behind children with no such addiction, variant GO/NO-GO (GNAT) paradigm of implicit association test (IAT) and a single-factor 2 level experimental design were adopted to test sixty participants (14 years of age) who were selected from two junior middle schools in Chongqing, China. This study results showed that compared with urban non-addicted left-behind children, urban Internet-addicted left-behind children gave more preference to negative emotion and poorer evaluation on their egos.

Keywords: Internet addiction; Urban left-behind children; Facial expression recognition; Implicit preference

Introduction

Emotional image recognition of facial expression is an important and widely used measure and method for study of emotions. Standardized emotional image system carries out matching of emotional valence and emotional arousal towards emotional stimulation materials, increases possibility of equal positive and negative intensity from emotion elicitation and makes experimental results possess higher comparability and stability. After emotion elicitation, signal detection theory is a general method to detect recognition condition of participants against experimental materials. Variant GO/NO-GO (Go/No-go association test, GNAT) test of implicit association test (IAT) that is used to measure internal mental process of individuals against a kind of thing or phenomenon tests participants' hit rate and false alert rate under different unified tasks by adopting principles of signal detection theory. Response of participants to stimulus that represents target and attribute categories is named as hit rate (i.e. Go), and no response to other represented stimuli is referred to as false alert rate (i.e. No-go). The hit rate and false alert rate are converted to z-score and the difference value is taken as d'-score; then, through comparison of d'-score under different combinations of target concept and attribute concept, perceptibility, propensity and preference of participants are reflected [1].

In 1980s, China witnessed its social and economic transition period, and a large number of adults rushed from underdeveloped western regions to developed eastern regions for work opportunities. These adults left their children in native homes, bringing a group named "left-behind children" into existence. In the later period of 1990s, the left-behind children especially referred to rural children, below 18 years old, who were left in their rural native homes for over a half year and needed to be taken under tutelage of other adults because their mothers, fathers or both parents left for work and came back homes with an interval more than three months [2-9].

Due to various reasons, the number of urban left-behind children is increasing in recent years. There are nearly 20 million left-behind children based on results of the fifth population census, including approximate 2.7 million urban left-behind children, accounting for 13.5% of the total number [10]. As the only municipality directly under the central government in Western China, Chongqing has 1.07 million left-behind children, accounting for 34% of total number of students in compulsory education stage of the region [11].

Thus, with changes in meaning, left-behind children include urban left-behind children and rural left-behind children, and the urban left-behind children have attracted attentions from all sides. The urban left-behind children refer to children, below 18 years old, who live under cares or tutelage from nurses, grandparents, other relatives or non-relatives in cities or towns for a long time because their mothers, fathers or both parents leave for work or study for over a half year and cannot take care of them [12,13]. Such group of children are not poor and some are even affluent; however, they feel loneliness and emptiness due to lack of communication and exchange with their parents and are highly susceptible to deviations in personality and behavioral patterns under temptations from complex environments.

Internet addiction refers to loss of control over impulsion for surfing the internet in the absence of addictive substances, representing a compulsive behavior similar to gambling [14]. Adolescents are high-risk group of Internet addiction, and susceptible age to Internet addiction is between ages of 13 and 18 in China [15]. In general, occurrence rate of Internet addition is 6%-14%, while relevance ratio of urban left-behind children to Internet addiction is 6.83% [16]; therefore, it cannot be ignored that Internet addiction causes negative effects on urban left-behind children.

According to relevant studies [17-19], Internet addicts give preference to emotional words, especially to negative emotional information. A Study reported by Wu and Zheng [19] also indicates that Internet-addicted teenagers give preference and attention to negative emotional information. Therefore, the goal of this study was to discuss implicit preference in facial expression recognition of urban Internet-addicted left-behind children through adopting variant GO/NO-GO (GNAT) paradigm of implicit association test (IAT).

*Corresponding author: Ying Ge, Faculty of Psychology, Key Laboratory of Personality and Cognition, Ministry of Education, Southwest University, Beibei, Chongqing, China, E-mail: gy8620@163.com

Step	Experiment frequency	Practice/test	Q Response circumstance	P Response circumstance	No response
1	20	Practice	Positive picture	Negative picture	
2	20	Practice	Ego word	Non-ego word	
3	20	Practice	Positive picture + ego word		Negative picture + non-ego word
4	40	Test	Positive picture + ego word		Negative picture + non-ego word
5	20	Practice	Negative picture	Positive picture	
6	20	Practice	Negative picture + non-ego word		Positive picture + ego word
7	40	Test	Negative picture + non-ego word		Positive picture + ego word

Table 1: Steps of Implicit Association Test.

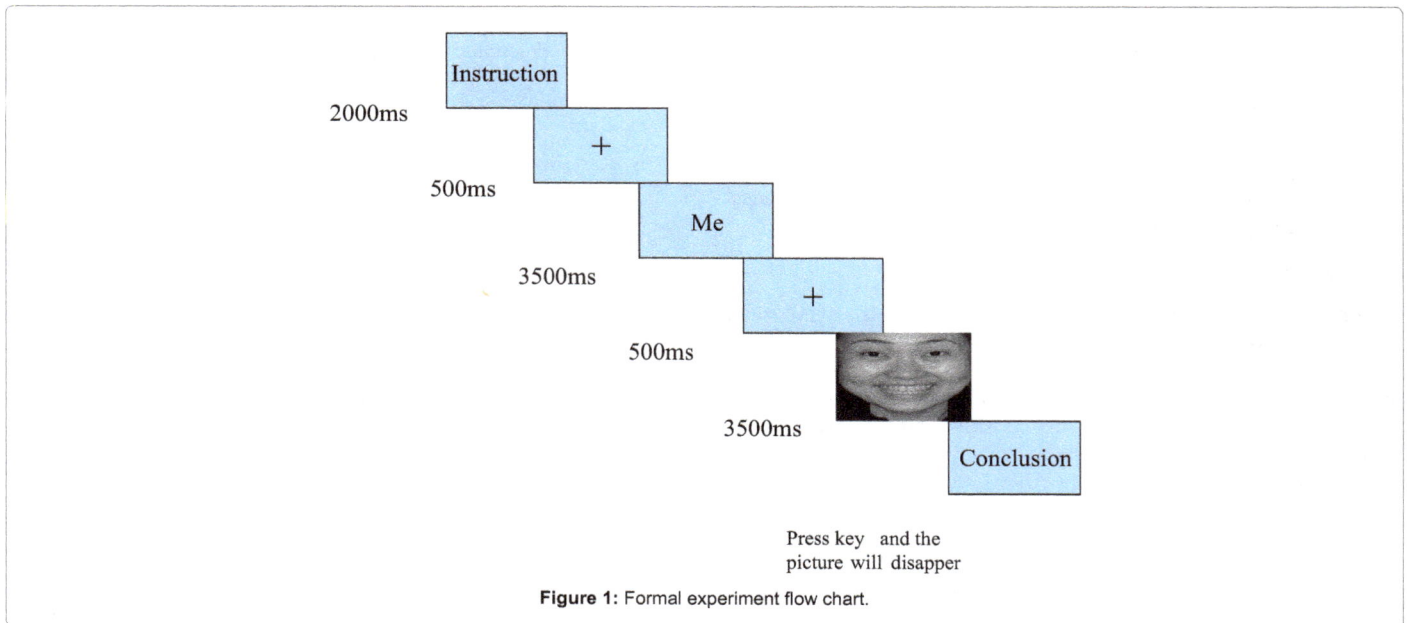

Figure 1: Formal experiment flow chart.

Method

Participants

Clue sampling was adopted in this study. Through mental health surveys in two middle schools with large proportions of urban left-behind children, we found that there existed internet use deviations among the students. Later than, we took children, below 18 years old, who, with registered permanent residences in cities or towns, are brought up by others because their mothers, fathers or both parents leave for work for over a half year as standard candidates for participants, conducted preliminary screening on urban left-behind children and selected out 500 urban left-behind children as the participants. Then, about one hour of interview was carried out aiming at the 500 children, and secondary screening was also conducted as per standards in Adolescent Pathological Internet Use Scale [20].

The scale has 38 questions in 6 dimensions: salience, social comfort, tolerance, compulsive surfing of the internet, withdrawal symptom and negative consequence. The scale adopts 5-point self-rating scale, ranging from "absolute inconformity" to "absolute conformity". With KMO index of 0.940 and Cronbach's Alpha coefficient of 0.948, the scale possesses relatively high reliability and validity. Participants with average item score no less than 3.15 points were defined as "Internet-addicted individuals", while those with average score less than 3.15 points were defined as "non-addicted individuals". Finally, 30 urban left-behind children with Internet addiction and 30 urban left-behind

children without Internet addiction (normal control group) were selected respectively as participants.

All participants were right handed with normal vision (with or without glasses) and euchromatopsy and without physiological maladies (such as heart disease and hypertension) or familial psychiatric history. The participants participated in the experiment voluntarily. Since the participants were all juveniles, the investigators obtained approval from the school and a signed consent from guardians prior to carrying out the experiment. Each of the participants was rewarded with a gift worth RMB 15 after the experiment.

Experimental design

A single-factor 2 level (urban left-behind children with Internet addiction and urban left-behind children without Internet addiction) experimental design was adopted for this study and the discriminability index d' in signal detection theory was adopted as the dependent variable.

Experimental materials and preparation

The affective pictures in Chinese face affective picture system [21] were used for this study. Ten pictures representing each emotional nature (positive and negative) were selected, five with male faces and five with female faces, so there–were 20 pictures in all, which were identified as attribute type. Target type was confirmed as the following words in the experiment: 10 ego words: I, my, me. mine, myself, oneself, my own, one's own, self and own; 10 non-ego words: he, his, outsider,

outsider's, other's, themselves, their own, they, their and other people. Then, the programs used for the implicit association test were developed with E-prime professional software (Psychology Software Tools, Inc., Pittsburgh, PA).

During the process of the experiment, quietness was maintained in the laboratory, and the experiment was carried out separately in the sound-proof cell. After knowing basic experimental requirements spoken by the experimenter, participants pressed keys and completed the test process independently according to experimental instructions. The experimental materials were presented by 19" flat-panel monitor with display refresh rate of 85Hz and resolution ratio of 1024 ×758 pixels.

Experimental procedures

Implicit association test was divided into seven steps (Table 1 and Figure 1 show the experimental process):

Step one: to present positive pictures and negative pictures at random (10 of each). Participants were required to classify the presented pictures and press the key as soon as possible, pressing key "Q" when positive pictures are presented and key "P" when negative pictures are presented (Practice).

Step two: to present ego words and non-ego words at random (10 of each). Participants were required to classify the presented words and press the key as soon as possible, pressing key "Q" when ego words are presented and key "P" when non-ego words are presented (Practice).

Step three: to present positive pictures and negative pictures (5 of each) and ego words and non-ego words (5 of each) at random. Participants were required to press the keys as soon as possible, pressing key "Q" when ego words and positive pictures were presented and not pressing any key when non-ego words and negative pictures were presented (Practice).

Step four: to present positive pictures and negative pictures (10 of each) and ego words and non-ego words (10 of each) at random. Participants were required to press the keys as soon as possible, pressing key "Q" when ego words and positive pictures were presented and not pressing any key when non-ego words and negative pictures were presented (Test).

Step five: to classify positive pictures and negative pictures presented at random. Participants were required to press the keys as soon as possible, pressing key "P" when positive pictures were presented and key "Q" when negative pictures were presented (Practice).

Step six: to present positive pictures and negative pictures (5 of each) and ego words and non-ego words (5 of each) at random. Participants were required to press the keys as soon as possible, pressing key "P" when non-ego words and negative pictures were presented and not pressing any key when ego words and positive pictures were presented (Practice).

Step seven: to present positive pictures and negative pictures (10 of each) and ego words and non-ego words (10 of each) at random. Participants were required to press the keys as soon as possible, pressing key "P" when non-ego words and negative pictures were presented and not pressing any key when ego words and positive pictures were presented (Test).

Pre-experiment and data processing

Four middle school students were selected at random as participants

of pre-experiment to demonstrate that the initial experimental design was favorable and can be directly applied in the formal experiment.

Data were combined by Emerge and then imported to SPSS13.0; gibberish was eliminated, leaving only correct response data in step four and step seven. Then, statistics was created on number of correct responses and wrong responses of each participant to different stimuli in step four and step seven. Thus, response matrixes of stage four and stage seven were obtained. d' of signal detection theory was acquired with the method below. Finally, comparison was performed on d'-score in both stages.

Analyze the two matrixes respectively:

1. with the matrix of stage four, positive d' to oneself and negative d' to others were obtained. Method for obtaining positive d' to oneself: calculate false alert rate and hit rate with number of false alerts equal to number of error items (oneself + negativity) and hit number equal to number of correct items (oneself + positivity), and then translate false alert rate and hit rate into Z-score; Z-score of hit − Z-score of false alert = positive d' to oneself. Method for obtaining negative d' to others: calculate false alert rate and hit rate with number of false alerts equal to number of error items (others + positivity) and hit number equal to number of correct items (others + negativity), and then translate false alert rate and hit rate into Z-score; Z-score of hit − Z-score of false alert = negative d' to others.

2. With response matrix of stage seven, negative d' to oneself and positive d' to others are obtained. Method for obtaining negative d' to oneself: calculate false alert rate and hit rate with number of false alerts equal to number of error items (oneself + positivity) and hit number equal to number of correct items (oneself + negativity), and then translate false alert rate and hit rate into Z-score; Z-score of hit − Z-score of false alert = negative d' to oneself. Method for obtaining positive d' to others: calculate false alert rate and hit rate with number of false alerts equal to number of error items (others + negativity) and hit number equal to number of correct items (others + positivity), and then translate false alert rate and hit rate into Z-score; Z-score of hit − Z-score of false alert = positive d' to others. Finally, import all the data above into SPSS13.0 and carry out independent samples t-test to get final results.

Results

After getting d' upon data processing, results (Table 2) were obtained through analysis on d' (implicit preference= positive d' − negative d'). Through independent samples t-test on participant type, it was found that there was very significant difference between the two groups of participants on positive attitude to oneself (p < 0.01), addicted group lower than non-addicted group; there was significant difference between the two groups of participants on negative attitude to oneself (p < 0.05), with addicted group higher than non-addicted group; there was significant difference between the two groups of participants on implicit preference to oneself (p < 0.05). However, there was no significant difference on positive attitude, negative attitude and implicit preference for others.

Discussion

d' index reflects preference to some kind of emotional pictures; d' of participants for unified task of ego words and positive emotional pictures is higher than that for unified task of ego words and negative

	Type of participant	Positivity	Negativity	Implicit preference
	Non-Internet addicted	2.26 ± 0.62	0.96 ± 1.25	1.31 ± 1.32
Oneself	Internet-addicted individuals	0.92 ± 1.46	2.39 ± 1.17	-1.40 ± 1.33
	t	2.83**	-2.77*	4.85*
	Non-Internet addicted	1.11 ± 0.74	2.06 ± 0.87	-0.96 ± 1.38
Others	Internet-addicted individuals	0.85 ± 1.14	1.18 ± 1.36	-0.32 ± 1.95
	t	0.62	1.84	0.36

Table 2: Sensitivity Index (d') and Difference Test.

pictures, which indicates that participants have implicit preference for positive emotional pictures, and vice versa [22]. This study results showed that the non-addicted group of urban left-behind children had implicit preference for positive emotional pictures, while the Internet-addicted group of urban left-behind children had implicit preference for negative emotional pictures, i.e. compared with non-addicted urban left-behind children, Internet-addicted urban left-behind children preferred negative emotions more. Implicit preference can reflect attitude towards oneself and others. In terms of attitude towards oneself, the non-Internet addicts behaved more positively while the Internet-addicted individuals behaved more negatively. Left-behind children may have problems due to specific growth environment: insufficient home education, indifferent family relations, insufficient guidance or excessive interference, protection or punishment given by parents or guardians to the children, and so on [23]. When all these problems cannot be appropriately solved, negative emotion of children will be increased, and when the negative emotion is increased to a certain level, many children will choose to surf the Internet to get rid of negative emotions; thus, they develop cognition-behavior model of pathological internet use and have many inappropriate negative cognitive schema [24]. Consistency of external stimulus and existing cognitive schema makes information processing easier [25]. As for Internet addicts, selection bias of individuals to emotional information was guided by negative schema in the brain, which decreased their positive evaluation of themselves and made them have implicit preference for negative emotions.

Conclusion

The results of this research suggest that compared with urban non-addicted left-behind children, urban internet-addicted left-behind children had more preference for negative emotions and poorer evaluation on their egos.

Suggestions and Countermeasures

Urban left-behind children are in the critical periods of physical and mental development and formation periods of their views of life, world views and values, and they greatly need attentions and guidance from adults. However, due to the particularity of their growing environments – their parents do not live together with them, when they face any problem that cannot be solved timely, they can only vent their negative induced emotions and handle their emotional disturbances by virtue of cyber world, which will finally make they rely on internet network and have instable emotions, anxieties, uncommunicative and eccentric dispositions and other negative personality characteristics. Aiming at the aforesaid current situation of the urban left-behind children, the following aspects shall be well done:

Establish good parent-child relationship

Although parents of the urban left-behind children work in other places, they shall often communicate with their children and care for their psychological needs. Moreover, they shall return homes at holidays

and festivals to accompany with their children, and communicate with the children in a heart-to-heart way and let the children feel concerns and warmth from families.

Strengthen school education responsibilities

Firstly, schools and teachers shall show more concerns on the unban left behind children and shall exchange with the children's parents or guardians more and cooperate to educate the children well. Secondly, schools shall strengthen education on internet morality, train correct view of internet of the urban left-behind children and enhance educators' internet qualities to guide internet behaviours of the urban left-behind children. Finally, schools shall strengthen campus network construction to build a civilized internet environment. As for urban left-behind children who have problems, schools shall ask them to go to psychological counselling rooms to tell their confusion and troubles to psychological counselling teachers and let the teachers help them solve their problems and guide their healthy psychological development.

Optimize social internet environment

First of all, monitoring towards illegal and harmful information of internet network shall be enhanced, so as to create a good cyberspace environment for urban left-behind children. In the second place, social attentions shall be paid to internet-addicted urban left-behind children because they not only need material satisfaction, spiritual fulfilment but also need the society to guide their ways out of internet addiction.

Declarations of interest

All authors declare no conflicts of interest.

Acknowledgement

This work was supported by the China, Chongqing Social Science Planning Project (2010YBJY40).We thank the many students from Zhongshan Middle School and Wolong Middle School. Finally, we thank the anonymous reviewers for their thoughtful comments.

References

1. Nosek BA, Banaji MR (2001) The Go/ No-go Association Task. Social Cognition 19: 625-664.

2. Chengrong D, Fulin Z (2005) A Study on Current Situation of Left-behind Children in China. Population Research 1: 29-30.

3. Fulin Z, Chengrong D (2006) Survey on Studies on Left-behind Children. Population Journal 3: 62-65.

4. Zhen H, Lijuan C (2007) Research on Defining the Standards of Left-behind Children. China Youth Study, 10: 40-43.

5. Chengrong D, Ge Y, Ying W (2008) A Study on Current Situation of Rural Left-behind Children in China. Population Research 5:15-25.

6. Jing L, Wei W, Wenbin G (2009) Review of the Studies on Rural Left-Behind Children in China. Advances in Psychological Science 17: 990-995.

7. Xinghua F, Xiaoyi F, Qinxue L, Yang L (2009) A Social Adaptation Comparison of Migrant Children, Rear Children and Ordinary Children. Journal of Beijing Normal University (Social Science Edition), 5: 33-40.

8. Jingxin Z, Xia L (2010) Rural Left-Home-Children's Depression and Antisocial Behavior: the Protective Role of Daily Pleasures. Psychological Development and Education 6: 634-640.

9. Hui L (2012) The Resilience and Adaptive Research on the Children Left Behind – Take the Children Left Behind in Changyang Tujia Autonomous County as an Example. Master Thesis. Wuhan: South-Central University for Nationalities.

10. Lin L (2008) The Study of Use Blog to Solve the Problems in Family Education of City Left Behind Children. Master Thesis. Changchun: Northeast Normal University.

11. The Education, Science, Culture and Health Committee of Chongqing Municipal People's Congress. (2012) Investigation Report on Education and Cultivation Situation of Rural Left-behind Children in Chongqing. Bulletin of Standing Committee of Chongqing Municipal People's Congress.

12. Zhi W, Qi J, Dajun Z (2008) A Study on Coding and Recognition of Internet Addicts. Psychological Development and Education 24: 106-112.

13. Dan Z, Yanjun C, Deng Jun D (2012) Effect of Family Education on Urban Left-behind Children and Countermeasure Analysis. Mental Health Education in Primary and Secondary Schools 11: 21-23.

14. Young KS (1998) Internet addiction: the emergence of a new disorder. Cyber Psychology and Behavior 3: 237-244.

15. Wenbin G, Zhiyan C (2006) A Study on Psychopathology and Psychotherapy of Internet Addiction. Advances in Psychological Science 14: 596 - 603.

16. Cancan J, Zhiyong Q, Xiaohua W (2010) On the Current Situation of Internet Addiction of Left-at-home Children and Migrant Children, Their Mental Health and Interpersonal Relationships. Chinese Journal of Special Education 7: 59-64.

17. Riesenhuber M (2004) An action video game modifies visual processing. Trends in Neuroscience 27: 72-74.

18. Shujuan L (2005) Research on Selective Cognitional Bias to Internet Related Stimuli in Heavy Internet Users. Master Thesis. Hangzhou: Zhejiang University.

19. Wenli W, Xifu Z (2012) Characteristics of Information Selection in Pathological Internet Adolescent Users. Chinese Mental Health Journal 26: 631-634.

20. Li L, Yang Y (2007) The Development and Validation of Adolescent Pathological Internet Use Scale. Acta Psychologica Sinica 39: 688-696.

21. Xu G, Yuxia H, Yan W, et al. (2011) Revision of the Chinese Facial Affective Picture System. Chinese Mental Health Journal 25: 40-46.

22. Ying Z, Junsheng L (2009) Using Eye-movement to Study Implicit Aggressiveness. Psychological Science 32: 858-860.

23. Min D, Xu C, Xuefeng Z, et al. (2010) Moderating Effects of Alienation between Coping Style and Social Adjustment for Left-behind Middle School Children. Chinese Journal of School Health 10: 1185-1187.

24. Davis RA (2001) A cognitive-behavioral model of pathological Internet use. Computers in Human Behavior 17: 187-195.

25. Beck AT, Clark DA (1988) Anxiety and depression: An information-procession Perspective. Anxiety Research 15: 23-26.

Study Type D Personality and Cognitive Strategies of Emotion Regulation as Predictors of Happiness and Quality of Life in Women with Breast Cancer

Mehrnosh Rabbani Zadeh[1] and Sareh Behzadi Pour[2]*

[1]Department of Psychology, Science and Research Branch, Islamic Azad University, Fars, Iran
[2]Department of Psychology, Shiraz Branch, Islamic Azad University, Shiraz, Iran

Abstract

Some personality traits, such as A and D, have great stress, anxiety, and negative emotions that causes the patients with breast cancer to be susceptible to more stress and negative perception of events. We aimed to investigate the association of type D personality and cognitive strategies of emotion regulation with happiness and QOL in women with breast cancer. The present cross-sectional study included 100 women with breast cancer referred to Shiraz Medical Centers in summer 2015 through purposive sampling method. Demographic information was recorded and they filled four questionnaires voluntarily, including type D personality scale, Cognitive emotion regulation questionnaire (CERQ), and Oxford happiness inventory and QOL (SF-36) questionnaires. The association between the variables were then tested by regression models. We found a significant negative association between type D personality and happiness and there was a positive association between type D personality and QOL (P<0.001), between positive cognitive strategies of emotion regulation, and QOL, and happiness (both P<0.001), but there was no significant relationship between negative cognitive strategies of emotion regulation and happiness and QOL (P=0.08). Type D personality and cognitive strategies could affect QOL and happiness in patients suffering from breast cancer.

Keywords: Type D personality; Happiness; Quality of life; Cognitive strategies of emotion regulation; Breast cancer

Introduction

Breast cancer, the most prevalent cancer in Iranian men and women, is among the three leading causes of death in Iran [1]. It is estimated that developing countries include half of the new cases and 60% of the world's deaths due to western life style and infections [2]. Therefore, cancer in developing countries requires greater attention.

Cancer is a crisis that anyone may encounter in life and causes many problems for the affected patients, including complicated treatment protocols, long treatment duration, and resistance to treatment that cause great stress and despair [3]. These complications are specifically difficult in the case of breast cancer, in which mastectomy may additionally cause psychosocial problems for the affected patients, including occupational and sexual problems [4]. In addition, patients suffering from breast cancer have increased rates of depression and anxiety in the first year after diagnosis [5].

Therefore, studies have focused on the effect of psychological factors on cancer [6]. Some studies have proven the effects of coping styles, hopelessness, and certain personality traits [7], although some others have found no association between personality traits and cancer risk [8]. Patients with personality traits D internally have a lot of stress and experience negative emotions and are at increased risk of cardiovascular disorders [9]. Studies have indicated that type D personality disorder increases the comorbidity and health burden in patients with cancer [10]. Cognitive emotion regulation is also associated with depression and emotional problems that are associated with various diseases [11,12]. Thus, these two factors may play a key role in prediction of the individual's happiness that interacts with the quality of life (QOL) in patients with breast cancer.

Due to the controversies, novelty, and significance of this issue, we aimed to investigate the association between type D personality and cognitive strategies of emotion regulation with happiness and quality of life in women with breast cancer.

Materials and Methods

Study design

The present cross-sectional descriptive study included 100 women with breast cancer who referred to Mottahari Clinic affiliated to Shiraz University of Medical Sciences for chemotherapy during summer 2015. One hundred women with breast cancer were selected as the study sample size through purposive sampling. We included patients whose diagnosis was made during one to five years prior to the study and had not underwent mastectomy. Any patient diagnosed more than 5 years prior to the study or had concurrent underlying diseases, including physical and psychological comorbidities, such as cardiovascular diseases, anxiety, bipolar and major depressive disorders was excluded. Incomplete questionnaires were also excluded from the study. The demographic data of patients were recorded and they were asked to complete the following questionnaires:

1. The questionnaire of quality of life (SF-36), designed by Ware and Sherbourne in 1992 [13], which contains 36 items depicting 8 different domains, including general health, physical functioning,

***Corresponding author:** Sareh Behzadi Pour, Department of Psychology, Shiraz Branch, Islamic Azad University, Shiraz, Iran, E-mail: sarebehzadi@gmail.com

limitation in role playing due to physical and emotional reasons, body pain, social function, vitality, and mental health. The scores range from 0-100 and higher scores show better QOL. The Persian version of the questionnaire has been previously validated by Montazeri and Colleagues [14] with an estimated internal reliability of 77-90% in all aspects, except delight (65%).

2. Oxford happiness inventory, designed by Argyl, Martin, and Crossland in 1989 [15], which contains 29 items in 5 domains, including satisfaction, positive mood, health, efficiency, and self-esteem. Each item has 4 choices, scored from zero to three, where never indicates zero, one few, two moderate, and three shows very much. The total scores ranges from 0-78, and scores less than 40-42 identifies depression and dissatisfaction, while scores greater than 42 shows happiness. The Persian version of the questionnaire has been previously validated by Hadinezhad and Zareei [16], reporting a Cronbach's alpha of 90% and test-retest reliability of 78%.

Type D personality scale, designed by Denollet [17], which evaluates the parameters of negative emotion and social inhibition. Each domain has 14 items, scored as "never, sometimes, often, and always" and is scored from 0 to 28; scores greater than 10 shows positive results and the total score ranges from 0-56. Reliability and Validity of Persian version of Type D personality Questionnaires (DS14) has been previously evaluated by Fakhari and colleagues in patients with coronary artery disease [18].

3. Cognitive emotion regulation questionnaire (CERQ), a multi-dimensional questionnaire, designed by Garnefski et al. in 2002 [19] that assesses the cognitive emotion regulation after an unpleasant event. The score ranges from 36-180. The Persian version of the questionnaire has been previously validated by Hasani [20], reporting a Cronbach's alpha of 0.76-0.92.

The participants completed the questionnaires without mentioning their names and under observation by the researcher who explained any vague points in the questionnaires to them.

Ethical considerations

The protocol of the study was approved by Shiraz University of Medical Sciences in 08.20.2015. The design and objectives of the study were explained to all participants and written informed consent was obtained from those who were willing to participate in the study and they were clarified that they were free not to take part in the survey and this would not affect their treatment protocol. The participants were ensured that their information will be kept confidential and anonymous in all phases of the study.

Statistical analysis

Quantitative variables were presented as mean ± standard deviation (SD) and categorical variables as frequency (percentage). The association between variables were defined by regression models and Pearson's coefficient. For the statistical analysis, the statistical software SPSS version 21.0 for windows (SPSS Inc., Chicago, IL) was used. P values of 0.05 or less were considered statistically significant.

Results

The mean ± SD age of patients was 50.39 ± 1.23 years. With respect to educational level, 9% were illiterate, 23% had primary school education, 21% had under high-school education, 29% high school education, and 18% had an academic education.

Mean scores of type D personality, happiness, quality of life, positive and negative strategies for cognitive emotion regulation were 27.31 ± 9.71, 51.5 ± 14.49, 49.19 ± 1.35, 69.6 ± 13.25, and 48.5 ± 10.74, respectively. Of all patients, 76% had personality type D, 80% had happiness, 93% used negative strategies and 15% used positive strategies for cognitive emotion regulation, and QOL was low in 53% of patients.

As shown in Table 1, we found a significant negative association between type D personality and happiness (P<0.001), and 39% of the patients' happiness could be predicted by type D personality. Also, there was a positive association between type D personality and QOL (P<0.001), and 19% of QOL could be predicted through type D personality.

There was also a significant positive association between positive cognitive strategies of emotion regulation and happiness and a negative association between positive cognitive strategies of emotion regulation and QOL (both: P<0.001), and 40% of happiness and -13% of impaired QOL could be predicted through positive cognitive strategies of emotion regulation (P<0.001); but the association between negative cognitive strategies of emotion regulation and QOL was not significant (P=0.08) and only 3% of QOL was predicted through negative cognitive strategies of emotion regulation.

Discussion

The QOL and happiness in patients suffering from cancer can have a significant role in their prognosis and general health. In addition, studies have indicated that patients with breast cancer had a worse social well-being than patients with other cancers [21]; therefore, considering the psychological factors in patients suffering from breast cancer is of great importance. The results of the present study indicated a significant negative association between type D personality and happiness and a positive association between type D personality and QOL (P<0.001), between positive cognitive strategies of emotion regulation and QOL and happiness (both P<0.001), and no significant relationship between negative cognitive strategies of emotion regulation and happiness and QOL (P=0.08).

Some of the findings of the current study are confirmed and some are rejected by other studies. Various studies have evaluated the association between personality type D and diseases, but seldom have they focused on patients with cancer. Personality is known as an independent factor in subjective well-being and happiness [22], which was confirmed by the results of the present study. Individuals with type D personality trait require to be confirmed by others and may therefore face problem coping with diseases [23], especially diseases that affect their body image, like breast cancer, which may ultimately lead to

	Type D personality trait	Negative cognitive strategies of emotion regulation	Positive cognitive strategies of emotion regulation	
Happiness	-0.63	0.11	0.63	Correlation coefficient
	0.0001	0.25	0.0001	p-value
Quality of life	0.44	0.17	-0.36	Correlation coefficient
	0.0001	0.08	0.0001	p-value

Table 1: The association between the study variables.

mastectomy. These complications strongly affect patients suffering from breast cancer, especially patients with type D personality trait, who face problems emotionally and have negative emotions; thus, type D personality trait is associated with social and emotional difficulties that predispose the patients to diseases [17,24].

Considering the association between type D personality and QOL, studies have obtained diverse results that might be due to the different nature of the diseases studied. Pederson and colleagues have established a significant negative association between type D personality and impaired QOL in cardiac patients [25]. Similarly have other researchers proven lower health-related QOL in cardiac patients with type D personality trait [26-28]. The results of the above-mentioned studies are inconsistent with the results of the present study, which might be due to the fact that patients with type D personality have difficulty in social relations and mostly choose loneliness [29] and patients with breast cancer have additional problems in social relations [4]; thus, they appear less in society and are less affected by the negative feedbacks of the society. In addition, most of the study population in the present study had breast cancer for 1-5 years, whereas social problems mostly appear in early stages of diagnosis (Burgess et al.) that could affect the results of the present study and cause higher QOL in patients with type D personality.

Some studies have also proposed that type D personality trait affect the neuro-endocrine system through stress [9]. Thus, type D personality trait may not only have psychological effects on patients' health, but it may also induce physiological changes in the body that affect patients' health status that require further investigation in the field of breast cancer.

Few studies have considered cancer, but they have also not focused on type D personality in patients with breast cancer. Denollet have previously proposed type D personality and age as independent risk factors for cancer development in men [27]. Carver et al. have also associated optimism and psychological well-being to survival of patients with breast cancer [7]. Similarly, Epping-Jordan et al. have assessed psychological adjustment in patients suffering from breast cancer at three and six months' follow-up and have indicated optimism as an important factor in these patients [30]. As long as pessimism is one of the characteristic of individuals with type D personality, the above-mentioned studies also confirms the results of the present study. Mols et al. have evaluated patients with colorectal cancer and have reported that patients with type D personality trait have a significantly higher psychological distress and concern about the disease [31] that generally confirms the results of the current study, although the above-mentioned studies have not focused on the variables discussed in the present study.

Similar to the results of the current study, Giese-Davis et al. have reported changed emotion regulation strategies in patients with metastatic breast cancer and have proven the efficacy of emotion-focused therapy [32] that is in line with the results of the present study, indicating that positive cognitive strategies of emotion regulation predict patients' happiness. In addition, emotion regulation strategies have also been associated to different diseases by other researchers. Kinnunen et al. have associated emotion regulation with metabolic syndrome [12] and Karademas et al. have associated emotion regulation strategies to illness-related emotions [33-35], which suggest that emotion regulation strategies have physiological effects in the body that require greater attention, especially in patients suffering from cancer. Therefore, it is suggested that future studies assess the psychological and physiological effect of personality traits and emotion regulation

strategies on patients suffering from breast cancer.

The strengths of the present study included evaluating this novel issue in patients with breast cancer that is the first most prevalent cancer in Iran and the results of the present study guide the researchers to focus the psychological state of patients suffering from breast cancer. But it also had some limitations, including not considering the prognosis of patients, which was not within the objectives of the study. Besides, as the results of the present study suggested, psychological treatment of patients with breast cancer may play a role in prognosis of patients. Thus, it is suggested that future studies evaluate the efficacy of psychotherapy in two aspects of personality traits and emotion regulation strategies in prognosis and treatment of patients suffering from breast cancer.

Conclusion

In conclusion, the results of the present study indicated a significant association between type D personality and cognitive strategies with QOL and happiness in patients suffering from breast cancer.

References

1. Mousavi SM, Gouya MM, Ramazani R, Davanlou M, Hajsadeghi N (2008) Cancer incidence and mortality in Iran. Annals of Oncology 20: 556-563.

2. Jemal A, Center MM, DeSantis C, Ward EM (2010) Global patterns of cancer incidence and mortality rates and trends. Cancer Epidemiology Biomarkers & Prevention 19: 1893-1907.

3. Gonzalez-Angulo AM, Morales-Vasquez F, Hortobagyi GN (2007) Overview of resistance to systemic therapy in patients with breast cancer. Breast Cancer Chemosensitivity, pp: 1-22.

4. Avis NE, Crawford S, Manuel J (2004) Psychosocial problems among younger women with breast cancer. Psycho-Oncology 13: 295-308.

5. Burgess C, Cornelius V, Love S, Graham J, Richards M (2005) Depression and anxiety in women with early breast cancer: five year observational cohort study. BMJ 330: 702.

6. Leshan LL, Worthington RE (1956) Personality as a factor in the pathogenesis of cancer: A review of the literature. British Journal of Medical Psychology 29: 49-56.

7. Carver CS, Smith RG, Antoni MH, Petronis VM, Weiss S (2005) Optimistic personality and psychosocial well-being during treatment predict psychosocial well-being among long-term survivors of breast cancer. Health Psychology 24: 508.

8. Temoshok L (1986) Personality, coping style, emotion and cancer: towards an integrative model. Cancer surveys 6: 545-567.

9. Habra ME, Linden W, Anderson JC, Weinberg J (2003) Type D personality is related to cardiovascular and neuroendocrine reactivity to acute stress. Journal of psychosomatic research 55: 235-245.

10. Mols F, Oerlemans S, Denollet J, Roukema JA, van de Poll-Franse LV (2012) Type D personality is associated with increased comorbidity burden and health care utilization among 3080 cancer survivors. General hospital psychiatry 34: 352-359.

11. Garnefski N, Kraaij V (2006) Relationships between cognitive emotion regulation strategies and depressive symptoms: A comparative study of five specific samples. Personality and Individual differences 40: 1659-1669.

12. Kinnunen ML, Kokkonen M, Kaprio J, Pulkkinen L (2005) The associations of emotion regulation and dysregulation with the metabolic syndrome factor. Journal of Psychosomatic Research 58: 513-521.

13. Ware Jr JE, Sherbourne CD (1992) The MOS 36-item short-form health survey (SF-36): I. Conceptual framework and item selection. Medical Care 30: 473-483.

14. Montazeri A, Goshtasebi A, Vahdaninia M, Gandek B (2005) The Short Form Health Survey (SF-36): translation and validation study of the Iranian version. Quality of Life Research 14: 875-882.

15. Argyle M, Martin M, Crossland J (1989) Happiness as a function of personality and social encounters. Forgas JP, Innes JM (eds.). Recent Advances in Social Psychology: An International Perspective, pp: 189-203.

16. Hadinezhad H, Zareei F (2009) Reliability, validity, and normalization of the Oxford Happiness Questionnaire. Psychological Research 12.

17. Denollet J (2005) DS14: standard assessment of negative affectivity, social inhibition, and Type D personality. Psychosomatic medicine 67: 89-97.

18. Fakhari A, Norouzi S, Pezeshki MZ (2014) Reliability and Validity of Type D Personality Questionnaires (DS14 Persian Version) in Coronary Artery Patients. Medical Journal of Tabriz University of Medical Sciences and Health Services 36: 78-85.

19. Garnefski N, Kraaij V, Spinhoven P (2001) Negative life events, cognitive emotion regulation and emotional problems. Personality and Individual differences 30: 1311-1327.

20. Hasani J (2010) The psychometric properties of the cognitive emotion regulation questionnaire (CERQ). Journal of Clinical Psycology 2: 73-84.

21. Üstündag S, Zencirci AD (2015) Factors affecting the quality of life of cancer patients undergoing chemotherapy: A questionnaire study. Asia-Pacific Journal of Oncology Nursing 2: 17-25.

22. Steel P, Ones DS (2002) Personality and happiness: a national-level analysis. Journal of Personality and Social Psychology 83: 767.

23. Denollet J (2000) Type D personality: a potential risk factor refined. Journal of psychosomatic research 49: 255-266.

24. Pedersen SS, Denollet J (2003) Type D personality, cardiac events, and impaired quality of life: a review. European Journal of Cardiovascular Prevention & Rehabilitation 10: 241-248.

25. Aquarius AE, Denollet J, Hamming JF, Henegouwen DPVB, De Vries J (2007) Type-D personality and ankle brachial index as predictors of impaired quality of life and depressive symptoms in peripheral arterial disease. Archives of Surgery 142: 662-667.

26. Denollet J, Vaes J, Brutsaert DL (2000) Inadequate response to treatment in coronary heart disease adverse effects of Type D personality and younger age on 5-year prognosis and quality of life. Circulation 102: 630-635.

27. Pedersen SS, Holkamp PG, Caliskan K, van Domburg RT, Erdman RA, et al. (2006) Type D personality is associated with impaired health-related quality of life 7 years following heart transplantation. Journal of Psychosomatic Research 61: 791-795.

28. Denollet J (1998) Personality and risk of cancer in men with coronary heart disease. Psychological Medicine 28: 991-995.

29. Williams L, O'Connor RC, Howard S, Hughes BM, Johnston DW, et al. (2008) Type-D personality mechanisms of effect: the role of health-related behavior and social support. Journal of Psychosomatic Research 64: 63-69.

30. Epping-Jordan JE, Compas BE, Osowiecki DM, Oppedisano G, Gerhardt C, et al. (1999) Psychological adjustment in breast cancer: processes of emotional distress. Health Psychology 18: 315.

31. Mols F, Denollet J, Kaptein AA, Reemst PH, Thong MS (2012) The association between Type D personality and illness perceptions in colorectal cancer survivors: a study from the population-based PROFILES registry. Journal of Psychosomatic Research 73: 232-239.

32. Giese-Davis J, Koopman C, Butler LD, Classen C, Cordova M, et al. (2002) Change in emotion-regulation strategy for women with metastatic breast cancer following supportive-expressive group therapy. Journal of Consulting and Clinical Psychology 70: 916.

33. Karademas EC, Tsalikou C, Tallarou MC (2011) The impact of emotion regulation and illness-focused coping strategies on the relation of illness-related negative emotions to subjective health. Journal of Health Psychology, p: 16.

34. Garnefski N, Kraaij V (2006) Cognitive emotion regulation questionnaire - development of a short 18-item version (CERQ-short). Personality and Individual Differences 41: 1045-1053.

35. Ma J, Jemal A (2013) Breast cancer statistics. Breast Cancer Metastasis and Drug Resistance. Ahmad A (ed.), Springer, pp: 1-18.

26

The Effect of Quality Accreditation Programs on Patient Safety Experiences in Nursing Services

Atilla Yaprak*

Sabuncuoğlu Şerefeddin Training and Research Hospital, Amasya University, Turkey

Abstract

Introduction: Ministry of Health has initiated Quality Accreditation studies with Transformation Project in Health in 2003. These studies have gained extensive momentum especially in the last decade, and have composed Quality Accreditation Programs (Quality Standards in Healthcare, associated guidelines), which are applied in all healthcare institutions and institutes. The status of achievement in applying the criteria, laid down by Quality Standards in Healthcare, is significantly affected by physical locations of institutions and institutes, technical facilities, and knowledge levels and experiences of personnel.

Purpose: This study has been conducted to assess the contributions of Quality Accreditation Programs to patient safety knowledge and practices in nursing services and to measure the effects of different variables on these practices.

Methods: The study has been conducted with 175 nurses in different age groups, at different educational levels, and working in hospital clinics, and having different durations of work experience. Data has been obtained by a questionnaire of 12 questions (two questions have sub-questions). Descriptive statistical methods have been used in data analysis, and Chi square test has been used in required sub-group analysis.

Findings: The half of the participants was in the age group of 25-34 years. 98.9% of nurses stated that they received patient safety training. 90.9% of participants thought that these trainings were sufficient. The ratio of the ones, indicating that they needed training on this subject, was 22.3%. The ratio of the participants, reporting on patient safety, was detected as 78.3%. The ratio of nurses, reporting on this subject, was found significantly high in the age group of 25-34 years (p=0.012). The rate of receiving training was low in nurses with work experience of less than one year (p=0.038). The rate of reporting on patient safety was significantly low in participants with work experience of less than one year and with work experience of more than 10 years (p=0.049).

Conclusion: Although the rate of receiving training on patient safety is high, the rate of participants, practically reporting on this subject, is low. This has led to the thought that training is not always fully effective in attitude change. We think that the implementation of short-term reminder trainings may be useful.

Keywords: Patient safety; Patient safety experience; Nursing services; Quality

Login

The Quality Accreditation Programs (Quality Standards in Health, linked guidelines) that have been established by the Ministry of Health with the Health Transformation Project in 2003 and the Quality Accreditation activities that have gained momentum in the last 10 years are being implemented in all health institutions and organizations. Success in implementing the criteria set forth by Health Quality Standards; The physical locations of the institutions and organizations, the technical possibilities and the level of knowledge and experience of the personnel are significantly influencing.

It is important that the staff reflect their level of knowledge, especially their knowledge, on their experience. Patient safety is one of the most important aspects of quality programs in health care. Patient safety is all the measures taken by healthcare organizations and employees in order to prevent damage to health care services, and constitutes the primary and indispensable condition of qualified health care. The purpose of patient safety is to provide safety by creating an environment that physically and psychologically affects patient and patient relatives and hospital employees positively. The main goal here is to prevent errors during service delivery, to protect the patient from possible damage due to errors, and to eliminate the possibility of error.

It is important that the staff reflect their level of knowledge, especially their knowledge, on their experience. The most important quality programs in health services The topic of patient safety is a subject that should be taken up by all personnel working in health services [1]. Although it is not possible to reduce the medical errors caused by the health workers while providing health services, it can be seen that these errors and risks can be reduced to a minimum with the adoption of patient safety culture in hospitals and at the same time by all employees. The first goal in ensuring patient safety is to reduce risks

The development of patient safety culture will also be significantly reflected in the experience. To protect patients from harm and to increase patient experience in the organization and to improve patient safety within the organization.

Patient safety-related events can cause harmful consequences for hospitalized patients and can bring an additional cost to the hospital. The damage suffered by the patient can cause serious injuries, prolonged hospital stay, disability, even death of the person. Human-

***Corresponding author:** Atilla Yaprak, Sabuncuoğlu Şerefeddin Training and Research Hospital, Amasya University, Turkey, E-mail: atiyaprak@hotmail.com

induced problems such as fatigue, inadequate training, communication problems, timelessness, wrong decision, and argumentative personality can cause medical errors. The reasons such as workplace structure, policies followed, administrative structure, wrong distribution of personnel, inability to solve problems constitute institutional problems. Technical factors such as inadequate automation, inadequate equipment and missing equipment also affect the staff experience and may be the cause of medical error [2-4].

Implementation of event reporting activity in health services provides a better service for the patient by revealing the missing side of the worker involved in the organization, recognizing their strengths, developing their creativity, leading the organization in determining the responsibility and duty to be assigned within the organization Kohn et al. [5], Dursun et al. [1], Altındish and Kunt [6,7].

The main objectives of error reporting are to collect qualitative information that can be used for the development of the student as well as the collection of epidemiological data. Because the goal here is to ensure that the whole organization can learn from the experiences of people about mistakes and unwanted events.

Nurses carry out a large part of the patient care phase and medical activities in patient safety. Due to the fact that the nurses are a group of health personnel with the highest number of patients and the most number of patients, the establishment of patient safety culture in nursing practice has a big precaution [8-10]; Nurses are nested with patient safety in all aspects of care. In order to talk about the culture of patient safety in an institution, it is necessary to increase the patient safety experience and the adoption and continuity of patient safety applications by the nurses.

Goal

This study was conducted to evaluate the contribution of Quality Accreditation programs to patient safety knowledge and practice in nursing services and to measure the effects of different variables on these applications.

Research Questions:

- What are the conditions for receiving patient safety training? What are the training requirements?

- What is the status of nurses reporting incidents related to patient safety?

- Is there a relationship between nurses' status of patient safety education and patient safety practices at the institution?

Methods

Type of study

The study was carried out in a descriptive design.

Sample of the study

The study was conducted with 175 nurses working in different age groups, different education levels, hospital clinics and with different work experience periods.

Data collection tools

"Survey Form" was used to collect research data. The data were obtained through a questionnaire consisting of 12 questions (there are subdivisions of the two problems).

Collection of data

The research was conducted on April 2016. The questionnaire forms were distributed from the hands after the necessary explanations were made to the nurses by the investigator. The nurses were given 3 days to fill out the forms and after this time the questionnaires were collected again and collected from the hand.

Data analysis

The data obtained from the nurses participating in the study were transferred to the computer environment and evaluated in the SPSS 16.0 program. In the analysis of the data, descriptive statistical methods and square test in necessary subgroup analyzes were used. Analysis was made by CO Medical Research Consulting Company.

Results

When the distribution of nurses according to their personal and professional characteristics was examined (Table 1); 49.1% of them were between 25-34 years of age, 90.9% of them were associate and undergraduate graduates and 41.1% were 2-5 years in the institution. The rate of receiving education in nurses who had less than one year of working time was low (p=0.038). The rate of reporting on patient safety was significantly lower (p=0.049) in participants with less than one year and more than 10 years of study time.

When the findings of nurses regarding patient safety were evaluated (Table 2); Nurses reported that 98.9% had received patient safety training. 90.9% thought this training was sufficient. The rate of those who stated that they need education in this subject is 22.3%. 14.3% (n=25) and 8.6% (n=15) of those who stated that they were in need of training expressed their need for medical device safety training. The rate of participants reporting on patient safety was 78.3%. 62.9% (n=110) reported that they reported on "falling". The proportion of nurses who report in this issue between 25-34 age group was found to be significantly higher (p=0.012). In the study, 76.0% of the nurses stated that patient safety applications were adequate and 79.4% of the nurses said that quality programs contributed to their experience in Patient Safety [11].

Discussion

This research was carried out in a descriptive design to determine the factors that affect the patient's experience in patient care in nursing services.

When the distribution of nurses according to their personal and occupational characteristics was narrowed, it was determined that 49.1% of the nurses were between 25-34 years of age, 90.9% of them were associate and undergraduate graduates and 41.1% were 2-5 years of institutional work. The rate of receiving education in nurses who had less than one year of working time was low (p=0.038). The rate of reporting on patient safety was significantly lower (p=0.049) in participants with less than one year and more than 10 years of study time.

It was determined that 98.9% of the nurses stated that they had been educated about the patient safety and 90.9% of the training areas were sufficient. The training needs of employees for patient safety were 22.3% and they were found to have the most and the same (22.9%) training needs in terms of Radiation Safety and medical device safety. These findings show that the nurses in the investigated hospital are given trainings for patient safety but there are still training needs in some cases. In line with these findings, the training needs of the nurses

		Sıklık	%
Age	20-24	11	6.3
	25-29	44	25.1
	30-34	42	24.0
	35-40	36	20.6
Education	High school	11	6.3
	Pre-license	82	46.9
	License	77	44.0
	Graduate	5	2.9
Department that works	Emergency	16	9.1
	Operating room	14	8.0
	Cardiology	13	7.4
	Infection Service	12	6.9
	Neurology	11	6.3
	Internal medicine	10	5.7
	General Surgery	10	5.7
	KBB - Eye	10	5.7
	Chest Hst.	9	5.1
	Orthopedics	9	5.1
	General intensive Care	8	4.6
	Hemodialysis	8	4.6
	Female Birth	7	4.0
	Plastic surgery	5	2.9
	Other*	33	18.9
Total working time at the ınstitution	Less than a year	6	3.4
	2-5 years	72	41.1
	6-10 years	44	25.1
	Over 10 years	53	30.3

*Child services, neonatal intensive care unit, remote treatment unit, child emergency, child surgery, coronary intensive care, intensive intensive care, neurology intensive care, diabetes education, ekk nursery, quality unit, psychiatry, dialysis, education,

Table 1: Personal and Occupational Characteristics of Nurses (n=175).

and nurses should be assessed with certain intervals and the training programs should be arranged and the training should be repeated

In the study, the reporting rate for patient safety practices was low (78.3%) and the reporting of the highest decrease was reported, the percentage of nurses reporting this issue between 25-34 age group was significantly higher (p=0.012) (P=0.049) at a significantly lower level during the study period of less than 10 years. Is a subject that needs to be emphasized. Reporting of faults is considered one of the most important indicators of patient safety culture in an institution. Although the rate of nurses receiving training on patient safety practices was high, the reporting rate was low. This shows us that the attitudes and behaviors of the nurses regarding the safety reporting system are inadequate or have problems. Authority managers should take care of this issue, organize short-term reminder trainings other than the routine trainings related to the safety reporting system, make employees aware of the problems, produce solutions for the problems experienced in implementation and strive to reflect the trainings given to practice. In the study, 76.0% of the nurses stated that patient safety

practices were adequate and 79.4% thought that quality programs contributed to their experience in Patient Safety, but the inadequate level of reporting suggests that patient safety culture has not developed sufficiently and that studies have to be done in this regard

Conclusions and Recommendations

In this study, 49.1% of the nurses stated that they were in the age range of 25-34, 90.9% of them were associate and bachelor graduates, 41.1% were 2-5 years in the institution, and 98.9% 90.9% of the respondents were satisfied that these trainings were adequate. In addition, 22.3% of the respondents indicated that they need education in this area. In the study, reporting on patient safety was reported at 78.3% and reporting of the highest falls was reported. It was determined that the rate of education in nurses who had less than one year of working time was low (p=0.038) and the rate of reporting of patient safety was significantly lower (p=0.049) in participants who had less than one year and more than 10 years of study time.

As a result;

➢ Despite the high rate of patient safety training, the low proportion of participants reporting in this regard in practice suggests that education is not always fully effective in changing attitudes.

Are you trained in patient safety?	Yes	173	98.9
Hasta güvenliği ile ilgili aldığınız eğitim sizce yeterli mi?	Yes	159	90.9
Is your education safe enough for your patient safety?	Yes	39	22.3
On what issues do you need training?			
	Safe drug applications	11	6.3
	Transfusion safety	11	6.3
	Safe surgical applications	10	5.7
	Reducing the risks of falling	8	4.6
	Contact	14	8.0
	Radiation safety	25	14.3
	Medical device safety	15	8.6
	Proper identification of patients	6	3.4
Do you report on patient safety practices?	Yes	137	78.3
On which issues are you reporting?			
	Identification	104	59.4
	Fall	110	62.9
	Drug Safety	103	58.9
	Surgical Safety	103	58.9
	Transfusion Security	106	60.6
Do you think that quality programs contribute to your experience in Patient Safety?	Yes	139	79.4
	No	5	2.9
	partially	31	17.7
Is it enough for you to apply patient safety?	Yes	133	76.0
	No	12	6.9
	partially	30	17.1

Table 2: Distribution of nurses situations related to patient safety (N=175).

➤ We believe that the implementation of short-term reminder training may be beneficial.

As a result of the research findings;

- Regular control tactics on patient safety experiences in institutions and evaluation of the current situation and the realization of the improvements in this way,

- As a result of these evaluations, it is necessary to organize training programs and raise awareness of employees,

- Emphasizing that in the trainings given for reporting on all aspects of patient safety, error reporting should not be regarded as punishment and should be regarded as an important part of the system,

- In order to improve the patient safety experience in the institution, it is recommended that the patient safety culture should be placed in the institution first and the administrators should continue their beliefs and attitudes in this subject with determination.

References

1. Dursun S, Bayram N, Aytaç S (2010) An application on the culture of patient safety. J Social Sci 8: 1-14.

2. Akalin E (2004) Culture of patient safety: How can we improve? Ankem Magazine 18: 12-13.

3. Ertem G, Oksel E, Akbiyik A (2009) A retrospective review with incorrect medical practices (malpractice). Dirim Tip Gazetesi 84: 1-10.

4. Karatas M, Hosci C (2010) Medical error causes and solutions. Inonu University Medical Faculty Journal 17: 233-236.

5. Kohn LT, Corrigan JM, Donaldson MS (2000) To err is human: building a safer health system. Volume 6. National Academies Press.

6. Karaca A, Arslan H (2014) A Study for Evaluation of Patient Safety Culture in Nursing Services. J Health Nurs Manag 1: 9-18.

7. Altindis S, Kurt M (2010) A research on the effect of knowledge management practices on patient safety: an application in Afyonkarahisar province. Selcuk University Institute of Social Sciences Dergis 24: 45-61.

8. Mitchell PH (2008) Defining Patient Safety and Quality Care.

9. Çirpi F, Dogan Merih Y, Yasar Kocabay M (2009) Determination of nursing practices and nurses' opinions on patient safety. Maltepe University Journal of Nursing Science and Art 2: 26-34.

10. Fearnot O (2012) Nurses' perception of the attitude of the administrators about patient safety. Dokuz Eylül University Journal of Social Sciences Institute 14: 91-112.

11. Cebeci F, Gürsoy E, Tekingündüz S (2012) Determining the tendency of nurses to make medical errors. Changes in Anatolian Nursing and Health Sciences 15: 188-196.

27

The Impact of Sociological Factors on Nurse Educators' Use of Information Technology

Ayala Gonen[1]* and Lilac Lev-Ari[2]

[1]*Nursing Department, School of Social and Community Science, Ruppin Academic Center, Israel*
[2]*Behavioral Department, School of Social and Community Science, Ruppin Academic Center, Israel*

Abstract

Background: Today, as the rapid progress of Information Technologies (I.T) in health care continues, it is crucial to find out more information about the factors that might advance or hinder the nurses' educators' acceptance of technological changes. The main goal of this study was to explain the use of using I.T, by focusing on sociological factors like the impact of support and influence. The study design was a quantitative research, using a written and online survey. One hundred and nine academic nurse educators from ten different academic nursing schools in Israel participated.

Results: support and influence predict actual use of I.T. The Chi-square Goodness-of-Fit index presented an excellent fit for the data *(p*=0.46; Normed Fit Index (NFI)=0.96; Root Mean Square Error of Approximation (RMSEA)=0.00). The relationship between sociological factors from significant others and the actual use of IT was mediated by personality characteristics such as self-efficacy, and innovativeness.

Conclusion: Management should ensure that sociological factors (such as support and influence) and personality characteristics (such as self-efficacy, attitudes toward I.T, and innovativeness) are considered when preparing to introduce new technologies to nurse educators. Enhancing support and influence and self-efficacy should be considered in the organization, in order to encourage favorable use among healthcare professionals.

Keywords: Social support; Nurse educators; Use of information technology; Attitudes; Self-efficacy; Innovativeness

Introduction

The twenty-first century is an age of new technologies, in which technology is used almost everywhere, mostly for information sharing. Smartphones, laptops, electronic devices, and social online communities are a few examples of nurses' constant immersion in technology [1]. As technology has become more powerful, it has provided educators with a valuable tool to support learning by advanced technology that has made learning more accessible, and offered educators a way to support learning inside and outside the classroom. Information technology (I.T) is the application of computers and internet to store, retrieve, transmit, and manipulate data, or information, often in the context of a business or other enterprise [2]. Information Technology (I.T) uses computers, networking, and software to manage information, in a way in which students are no longer tied to their desks and can interact with learning objects [3].

Informatics education in the nursing career has direct impact in training and future development of nurses in the professional field [4]. The exception to this constant exposure to I.T can be found in nursing education, and the big question is how faculty staff can integrate technology into their daily activities and into the curriculum in order to enhance their way of teaching.

In the contemporary information systems literature, research on I.T acceptance focuses mainly on the examination of attitudes towards using I.T [5,6]. On the other hand, behavioral sciences and individual psychology literature suggests that social influences and personal traits are potentially important and can be explanatory variables in technology adoption as well [7].

The ministry of health/nursing division, in Israel is characterized by a global trend of growing recognition in the importance of the academization of nurses. Today, there are in Israel more than 20 Institutions for training academic registered nurses that are entitled to

enrich the study program required for register nurses [8]. The required courses in the learning program contains 126 academic credits, 100 of which are theoretical academic credits and 26 are clinical experience academic credits.

With this in mind, the authors chose to build a research model that would explain the behavior process of using I.T, by nurses' educators, focusing on the impact of support and influence. A S.E.M (Structural Equation Modeling) model-a statistical technique embodying multiple linear regressions, will be used to explain the relationship between influence and support received by the nurse educators and variables concerning the use of Information Technology (I.T), including a number of variables such as self-efficacy, innovativeness, attitudes, and actual use of I.T.

Theoretical Framework

Over the years, many models and theories have been developed and have been tested in order to identify variables affecting the acceptance and use of I.T provided to end-users. Among them, the classical Theory of Reasoned Action (TRA) [9] is based on the subjective norms and attitudes that determinate the intention to change a behavior and the behavioral response, (i.e., their actual use of the system). The Ajzen [10] developed the TPB (Theory of Planned Behavior) model that explains

---

*Corresponding author: Ayala Gonen, Nursing Department, School of Social and Community Science, Ruppin Academic Center, Emek Hefer, Israel, E-mail: ayala.gonen@gmail.com

various human actions by integrating subjective norms, attitudes, self-efficacy, and use. In this study, our theory is based on the Theory of Planned Behavior, and we hypothesized that subjective norms, attitudes, self-efficacy, and innovativeness, all serve as antecedents to a mediating process that results in the actual behavioral use of I.T.

Subjective norms

The second determinate of the theory of reasoned action [9] is subjective norm-one's perception of the social pressures put on one to perform or not to perform the behavior in question. Subjective norm was found to be the most important antecedent of user intention towards use of e-learning [11]. Subjective norm is influenced by the judgment of significant others, people that are important to the person such as parents, spouse, friends, and direct manager. These people can influence and support the behavior, and one might feel social pressure (subjective norm) regarding performance or non-performance of a certain behavior.

In addition to teaching at an academic nursing school, the nurse belongs to multiple other groups, such as family, friends, and organizations, and this fact highlights the demand from the manager to consider the vitality of the nurse environment. One of the important benefits that a person receives from the environment is social support. The literature extensively indicates the main role and impact of social support [12,13]. Altogether, it is surprising to find out that the relationship between supports from significant others and the level of influence that the nurse educator feels concerning using I.T has received so far very little attention.

Social support may yield a wide range of functions, including empathy, encouragement, assistance, and sense of sharing. Koivunen et al. [6] claim that nursing directors have a significant role, because their important task is management of change in many areas including innovative I.T implementation processes. Significant others, such as family and friends, have an important role that can be seen when the nurse educators seek their support, and the influence they have on them can be seen in the nurse educators' attitudes and behavior. Yang et al. [14] found that behavioral beliefs in combination with social influences are all important determinants for services adoption and use, but their impacts on behavioral intention do vary across different stages. Therefore, the need for social support in nursing education is very important. By reinforcing support, I.T can increase the nurse educator's self-efficacy, and possibly lead to increased academic performance [15], which can also be related to beliefs in one's ability to accomplish and use I.T. [16] found that social influence had direct influence on using I.T.

IT use

I.T use is the technology hardware and software that everyone is using in daily work in the healthcare and education surrounding-this term includes using the servers, networks, computers, software programs and other equipment used to manage information. Using I.T, is the most significant change to occur in nursing education since the move from hospital training to academic teaching [17]. Most nurses use information and communication technology, and the Internet is part of their daily work. A number of factors have been associated with acceptance and use of I.T [6]. These include the level of I.T skills, and managers' support. Usually, the nurse educators already have years of hands-on experience, and it may be quite difficult for them to change their way of teaching without providing them with substantial support and guidance. Duncan et al. [18] claim that the world has indeed changed, and these changes will shape the way nursing should be

prepared for the next generation of nurses. Task forces and research reports sheds light on strategies needed to support nurses to address today's challenges in nursing practice and education. Today, nurse educators have taken steps to transform their curriculum and make use of a variety of educational technologies to facilitate learning, and that is so important to advance nurses' motivation to use I.T.

Nurse educators must keep in pace with technological changes not only in the classroom but also in the practical arena. Members of the academic staff have to use the power of I.T tools to create learning communities for sharing and exchanging ideas, research, and knowledge about nursing education. Nguyen et al. [19] conducted a survey about nursing faculty needs for training in the use of new technologies for education and practice. Their findings suggest that nursing faculty perceive a need for training and support to effectively use educational technologies in nursing education, and this leads to the main aim of the research. For this reason, it is important to investigate whether there is a connection between the nurses' educators' use of I.T, and other variables such as self-efficacy, sense of innovation, attitudes and whether the level of influence and support received by them is also linked to using I.T use.

Attitudes

Users' beliefs and attitudes have been shown to have a major influence on the acceptance of new technology [20]. A number of models and frameworks have been developed to measure these influences on users' acceptance and model adoption. Concerning the use of I.T in the education field [21], who studied teacher adoption of technology, claim that positive attitude toward technology and having the skill to use the technology in the classroom are important in the level of integration of technology into the teaching process. Individual nurse's attitudes toward I.T use may be effected by attitudes among other nurses on the ward, due to normative beliefs related to social pressures that may hinder the intention to use I.T [22].

Self-efficacy

Another important dimension in computers' use is self-efficacy. Self-efficacy is defined as peoples' beliefs about their capabilities to produce performance that influence over events that affects their lives. The term was coined by the classical Social Learning Theory of Bandura (1977). Teachers' self-efficacy influences their level of enjoyment and feeling of control when using technology in the classroom [23]. Studies conducted in healthcare settings have found that self-efficacy has a significant influence on using I.T [15,24,25]. Nurse educators that have high levels of self-efficacy are more confident, they tend to use new teaching approaches, and have more motivated students. When self-efficacy is extended to the context of integrating IT into teaching, it describes teachers who view technology as an effective way to enable student learning and perceive I.T as a useful means to support their teaching.

Innovativeness

Innovativeness is the nursing educators' willingness to use new technology. Innovativeness is not defined as a part of the TPB Theory, but was added due to its importance. Innovativeness is the capacity to be enthusiastic about new ideas, to initiate new projects, to innovate new ideas or methods and to plan to what extent this new idea or invention can be useful. Innovativeness can be expressed in various ways such as interest in technological innovation, intention to buy new gadgets, etc. A tendency to innovativeness should have a positive relationship with attitudes towards computer use, as was presented by Reference [26,27].

In summary, according to the TPB theory [10], Subjective norms as it is expressed in variables such as social support and significant other' influence, are parts of the whole model. Attitudes toward using I.T, subjective norms, self-efficacy and the addition of innovativeness, will be tested for their relationship with nurses' educators' use of II.

Aims of this research

This study's main goal was to examine the correlation between nurse educators' perception of the degree of influence and support they get from their significant others (close family, friends, and managers) concerning the use of I.T, as well as examining a number of variables such as self-efficacy, innovativeness, attitudes, and use of I.T.

Research hypotheses

The following research hypotheses were derived from the aims of this research:

  a) A positive correlation will be found between the nurse educators' sense of influence and support from their significant others and their attitudes toward using I.T, use of I.T, self-efficacy, and innovativeness.

  b) The nurse educators' perception of their sociological factors (such as support and influence) and personality factors (such as attitudes, innovativeness, and sense of efficacy) will predict actual I.T use.

The importance of the research

This study attempts to contribute a better theoretical understanding of the antecedents of adoption of I.T by nurse educators, focusing on the influence and support of their significant others. The degrees of support and the amount of influence by significant others will point to the characteristics of the relationship between using I.T and specific personal and professional factors. Knowing what sociological factors are related to the I.T use is important and can be used to assist education and to develop better attitudes toward I.T use. A good number of I.T projects around the world have failed or have been abandoned, due to their discrepancy for the nurses, therefore, it is critically important that factors influencing healthcare professionals' acceptance and use behavior of I.T and related technology be investigated [28].

Methods

Nurse educators are an important group in the nursing field. They build, design, and mold the future nurses. This study will examine different angles of the nurse's behavior: the relationship between the level of nurse educators' I.T use and three groups of human factors: **a)** Sociological factors-subjective norms (the current study), **b)** Environments factors-work climate [25], and **c)** Emotional factors-perceived level of threat and challenge (in process). Each of these factors is important, and its discussion can be of great benefit to the nursing profession. Each part is individual, and the insights from the entire three parts will provide a comprehensive perspective of the issue. For the avoidance of any doubt, the present study, examining the impact of the support and influence of the significances others, was carried out using it to the same participants at the same time. Every issue was presented in the questionnaire with the appropriate questions.

Design, population and research tools

Design: This study is a correlative, quantitative research.

Population: A convenience sampling was done, 109 nurses educators, working at 10 different academic institution around Israel (out of 20 nursing academic institutions), participated in the survey. These institutions differs by their sizes; the bigger the institution, the greater the number of nurses educators employed. The sample was made up of female nurses because the number of male educators nurses during the study period was less than 8% of the total number of nurses educators. The age range of the participants is 20 to 65 years. A nurse educator in Israel must have the minimum academic degree, a Master's degree, which explains why their average years of experience were 16, and the average age was 46.

Research tools: An online survey and hardcopy questionnaires were prepared. The main aim of using hardcopy questionnaires was to encourage those who were deterred by technology to participate. Both the online survey and the questionnaire were accompanied by an introductory letter including information about the purpose of the study, assurance of confidentiality, and each nurse was asked to sign informed consent.

Data collection: The survey that was conducted during 2015. The managers of the nursing academic institution were asked to help the authors by approaching the nursing staff faculty in each institution and ask them to participate. Participation was voluntary and the data was collected anonymously. Out of the 150 questionnaires, 109 were returned (71 hand written+38 online), and the total response rate 72.5%.

Ethical consideration: The research was approved by the Ethics Committee of the Academic Institution. Health professionals participated on a voluntary basis, and their rights to anonymity and confidentiality were ensured.

Measures

A questionnaire with a total of 66 questions was constructed by the authors to examine factors that support and influence nurse educators' use of technology. Most of the questions were adapted from [26] questionnaire, except the I.T use's part that was developed by the current authors. The whole questionnaire included the following sections: "background demographic factors such as age, seniority, and religion; Sociological factors such as support and influence from significant others and Personality factors such as attitude toward using I.T, self-efficacy, a innovativeness and I.T use.

Measurement of Significance others: The nurses were asked to state their opinion, about if and how they believe they were influenced by the significance others such as their manager, their direct family (spouse and children) and their colleagues. They were also asked what the level of support they believed they received from significance others concerning the concept of their use of I.T during the daily work, all these on a scale of 1-4: from 1- not influenced at all to 4 totally influenced, or 1-totally non-supportive to 4-totally supportive. An example of the influence from significant others' scale: "To what extent do you believe that you are influenced by the opinions of the listed below: (direct manager, peer group, close family)", and another example of the support variable: "Do you believe that your direct manager thinks that it is important for you to use Technological tools in teaching?".

Measurement of Attitudes: The questionnaire of Attitude toward using I.T consists of 19 questions on a Likert scale, was based on the classic attitudes scale by Ref. [29]. The scale has good reliability; Cronbach's alpha=0.89. Factor analysis confirmed a one-factor solution explaining 34% of the variance. Sense of innovativeness scale consists of three questions on a Likert scale, and has good psychometric properties; Cronbach's alpha=0.78. Factor analysis confirmed a one-factor solution explaining 70.51% of the variance. Sense of self-efficacy scale consists of two questions on a Likert scale, and has good psychometric properties; Cronbach's alpha=0.41. Factor analysis confirmed a one-factor solution explaining 63.80% of the variance.

Measurement actual I.T use: The scale of actual I.T use was constructed for this study by the authors. It is not simple to measure the actual I.T use due to the fact that there are some levels of use in the nurse's education pattern of I.T uses. The whole process of building this scale included consulting with 2 senior nursing educator experts. They revised the questions and approved them. The next step involved a pilot questionnaire for five nursing educators. In sum, this scale starts with very basic tools like the MS-Office (Word, Excel, Power Point, Outlook). Since the nurses' educators average age was 46, the assumption was that not all of them are familiar with such competencies. There were 4 items and the Cronbach's alpha was=0.82.

Another dimension of using I.T is reflected by the way the nurses' educators are using the internet and working with emails. We used 2 items and the Cronbach's alpha was=0.83.

The more advanced way of using I.T is reflected by the way they use more complicated educational and healthcare software in class like Moodle (a free and open-source software learning management system), or Poll everywhere app (Poll Everywhere is a mobile app, for responding to polls, presenting polls, and clicking through PowerPoint presentation)-this stage included two items; and the Cronbach's alpha was 0.83. The reliability of the combined three scales of I.T use was 0.83 [30].

5.2.4 Data analysis: In order to assess the relationship between sociological, personality and behavioral factors, Pearson correlations were conducted. In order to assess the direct and indirect influence of sociological factors such as support and influence from significant others on actual I.T use, a Hierarchical Regression analysis was used. In order to understand the mediated effect of sociological factors on actual I.T use (mediated by personality factors) a Structural Equation Model (SEM) was used. The SEM model adds to the regression model in that it assesses direct and indirect paths simultaneously.

Results

The first research hypothesis referred to possible correlations between influence and support and attitudes toward using I.T, use of I.T, self-efficacy, and innovativeness. As can be seen, Table 1 shows the correlations between the indices. Positive correlations between support, influence, self-efficacy, attitudes towards I.T, meaning that the higher support, the higher the influence and the more positive the attitudes, the sense of efficacy. No correlations between influence and the other indices emerged. Sense of efficacy, positive attitudes towards using I.T, and actual use were all highly inter-correlated.

The second research hypothesis intended to check which variables would best predict the actual use of I.T. The variables were divided into two factors: sociological factors (such as support and influence) and personality factors (such as attitudes, innovativeness, and sense of self-efficacy). This hypothesis was tested using a hierarchical regression model in which actual use was the dependent variable; personal factors were entered in the first step, followed by personality factors. The Table 2 shows the outcomes of the regression analysis.

As can be seen in Table 2, support and influence predict actual use. Support predicts it positively, while influence predicts use negatively. This means that the more support you have the higher the actual use of I.T is, but the more influence you have, the less actual use there is.

Sense of self-efficacy and innovativeness both fully mediated this result, meaning that support and influence predict actual use of I.T through personality factors. The study tried to build a research model that would explain the behavior process of using I.T, focusing on the influence and impact of the support and influence. We hypothesized that personality characteristics (innovativeness, attitudes and self-efficacy) would mediate the relationship between personal factors and actual use. The Figure 1 depicts our SEM model. The Chi-square Goodness-of-Fit index presented an excellent fit for the data (p=0.46; Normed Fit Index (NFI)=0.96; Root Mean Square Error of Approximation (RMSEA)=0.00). The statistically significant path coefficients are provided as standardized estimates in Figure 1.

The SEM model shows that influence does not directly predict any of the other variables. Its only influence is through its positive correlation with support. This may explain the negative predictive strength it had in our regression model. Support positively predicted self-efficacy, attitudes toward I.T, and innovativeness, but did not predict actual use directly. This supports our regression model in the understanding that personality characteristics fully mediate the relationship between sociological factors and actual use of I.T.

Discussion

The main aim of this study was to provide information regarding the impact of significant others on the nurse educators' actual I.T use. The first research hypothesis about correlation between influence and support and attitudes toward using I.T, actual use of I.T, self-efficacy, and innovativeness was supported. We have evidence to support the importance of the influence and support variables in connection with the significance other. Burke et al. [31] who collected Data from 2104 nurses in Spain concerning job demands, social support, and work satisfaction, found that lack of social support, particularly from supervisors and co-workers, were associated with d more unfavorable work/organizational outcomes.

The impact of the significant others (social support) on the nurse educators use of I.T was substantiated, and it is quite important. Sources of social support can be colleagues, subordinates or superiors, as well as factors outside the workplace such as family and friends. The support pattern can be emotional, functional, and informative or appreciation. It can be assumed that social support would help the nurse educator to face workplace pressure [31]. Poelmans et al. [32] showed that the enrichment of family or work have a positive effect on satisfaction from both work and family life, and produce a feeling of well-being, physically and mentally. Job satisfaction increases the possibility that work will enrich the family, and family satisfaction increases the likelihood that the family will enrich the work system [33]. Accordingly, when the needs of the nurse educators' job are suitable to the close family environment, there will be less conflicts between the significant others and work, and the nurse educator's attitude toward the workplace would be more positive. The significant correlation between social support and intention to use I.T was found also by Ref. [28,34,35]. The variable of behavioral intention toward accepting and integrating I.T was less relevant in this study because the subjects were already (more or less) using the new technology.

The research model explained the behavior process of using I.T, focusing on the effect and impact of support and influence. Support positively predicted self-efficacy, attitudes toward I.T, and innovativeness, but did not predict actual use directly. This strengthens our regression model in the understanding that personality characteristics fully mediate the relationship between sociological factors and actual use of I.T.

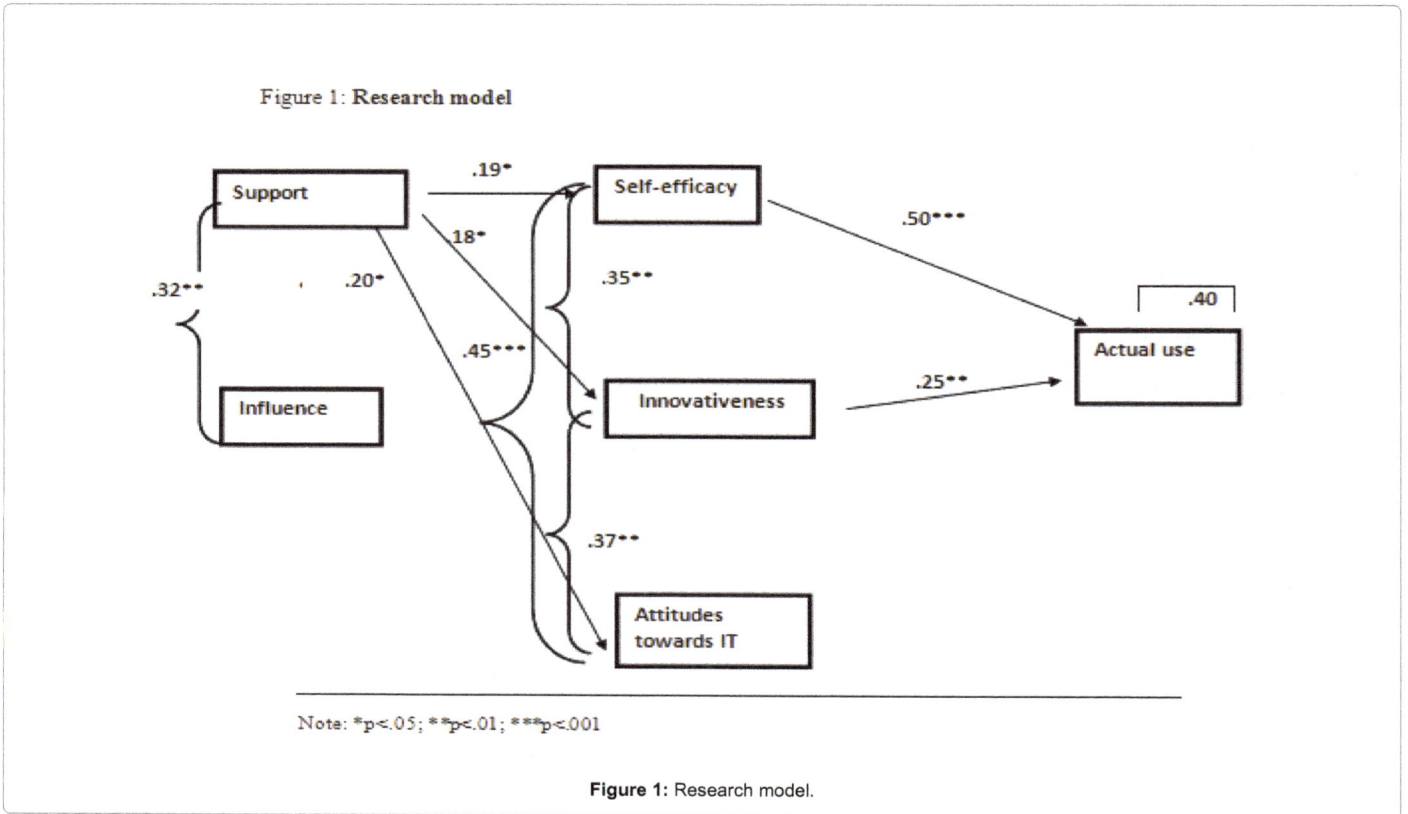

Figure 1: Research model

Note: *p<.05; **p<.01; ***p<.001

Figure 1: Research model.

	Influence	Self-efficacy	Attitudes toward IT	Intention to use IT	Actual IT use
Support	0.32***	0.19*	0.20*	0.20*	0.15
Influence		-0.10	-0.009	-0.01	-0.13
Self-efficacy			0.47***	0.34***	0.59***
Attitudes toward IT				0.60***	0.27**
Intention to use IT					0.11

Note: *P<0.05; **P<0.01; ***P<0.001

Table 1: Pearson correlations between subjective norms, personality characteristics, intention to use IT, and actual use of IT.

	R²	Adj. R²	ΔR²	F	B	T
Step 1	0.06	0.04		(2,103)=3.12*		
Support					0.20	2.02*
Influence					-0.21	-2.03*
Step 2	0.41	0.38	0.35***	(5,100)=13.65***		
Support					0.04	0.52
Influence					-0.10	-1.16
Self-efficacy					0.51	5.61***
Innovativeness					0.27	3.10**
Attitudes toward IT					-0.09	-0.98

N=109; *p<05; **p<01; ***p<001

Table 2: Hierarchical Regression Analysis predicting actual IT use from demographic data, personality characteristics and intention to use.

Computer self-efficacy has been proven an important variable concerning attitudes and acceptance of I.T [36]. The nurse educator who has a sense of self-efficacy is more confident and believes in her ability to cope successfully with I.T. Consequently, the nurse has positive attitudes and is more willing to use new technology. A sense of innovativeness is also a valuable factor [37]. A sense of innovativeness is a very important value for nurse educators and for their students, because innovativeness helps to find novel ways of virtual teaching for the benefit of the profession. Innovative teaching/learning strategies are needed, because the virtual world provides a big opportunity for nurse educators to develop meaningful, simulated learning that may then be transferred to the real world of the nursing practice.

Findings of this study, especially the model, may be applicable to other research dealing with human behavior, and may serve as a useful base for comparisons in future studies.

Finally, the uniqueness of this study's results is proof of sociological factors' importance and how they affect the nurse educators' personality characteristics, namely attitudes, computer self-efficacy, and innovativeness. These insights should be used by policymakers and managers, who should ensure that when introducing new I.T to nurse educators, sociological factors are taken into consideration in order to encourage favorable use behavior among them [38-40].

Limitations

a) The study was conducted in one country. Israel is a multicultural country, and there might be differences in generalization of the study's findings to other countries.

b) The authors used a sample that is really not big enough for a SEM.

c) The questions about I.T use was developed by the authors and it would be interesting to check it with further more research.

Conclusions

This study is an interesting approach to outline the factors that are involved in the adoption/acceptance and use of certain I.T. Today, as the rapid progress of Information Technologies (I.T) in health care continues, it is crucial to find out more information about the factors that might advance or hinder the nurses' educators' acceptance of technological changes. The relationship between sociological factors from significant others and the actual use of I.T was mediated by personality characteristics such as self-efficacy, and innovativeness.

The managers should ensure that sociological factors (such as support and influence) and personality characteristics (such as self-efficacy, attitudes toward I.T, and innovativeness) are taken into account when introducing new technologies to the nurse educators. Enhancing support and influence and should be considered in the organization, in order to encourage favorable use among healthcare professionals.

In the field of nursing education, the findings of this study contribute to expanding the knowledge of the sociological factors that affect nurse educators' behavior concerning I.T use. Activating and implementing the research insights, concerning the relationship with significant others, could help to provide nurses' educators with the relevant skills that would act to improve the quality of the nursing education and profession.

Conflict of Interest

There are no possible conflicts of interest in the manuscript including financial, consultancy, institutional or other relationships that might lead to bias or conflict of interest.

References

1. Crews TB, Miller JL, Brown CM (2009) Assessing faculty's technology needs. Educause Quarterly 32.

2. Daintith J (2009) A Dictionary of Physics. Oxford University Press, UK.

3. Mac Callum K, Jeffrey L, Kinshuk K (2014) Factors impacting teachers' adoption of mobile learning. J Inf Technol Educ 13: 141-162.

4. González ZA, Schachner MB, Tattone MA, Benítez SE (2016) Changing Educational Paths in an Informatics Course According to the Needs and Expectations of Nursing Degree Students. Stud Health Technol Inform 225: 324-328.

5. Kaya N (2011) Factors affecting nurses' attitudes toward computers in healthcare. Computers Informatics Nursing 29: 121-129.

6. Koivunen M, Anttila M, Kuosmanen L, Katajisto J, Välimäki M (2015) Team climate and attitudes toward information and communication technology among nurses on acute psychiatric wards. Inform Health Soc Care 40: 79-90.

7. Wu J, Lederer A (2009) A meta-analysis of the role of environment-based voluntariness in information technology acceptance. MIS Quarterly 33: 419-432.

8. Ministry of Health (2016) Israeli Ministry of Health, Nursing Division, Israel.

9. Fishbein M, Ajzen I (1977) Belief, attitude, intention, and behavior: An introduction to theory and research.

10. Ajzen I (1991) The theory of planned behavior. Organizational Behavior and Human Decision Processes 50: 179-211.

11. Mohammadi H (2015) Social and individual antecedents of m-learning adoption in Iran. Comput Human Behav 49: 191-207.

12. Chenot D, Benton AD, Kim H (2009) The influence of supervisor support, peer support, and organizational culture among early career social workers in child welfare services. Child welfare 88: 129-147.

13. Lietz CA (2009) Critical thinking in child welfare supervision. Administration in Social Work 34: 68-78.

14. Yang S, Lu Y, Gupta S, Cao Y, Zhang R (2012) Mobile payment services adoption across time: An empirical study of the effects of behavioral beliefs, social influences, and personal traits. Comput Human Behav 28: 129-142.

15. Tenaw YA (2013) Relationship between self-efficacy, academic achievement and gender in analytical chemistry at Debre Markos College of Teacher Education. Afr J Chem Educ 3: 3-28.

16. Maillet É, Mathieu L, Sicotte C (2015) Modeling factors explaining the acceptance, actual use and satisfaction of nurses using an Electronic Patient Record in acute care settings: An extension of the UTAUT. Int J Med Inform 84: 36-47.

17. Button D, Harrington A, Belan I (2014) E-learning and information communication technology (ICT) in nursing education: A review of the literature. Nurse Educ Today 34: 1311-1323.

18. Duncan S, Rodney PA, Thorne S (2014) Forging a strong nursing future: insights from the Canadian context. J Res Nurs 19: 621-633.

19. Nguyen DN, Zierler B, Nguyen HQ (2011) A survey of nursing faculty needs for training in use of new technologies for education and practice. Journal of Nursing Education 50: 181-189.

20. Cheung R, Vogel D (2013) Predicting user acceptance of collaborative technologies: An extension of the technology acceptance model for e-learning. Computers & Educ 63: 160-175.

21. Zhao Y, Cziko GA (2001) Teacher adoption of technology: A perceptual control theory perspective. J Technol Teacher Educ 9: 5-30.

22. Van Achterberg T, Schoonhoven L, Grol R (2008) Nursing implementation science: how evidence-based nursing requires evidence-based implementation. J Nurs Scholarsh 40: 302-310.

23. Hammond M, Reynolds L, Ingram J (2011) How and why do student teachers use ICT? J Comput Assist Learn 27: 191-203.

24. Liang JC, Wu SH, Tsai CC (2011) Nurses' Internet self-efficacy and attitudes toward web-based continuing learning. Nurse Educ Today 31: 768-773.

25. Gonen A, Sharon D, Offir A, Lev-Ari L (2014) How to enhance nursing students' intention to use information technology: The first step before integrating it in nursing curriculum. Computers Informatics Nursing 32: 286-293.

26. Shoham S, Gonen A (2008) Intentions of hospital nurses to work with computers: based on the theory of planned behavior. Computers Informatics Nursing 26: 106-116.

27. Hsu HM, Hou YH, Chang IC, Yen DC (2009) Factors influencing computer literacy of Taiwan and South Korea nurses. J Med Syst 33: 133-139.

28. Princely I (2014) Factors influencing nursing professionals' computer-based information systems (CBIS) use behavior. In: Encyclopedia of Information Science and Technology. Khosrow-Pour M (Editor). 3rd edn. IGI Global, Hershey, PA, USA, pp: 3332-3343.

29. Stronge JH, Brodt A (1985) Assessment of nurses' attitudes toward computerization. Comput Nurs 3: 154-158.

30. Burke RJ, Moodie S, Dolan SL, Fiksenbaum L (2012) Job demands, social support, work satisfaction and psychological well-being among nurses in Spain. ESADE Business School Research Paper 233.

31. Hsiao JL, Chang HC, Chen RF (2011) A study of factors affecting acceptance of hospital information systems: a nursing perspective. J Nurs Res 19: 150-160.

32. Poelmans SA, Kalliath T, Brough P (2008) Achieving work–life balance: Current theoretical and practice issues. J Manag Organ 14: 227-238.

33. Carlson DS, Hunter EM, Ferguson M, Whitten D (2014) Work-family enrichment and satisfaction mediating processes and relative impact of originating and receiving domains. J Manag 40: 845-865.

34. Lee CC, Lin SP, Yang SL, Tsou MY, Chang KY (2013) Evaluating the influence of perceived organizational learning capability on user acceptance of information technology among operating room nurse staff. Acta Anaesthesiol Taiwan 51: 22-27.

35. Holden RJ, Brown RL, Scanlon MC, Karsh BT (2012) Modeling nurses' acceptance of bar coded medication administration technology at a pediatric hospital. J Am Med Inform Assoc 19: 1050-1058.

36. Leblanc G, Gagnon MP, Sanderson D (2012) Determinants of primary care nurses' intention to adopt an electronic health record in their clinical practice. Computers Informatics Nursing 30: 496-502.

37. Tsai HM, Liou SR, Hsiao YC, Cheng CY (2013) The relationship of individual characteristics, perceived worksite support and perceived creativity to clinical nurses' innovative outcome. J Clin Nurs 22: 2648-2657.

38. Bandura A (1977) Social Learning Theory. Englewood Cliffs, Prentice Hall, NJ, USA.

39. Gonen A, Lev-Ari L (2016) The relationship between work climate and nurse educators' use of information technology. Nurse Educ Today 39: 1-6.

40. Wayne JH, Randel AE, Stevens J (2006) The role of identity and work–family support in work–family enrichment and its work-related consequences. J Vocat Behav 69: 445-461.

28

The Incredible Costs of Chronic Diseases: Why they Occur and Possible Preventions and/or Treatments

Knox Van Dyke*

Department of Biochemistry and Molecular Pharmacology, West Virginia University Medical School, Morgantown, WV 26506, USA

Abstract

The United States government spends 3 trillion dollars on disease treatment each and every year. Chronic diseases are responsible for 86% of these health care costs. Chronic diseases are linked to 70% of the deaths that occur each year. The costs worldwide are likely even greater. After the age of 50, at least 50% of the people from the US have at least one chronic disease. About 1/3 of the US population has some form of diabetes or pre-diabetes. Why does this continue and certainly it is a major factor in the debt of the United States which is approximately 20 trillion dollars. How can the government and our medical people including scientists allow this outrage to continue?

Is it because we do not understand the cause of chronic diseases? Certainly we have not developed effective medications and or treatments; so even if we knew what the root cause of chronic diseases could we prevent or reverse them?

Dr Peter Barnes, M.D., Ph.D. is the premier scientist in the world who studies acute and chronic lung diseases. He has found that acute diseases can be effectively treated with steroidal anti-inflammatory drugs e.g., asthma; but chronic diseases like chronic obstructive pulmonary disease are not effectively treated with those same steroidal anti-inflammatory drugs. The difference between the two diseases forms the blueprint of what causes chronic diseases other than those caused by genetic defects which are relatively rare. The major difference between acute (treatable diseases) and chronic (essentially untreatable or poorly treatable diseases) is the excessive generation of peroxide called peroxynitrite (OONO-). Chronic diseases produce excessive amounts of peroxynitrite and this can create massive biochemical damage to the cell particles (mitochondria) that allow life to continue and produce necessary energy and key enzymatic proteins are damaged as well as the DNA, and RNA-the master molecules of life. Excessive peroxynitrite is the linchpin of chronic diseases.

Therefore the key to controlling chronic diseases is to control excessive peroxynitrite. This prevents the damage to our bodies from nitration, nitrosylation and nitrosation all major damages caused by peroxynitrite. How do we control these diseases -we need to find suitable targets of peroxynitrite damage that are non-toxic and exist in a continuous state to fight this toxic chemical. There are peroxynitrite catalytic antagonists and some vitamins like vitamin C and different forms of vitamin E are targets which destroy peroxynitrite and these have been shown to be somewhat effective against chronic diseases. We must introduce the peroxynitrite antagonists early in the disease state before the diseases become irreversible.

The excessive peroxynitrite actually damages the epigenetic mechanism (histone deacetylase) by which steroids exert their anti-inflammatory action. But, if we can suppress peroxynitrite early in the chronic disease state -chronic diseases can be become acute and very treatable diseases.

Keywords: Acute; Chronic diseases; Peroxynitrite; Nitration; Nitrosylation; Nitrosation; Mitochondria

Introduction

Each and every year the United States Government spends several trillion dollars to combat or treat chronic diseases with little change in the foreseeable future. Chronic diseases are responsible for 86% of our health care costs [1]. The cost worldwide must be even greater. Chronic diseases are responsible for the majority of deaths- probably in the area of 70% of the deaths. Why does this continue? It is because the basis of chronic diseases is not well understood so the treatments for these diseases are palliative or superficial and never getting to the actual basis of these diseases. If one believed the media it could be surmised that oxidants cause damage possibly by free radicals which could be prevented by eating or swallowing multiple antioxidants (cause gain of electrons). But biochemically oxidation is crucial to metabolize sugars and other nutrients so we can produce the energy to power our body. Oxidation (loss of electrons) is important in control or stimulation of a variety of important biochemical pathways. Siess of Germany developed the idea of oxidative stress which is the ratio of oxidants/antioxidants >1 or in other words there are more oxidants than antioxidants to oppose them [2].

There are a few problems with this basic concept because a person could have oxidative stress locally but not generally and it probably would be a transitory imbalance. The other problem with this idea is a person could take considerable amounts of antioxidants and see little to no result in a given chronic disease state. If antioxidants were at the basis for disease control why are they not more effective in disease states?

As we shall see from this review it is almost certain that nitrosative stress which includes, nitration of unsaturated organic structures, nitrosylation of sulfhydryls and nitrosation of amines are likely the real

*Corresponding author: Knox Van Dyke, Department of Biochemistry and Molecular Pharmacology, West Virginia University Medical School, Morgantown, WV 26506, USA, E-mail: kvandyke@hsc.wvu.edu

culprits in chronic diseases. They likely stem from the generation of peroxynitrite (OONO-) or one of its derivatives that when produced in excess makes acute (treatable diseases) to become chronic and mostly untreatable diseases. See cartoon Figure 1 of the likely chemical culprit in chronic diseases.

There have been trillions of dollars spent to treat chronic diseases and most treatments have been effective to a trivial extent or ineffective at all. For example multiple millions of dollars have been spent of treatment for cancer and for many people the chemotherapy or treatment often produces a few months of extra life but often they are in agony for much of the treatment. Most cancer chemotherapy is fairly non-selective for the cancer versus the normal cells. Since the normal cells die at a substantial rate, the side effects from these mostly poisonous substances are generally very substantial.

How effective have our medical and research community been in treating, arthritis, cancer, neurodegenerative diseases, brain damage, diabetes, diseases of the kidney, liver, pancreas, eye, hearing, lung, heart diseases which are chronic and the many vascular diseases, stroke etc. Answer-not very effective since these chronic diseases are the main causes of death.

There must be a defect in our basic understanding of chronic diseases. The key questions are the following:

- What causes acute and chronic diseases?

- How can we treat or prevent these diseases?

The major driving force in almost all disease states is inflammation. There are two major types of inflammation:

1. Acute

2. Chronic

How does acute inflammation happen? Two different types of inflammatory cells play major roles in inflammation. They are short lived neutrophils and long lived macrophages and these are both white cells that appear in both blood and tissues. The DNA of these cells is covered with positively charged histone proteins. When acute inflammation occurs a DNA transcription factor called nuclear factor kappa b (nf-kappa b) is activated which stimulates an enzyme called histone acetyl transferase (HAT). The histones are acetylated (with a two carbon acetate group similar to acetic acid) which changes the charge between the DNA and histones causing the histones to peel away from the DNA and the inflammatory genes of the DNA are stimulated to produce the gene products of inflammation.

This turn on process for inflammation is an epigenetic (non-gene regulation via a control histone-acetylated DNA on- switch).

How is acute inflammation stopped? The gold standard of anti-inflammatory drugs are steroidal anti-inflammatories which are used to inhibit or stop acute inflammation e.g., dexamethasone or prednisone etc.

How do steroids stop acute inflammation? They stimulate an enzyme called histone deacetylase 2 or (HDAC 2) linked to the nf kappa b-DNA transcription factor. This enzyme cuts off the acetate groups from the inflammatory- activated histones causing the positive histone proteins once again to be charged and is attracted to and covers the negative DNA, therefore shutting down the inflammatory process.

Therefore, the inflammatory off- switch is the deacetylation of histones from the inflammatory cell DNA which creates opposite charges between histones and DNA which causes acute inflammation to cease.

During this acute inflammatory process, the macrophages are also stimulated to produce a sufficient amount of superoxide (which is oxygen with an extra electron) which combines with available nitric oxide (.NO) which also carries a free electron. These two gaseous substances dissolved in bio-fluids react at diffusional speed (10^{-9} sec) to produce a strongly oxidizing/nitrating substance called peroxynitrite (OONO-) first in relatively small amounts in acute inflammation and therefore OONO- does not have a major effect on the acute inflammatory process mechanism. See standard Figures 2 and 3 for inflammation diagram and inflammatory cellular effects linked to peroxynitrite or its metabolites.

We were studying silicosis which is caused by inhaling fine sand particles into the lung and in our studies on rats so affected, we found a 10 fold jump in peroxynitrite based luminol luminescence 24 hours after silica placement- Antonini [3]. This is due to the nf-kappa b induction of nitric oxide (NO) synthase 2 (a highly inducible enzyme) which can produce large amounts of nitric oxide from macrophages. When dexamethasone was given acutely and simultaneously with the silica the induction of nitric oxide and thus peroxynitrite was stopped completely [4,5]. Therefore, when steroids are given during acute inflammation, they are very effective anti-inflammatory drugs stopping the acute inflammatory process.

Steroids are ineffective for chronic inflammation. After the silica remained in rat lung for 6 weeks and rat lung macrophages were assayed for peroxynitrite, we observed a 1000 fold increase in peroxynitrite-luminol luminescence compared to the control without silica [4]. This is a superior model of both acute and chronic inflammation. Later, it was shown by us that the actual source of inflammation is actually calcium ions which use silica as a carrier. When the calcium is removed or chelated using the membrane permeable INDO 1-AM, the inflammatory killing capacity is thwarted completely. This is a portion of the proof that black lung disease or coal worker's pneumoconiosis is actually caused by silica contaminated with calcium in the coal dust which can be easily viewed by silica examination via X-ray microanalysis [6].

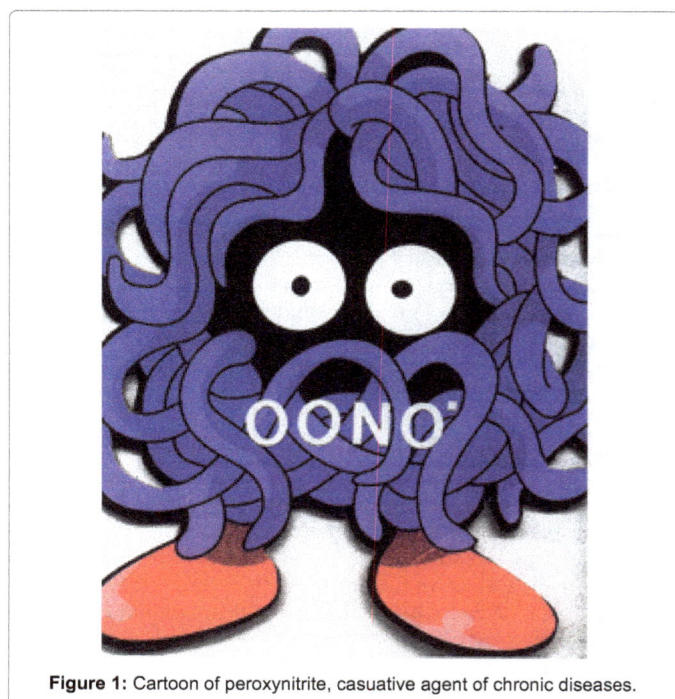

Figure 1: Cartoon of peroxynitrite, casuative agent of chronic diseases.

Toxic Mechanisms Caused By Peroxynitrite (OONO⁻) or Derivatives Creates Nitrosative Stress

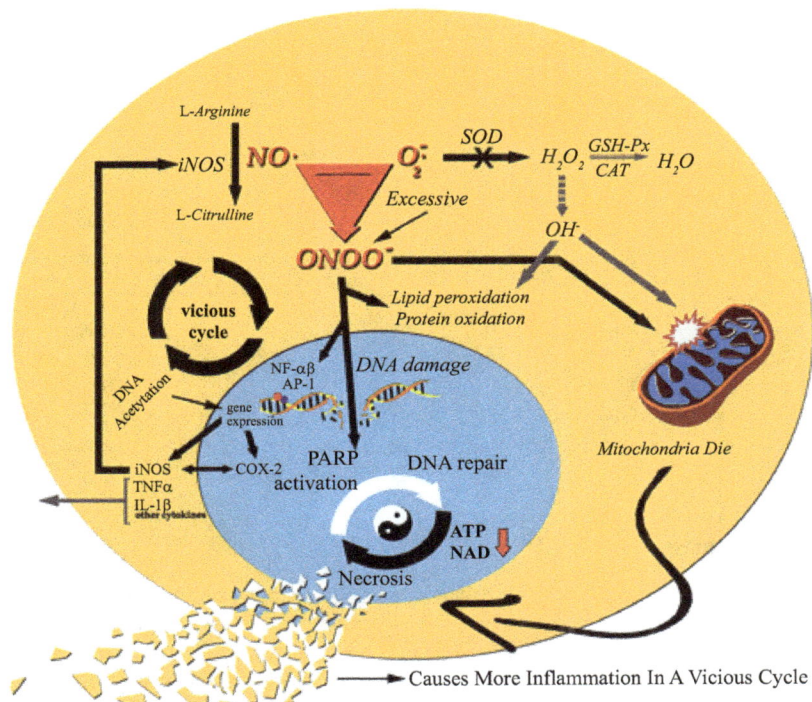

Oxidation stress is often an early and key event that activates numerous pathways involved in several cancer and development of chronic diseases. If the causative agent (e.g, hyperglycemia, cigarette smoking, UV lights and chemical toxicants) persists, eventually iNOS is activated and ONOO⁻ is formed. By then, cellular stress is transformed from oxidative only to nitro-oxidative. ONOO⁻ exerts its harmful effects directly and indirectly. It causes activation of transcriptional factors leading to pro-inflammatory gene expression. During this process, nitro oxidative stress also involves an inflammatory response. Interactions between transcriptional factors and pro-inflammatory products lead to a vicious cycle of damage. The cytokines spread the inflammatory signals through the circulation. Unless excess O₂⁻ and iNOS⁻ derived NO production are terminated, this mechanism continues to propagate damage within cell. Moreover ONOO⁻ directly damage all macromolecules including lipids, proteins and DNA. ONOO⁻ induced DNA damage is sensed by DNA repair enzymes, in particular poly (ADP ribose) polymerase (PARP). In presence of severe genomic damage, overactivation of PARP causes cellular NAD⁺ and ATP depletion by attempting a repair process. This drives cells into an energy crisis eventually leading to necrosis. This futile mechanism, so called suicide hypothesis of PARP activation, is reportedly involved in many diseases relative to nitro-oxidative stress. Since mitochondrion has its own DNA and PARP enzyme, this pathophysiologic process also takes place within the mitochondrion. It is well known that, both oxygen and nitrogen based radicals are prone to directly damage this organelle. Consumption of the majority of NAD⁺ by PARP also slows the rate of glycolysis and mitochondrial respiration, and eventually leads to cellular dysfunction and death.

Figure 2: Basic machanism of peroxinytrite-induced toxicity and related pathways (As described by Korkmaz in the year 2008).

At this time, in chronic silicosis, anti-inflammatory steroids do not inhibit peroxynitrite-based luminol luminescence since this is chronic inflammation.

This occurs because the silicosis over a prolonged period of time caused the inflammation to be activated from acute to chronic inflammation [6]. Why is chronic inflammatory disease insensitive to steroidal anti-inflammatory drugs?

Peter Barnes et al. have explained this unusual phenomena with great clarity and they have written many articles after the major one cited here [7]. He or they demonstrated that excessive nitration by peroxynitrite attacks key tyrosines in the enzyme histone deacetylase 2 (HDAC-2). This destroys the HDAC-2 enzyme activity and prevents its anti-inflammatory action which is necessary for the actions of steroidal glucocorticoids (steroids). If histone deacetylase 2 has its active sites damaged via nitration, the enzyme cannot strip the acetates from the histones and steroid action becomes ineffective. The key to understanding chronic inflammation is to know that peroxynitrite in high chronic doses destroys the epigenetic mechanism used by the cell to create steroidal anti-inflammatory action. If steroids are ineffective in treating chronic inflammation there are limited options to inhibit chronic inflammation; although tumor necrosis alpha inhibitors have proven somewhat effective; however, they can cause lymphoma and other cancers in some people and these drugs complicate treatment of tuberculosis and other diseases. Chronic inflammatory diseases are caused by excessive peroxynitrite generation, and HDAC-2 gene silencing then occurs from excessive peroxynitrite. Inactivation of the steroidal epigenetic gene mechanism renders steroids ineffective causing steroid resistance. Excessive peroxynitrite caused DNA damage/repair and cellular necrosis via PARP activation /DNA repair and necrosis. When cells die from necrosis they disintegrate into unusual particles that are basically un-recyclable. Furthermore necrosis causes a chronic cycle of chronic inflammation. Therefore, chronic diseases are creating a non-ending cycle of cell death that ends in the demise of the individual so affected.

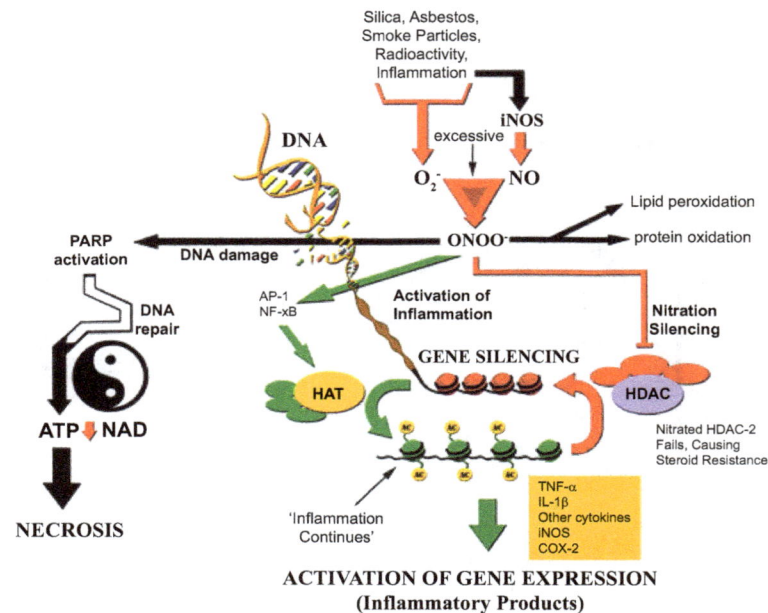

Figure 3: Lessons-learned from treatment of patients with COPD and proposed overall mechanism of ONOO⁻ induced cell toxicity. NF-kB and AP-1 switch on inflammatory genes by inducing several co-activators (e.g., p300/CBP) that have intrinsic HAT activity. Gene transcription only occurs when the chromatin structure is opened up, with unwinding and acetylation of Histones/DNA so that RNA polymerase II and basal transcription complexes can now bind to the naked DNA to intiate transcription. Glucocorticoids switch off multiple inflammatory genes that have been activated by NF-kB and AP-1 during the chronic inflammatory process. Both activation of HDAC and inhibition of HAT may be involved in glucocorticoid-depending gene silencing. As found in patients with COPD, ONOO⁻ may block the HDAC activity, thereby cause glucocorticoid resistance. This mechanism may partly explain the controversy that antioxidants that only have the capability of scavenging superoxide, but not peroxynitrite may fail in a variety of chronic oxidative stress.

Are there alternative treatments for chronic diseases and brain damage diseases, chronic traumatic encephalopathy (cte) and/or trauma? Since excessive peroxynitrite or its derivatives are a major root cause of chronic diseases, it seems likely that controlling the excessive amount of peroxynitrite would be a logical step particularly if done early in the disease state before major chronicity occurred.

The key is to control the action of peroxynitrite to prevent or treat chronic diseases before they become untreatable with steroids.

There have been over 14,000 papers on various aspects of peroxynitrite generation, control etc., However, excessive peroxynitrite has been demonstrated to be very difficult to control- particularly in the brain- since 98% of drugs do not cross the blood-brain barrier. In addition, a drug that controls the peroxynitrite very effectively could cause immunosuppression, since it plays an important role in killing invaders e.g., bacteria, virus, fungus, parasites etc. A key problem is that peroxynitrite is made continuously and therefore any drug which destroys it must be there and working in a continuous manner. In addition, it must be in a useful concentration everywhere macrophages occur which essentially is in all major vascular and tissue portions of the body. Further, this drug or supplement must produce very little toxicity of its own or it would not be very effective.

Since peroxynitrite is made in macrophages which are found both in blood and tissues-The anti-nitration protein target must occur in a continuous manner and in an active state everywhere. Does such a compound exist without causing major toxicity?

This narrows the field down to very few substances. Some of the most effective substances which destroy OONO- are known peroxynitrite-decomposition catalysts and several have been used and have been found to be effective in animal models of pain and brain damage. Iron porphyrinate (FeTPPS) has shown to be effective in an early model of brain damage associated with Huntington's disease model in rats [8]. Stavniichuck [9] has demonstrated that FeTMPS inhibited diabetic peripheral neuropathy [10,11] demonstrated that SR 110 and SR135 peroxynitrite decomposition catalysts inhibited diabetes and enhanced beta cell production of insulin in diabetic mice.

Salvemini [12] used peroxynitrite decomposition catalysts to lessen peroxynitrite and inhibit opiate antinociceptive tolerance. Van Dyke [13,14] prevented diabetes 1 and 2 using carboxy PTIO, and nitration targets to lower nitric oxide and peroxynitrite in a short term diabetes model using streptozotocin- treated rats.

Since peroxynitrite is composed of superoxide ($.O_2$-) and nitric oxide (.NO) and when both gases with free electrons react together at tremendous speed by having the two free electrons pair-peroxynitrite (OONO-) forms. Theoretically one could limit the peroxynitrite production by delimiting production of nitric oxide and/or superoxide but since both molecules have important physiological roles that would likely be ineffective and counterproductive. However, it has been found that producing excessive nitric oxide relative to the amount of superoxide can inhibit formation of peroxynitrite- likely from a feed–back like mechanism.

Could we treat chronic diseases early before the disease gets into an irreversible state causing death?

Is it possible to detect diseases early before a chronic state is reached so that a cure is possible? Diseases like diabetes type 1 and 2, Parkinson's disease, Alzheimer's disease, cancer, heart and other chronic inflammatory diseases like neurodegenerative diseases are certainly more treatable if they can be detected before they go into an irreversible state. All of these diseases are linked to excessive nitration-- and therefore, excessive nitration could be used to detect the disease early. Therefore a sensitive and selective protein nitration assay for a key inflammatory protein, which might be detected early in the disease state, and before the diseases greatly progress to produce massive nitration damage would likely be effective before major irreversible damage is done.

Further, if effective non-toxic nitration inhibitors could be found, the extent of nitration for a given protein would decrease, which would become a measurement of effectiveness of disease treatment. We are developing such an assay using the principles of luminescence which we have developed for a variety of diseases.

In addition, the vascular system is very dependent on the production of nitric oxide in the inner cellular walls formed from epithelial cells. In order to maintain healthy blood vessels it is necessary to produce sufficient nitric oxide which is a major vasodilating substance in the vascular walls themselves- in order to prevent hypertension or high blood pressure. This can be also helped by ingesting sustained release 6-8b grams/day in divided doses of L-arginine, L-citrulline or lesser dses of nitrates from foods like raw spinach, dark green lettuce or beets or beet juice. See Figure 4 which depicts peroxynitrite chronic disease chemistry occurring in blood vessels.

In addition, in the diseases of type 1 and 2 diabetes it has been shown by us and many other researchers [15-26] that the death and illness of these diseases is linked to both excess sugar but also by excess nitration since even when blood sugar is well maintained diabetes of either type continues to persist. The pathological consequences of diabetes are depicted in Figure 5.

Why Hasn't Science Done a Better Job in Conquering These Chronic Diseases? Much of the money spent on disease states is done by scientists and physicians who generally have been taught to think with a group mentality. The National Institutes of Health and other Health Organizations get caught up in the complexities and the politics of science. Money is spent on projects that cannot make any major impact on prevention or understanding the mechanisms of how the disease toxicity is actually occurring. Chronic diseases are the result of overactive immunity greatly linked to macrophage stimulation. Chronic stimulation of macrophages causes chronic inflammation to occur. We can control this situation but it will take properly directed funding and courageous people that actually have an interest in preventing diseases rather than treating diseases after the die is cast. I believe that politics and ignorance has led us to support the NIH rather blindly without asking why haven't these chronic problems been mostly solved? Certainly the FDA and the major drug companies need to have an adjustment in attitude. What is needed is to focus on what is important to human health and not how do we make the most money with drugs that barely make a difference to the health of most humans. I predict that if we take the correct route to discovery, it is certainly possible for almost all humans to live a long, heathy, productive and happy lives.

Summary

Excessive efforts have been expended on the belief that the basis of chronic diseases is linked to gene defects or deficiency of antioxidants which disallow the control of toxic free radicals and the production of aging itself. Based on data presently available, these concepts are far

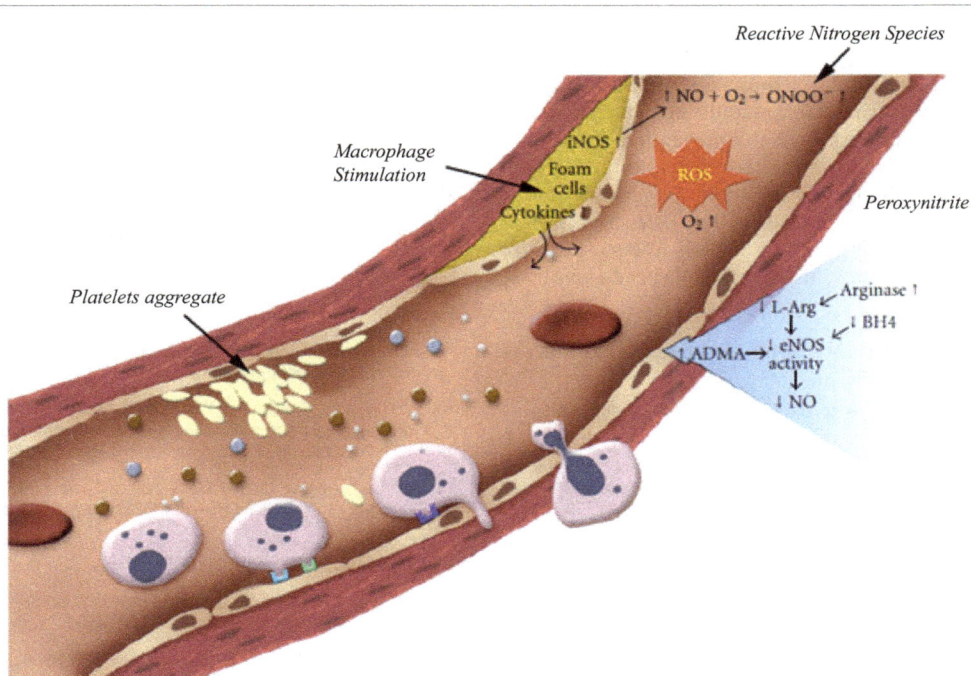

Figure 4: Vascular inflammation associated with chronic diseases.

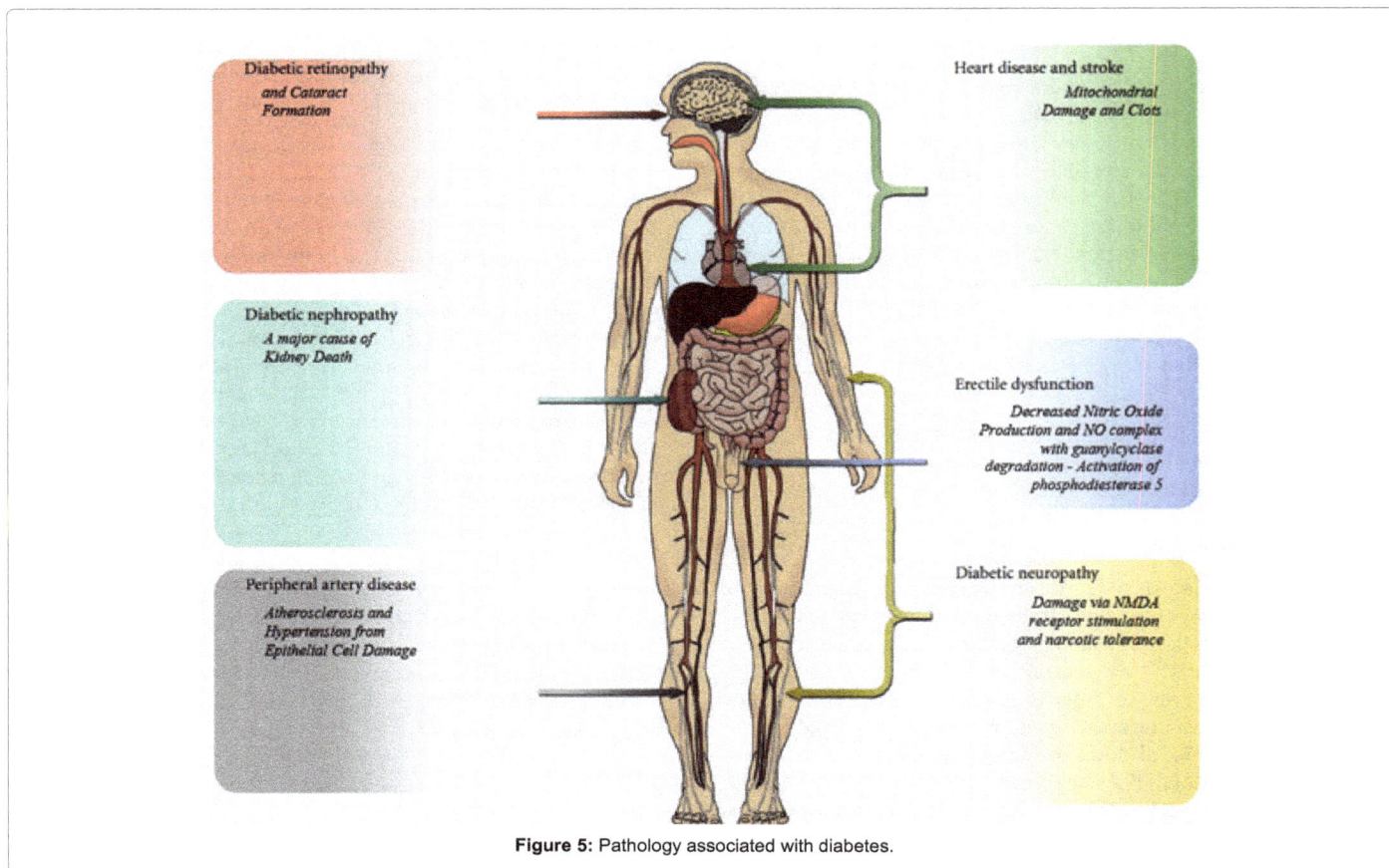

Figure 5: Pathology associated with diabetes.

from the important toxic mechanisms which actually control most untreatable chronic diseases.

Clearly, it is a chemical attack on epigenetic regulatory systems which renders our best anti-inflammatory drugs useless. Since chronic diseases are mostly caused by chronic inflammation, we must focus our attention on the chemistry causing damage to the epigenetic- control mechanism namely histone deacetylase 2 and prevention of nitration by peroxynitrite damage to this key enzyme as well as nitration damage to DNA, RNA, proteins containing tyrosines and tryptophans as well as key lipids and sulfhydryl containing molecules. It is excessive nitration that causes most of damage causing chronic diseases. We must control this excessive nitration to live happy, healthy and long productive lives.

References

1. CDC (2016) United States Department of Health and Human Services. Center for Disease Control and Prevention.

2. Siess H (2015) Oxidative Stress: a concept in redox biology and medicine. Redox Biology 4: 180-183.

3. Antonini J, Van Dyke K (1994) Introduction of Luminol –dependent Chemiluminescence as a Method to Study Silica Inflammation in the Tissue and Phagocytic cells of Rat Lung. Environmental Health Perspectives 102: 37-42.

4. Castranova V (2002) Effect of inhaled crystalline silica in a rat model-time course of pulmonary reactions. Mol Cell Biochem 37: 177-184.

5. Vandyke K, Gutierrez J, Vandyke C, Nowack C (1993) "Piggy Back" Mechanism with Calcium Explains How Silica Exerts Its Toxicity to Phagocytic Cells. Microchemical Journal 48: 34-41.

6. Van Dyke K, Antonini JM, Wu L, Ye Z, Reasor MJ (1994) The inhibition of silica-induced lung inflammation by dexamethasone as measured by bronchoalveolar lavage fluid parameters and peroxynitrite-dependent chemiluminescence. Agents and actions 41: 44-49.

7. Barnes PJ (2011) Glucocorticosteroids: current and future directions. British journal of pharmacology 163: 29-43.

8. Medina-Campos ON, Pérez-Severiano F, Ali SF, Santamaría A (2005) Excitotoxic brain damage involves early peroxynitrite formation in a model of Huntington's disease in rats: protective role of iron porphyrinate 5, 10, 15, 20-tetrakis (4-sulfonatophenyl) porphyrinate iron (III). Neuroscience 135: 463-474.

9. Stavniichuk R, Shevalye H, Lupachyk S, Obrosov A, Groves, et al. (2014) Peroxynitrite and protein nitration in the pathogenesis of diabetic peripheral neuropathy. Diabetes/metabolism research and reviews 30: 669-678.

10. Johns M (2016) Oral Administration of SR-110 Peroxynitrite Decomposition Catalyst Enhances Glucose Homeostasis, Insulin Signaling and Islet Architecture in B6DF1 Mice Fed a High Fat Diet. Arch Biochem Biophys 596: 126-137.

11. Johns M (2015) SR-135, A Peroxynitrite Decomposing Catalyst SR-135 Enhances Beta Cell Function and Survival in B6DF1Mice Fed a High Fat Diet. Arch of Biochem Biophys 49-59.

12. Salvemini D (2009) Peroxynitrite and opiate antinociceptive tolerance: a painful reality. Arch Biochem Biophys 484: 238-244.

13. Van Dyke K, Ghareeb E, Hoeldtke R, Van Dyke M, Van Dyke C, et al. (2011) Can diabetes I and early blindness be prevented using a tylenol combination which inhibits oxidative and nitrosative stress? ISRN toxicology 1-8.

14. Van Dyke, Knox (2014) Does Nitric Oxide and Superoxide Cause Type 2 Diabetes and Can It Be Prevented? Biology and Medicine J 6: 1.

15. Pacher P, Szabó C (2006) Role of peroxynitrite in the pathogenesis of cardiovascular complications of diabetes. Curr Opin Pharmacol 6: 136-141.

16. Pacher P, Beckman JS, Liaudet L (2007) Nitric oxide and peroxynitrite in health and disease. Physiol Reviews 87: 315-424.

17. Szabo C (2007) Peroxynitrite, Pathophysiology and Developmental Therapeutics. Nat Drug Discov 6: 662-680.

18. Rubino F, Moo TA, Rosen DJ, Dakin GF, Pomp A (2009) Diabetes surgery: a new approach to an old disease. Diabetes Care 32: 368-372.

19. Ponce J, Haynes B, Paynter, S, Fromm R, Lindsey B (2004) Effect of Lap-Band®-induced weight loss on type 2 diabetes mellitus and hypertension. Obes Surg 14: 1335-1342.

20. Kaplan M, Aviram M, Hayek T (2012) Oxidative stress and macrophage foam cell formation during diabetes mellitus-induced atherogenesis: Role of insulin therapy. Pharmacol Therap 136: 175-185.

21. Chait A, Bornfeldt KE (2009) Diabetes and atherosclerosis: is there a role for hyperglycemia? J Lipid Res 50: 335-339.

22. Diabetes Control and Complications Trial Research Group (1993) The effect of intensive treatment of diabetes on the development and progression of long-term complications in insulin-dependent diabetes mellitus. N Engl J Med 1993: 977-986.

23. Nakhjavani M, Khalilzadeh O, Khajeali L, Esteghamati A, Morteza A, et al. (2010) Serum oxidized-LDL is associated with diabetes duration independent of maintaining optimized levels of LDL-cholesterol. Lipids 45: 321-327.

24. Gylling H, Hallikainen M, Pihlajamäki J, Simonen P, Kuusisto J et al. (2010) Insulin sensitivity regulates cholesterol metabolism to a greater extent than obesity: lessons from the METSIM Study. J Lipid Res 51: 2422-2427.

25. Forbes JM, Mark CE (2013) Mechanisms of diabetic complications. Physiol Rev 93: 137-188.

26. Krishna KG, Shyamal BC, Christopher GK (2012) Endothelial dysfunction and diabetes: effects on angiogenesis, vascular remodeling, and wound healing. Int J Vascular Med 2012: 1-30.

29

The Influence of Exam Stress on Menstrual Dysfunctions in Saudi Arabia

Muneerah Khalid AlJadidi[1]*, Ohoud Oadah AlMutrafi[1], Rawan Othman Bamousa[1], Sarah Safar AlShehri[1], Anwar Sattam AlRashidi[1], Huda Abdullah AlNijadi[1], Arwa Abdulrhman AMousa[1], Alanoud Saleh AlNami[1], Norah Mohammad AlSubaie[1], Norah Abdulaziz AlMulhim[1], and Lamees Abdulla AlAbdulgader[1]

[1]College of Medicine, King Faisal University, Saudi Arabia
[2]Department of Biostatistics, College of Medicine, King Faisal University, Saudi Arabia

Abstract

Menstrual changes affect the quality of females' lives, it indicates some underlying problems. The purpose of this research is to determine the influence of exams' stress on menstrual dysfunctions. The objectives are to measure the common menstrual dysfunctions among girls during exams, find the most affected characteristics among the measured ones, hence figuring out any relation between the exams (as a source of stress) and the menstrual dysfunctions of 204 Saudi female college students between the age groups of 18 to 25 who matched the required criteria when completed the exam stress social networks questionnaire study on menstrual disorders. It was found that 80.9% of the sample had menstrual changes during exams. Regarding the characteristics; 59.3% had a change in the level of pain, 50% had a change in blood flow, and 54.9% had it in the menstruation timing. The dysmenorrhea was marked as the most common dysfunction within 57.4% of the students during exams. A more detailed research is highly required to explore the risk factors, the pathophysiological mechanisms underlying stress in female students during exams in contemplation to establish a modifying or abortive treatment modalities.

Keywords: Exam stress; Menstruation; Menstrual changes; Menstrual dysfunctions; Dysmenorrhea

Background

Adolescence and early adulthood are times of enormous physical and psychological changes for young women. Yet serious gynecological pathologies are rare in these age groups, but menstrual disturbances are not uncommon, it may also add further disruption to this difficult phase in young females' lives and their families'.

Stress is the body's reaction to any change that requires an adjustment or a response. The body reacts to these changes with physical, mental, and emotional responses, exam stress can cause a lot of problems to menstrual disorders and affect it.

Introduction

There are many women who suffer from menstrual disorders at some point in their life. This problem can significantly affect a woman's life with the exam stress as one of its causes. Stress has always been noted to play a major role as a cause of menstrual disorders.

So, a woman's menstrual cycle might be regular-about the same length every month and her period might be light or heavy, painful or pain-free, long or short, but still be considered normal within a broad range. But as a result of stress that would change to affect the menstruation and take it out from the normal to the abnormal.

Literature Review

Matteo 1987 showed the effect of job stress and job interdependency on the menstrual cycle length, regularity and synchrony, add to that the effect of the menstrual cycle phases on self-reported measures of daily stress. At the end, the study showed that women who experienced high levels of anxiety and job stress were less synchronized than women with low levels of these variables. As it was shown that longer menstrual cycles were associated with women who reported high levels of anxiety and those who had high scores on the Holmes-Rahe Schedule of Recent Events. Regular cycles were associated with lower levels of anxiety and lower scores on the Holmes-Rahe inventory. Self-reports of daily stress were greater during the late luteal and early menstrual phase of the cycle [1-10].

Harlow and Matanoski showed the association between weight, physical activity, stress and variation in the length of the menstrual cycle. They examined 166 college women, aged 17-19 years, who kept menstrual diaries during their freshman year. At the end it was shown that stressors, characterized by situations, which create a demand for performance or require adjustments to new demands, also increased the risk of a long cycle [2].

Fenster et al. showed the effects of psychological stress in the workplace and menstrual function among married women between 18 and 39 years of age. It was found that women who work in stressful jobs were classified as twice more to experience shorter cycles than those working in other jobs also they were slightly more likely to have an anovulatory episode, but the numbers were very small and the confidence interval included unity. In addition, the effect estimates decreases after adjustment [8].

Barsoma et al. showed the association between psychological stress and menstrual cycle characteristics in premenopausal women. The study population was drawn from participants of the Tremin Research Program on Women's Health (Tremin), a predominantly white, well-educated group of women. The results of this investigation suggested that, in the long term, stressful life events have little relationship to the length of menstrual cycle intervals and the duration of menstrual bleeding in premenopausal women. Though without data on the exact timing of stressful life events, however, these results were not conclusive, especially since there was some indication that marked increases in

---

*Corresponding author: Muneerah Khalid AlJadidi, College of Medicine, King Faisal University, Saudi Arabia, E-mail: muneerahkhalid@gmail.com

the level of stress may be related to the length of cycle intervals and duration of menstrual bleeding in the short term [6].

Allsworth et al. showed the influence of stress on the menstrual cycle among newly incarcerated women. At the end of the study, they were found to have high rates of amenorrhea and menstrual irregularity and the prevalence may be associated with certain stresses. Also, the menstrual dysfunctions were common in this population. 9% reported amenorrhea, while 33% reported menstrual irregularities. A number of stressors were associated with menstrual irregularities, including having a parent with a history of alcohol or drug problems, childhood physical or sexual abuse, race/ethnicity, smoking status and recent drug use. These effects were attenuated somewhat when excluding women who had reported with any hormonal contraceptive use in the past 3 months [1].

Sood et al. showed the poor correlation of stress levels and menstrual patterns among medical students. It was done on 359 female medical students from years one and two at the Faculty of Medicine, University Teknologi MARA. All students were between the age groups of 16-20 years with average height and weight and previous normal cycles. The results showed that there is no significant association between stress levels and menstrual changes among preclinical medical students [9].

The Need for the Study

The study is conducted to determine the effects of exam stress on menstrual disorders on Saudi educated females.

The Objectives of the Study

➢ To show the existence of exam stress's effect on menstruation.
➢ To determine the distribution of exam stress's effect among the characteristics (timing change, flow or pain) of menstruation.
➢ To measure the frequencies of the most common menstrual dysfunctions during exams.

Methodology

Research design and sampling

The sample of the study is designed to include female college students excluding physically less mature ones; those who haven't achieved an ovulatory cycle to have menarche. The study was targeting female sample between age groups of 18-25, single, healthy of any hematological disorders and studying in college.

This research is a descriptive cross-sectional, which consists of a comparison between one group to one subject to determine the most common change (dysfunction) which might be associated with exam stress.

The questionnaire is developed following an extensive review of which questions were more suitable to be asked and would give sufficient answers. Once developed it was reviewed and finalized. The questionnaire included 11 closed questions and 2 open ones. Questions included personal ones, including age, marital status and educational level to exclude undesired samples, others focused on the menstruations of the subjects in relation to the timing, the flow of blood, the level of pain and other characteristics during exams' stressful days. Finally, data have been collected from 204 girls who matched the criteria of the research through an online survey distributed on social networks.

Ethical consideration

Data was collected anonymously, there was no revealing of any personal information, the questionnaire identified the researchers, their purpose to the respondents, and hence no one but the team was allowed to look through the data.

Statistical analysis

By using SPSS version 21.0.0,0, data was entered and analyzed using the descriptive statistics (frequencies) and chi-square test of independence to measure the relations.

Results

A total of 204 girls responded as a match to the criteria of the research questionnaire. All were single college students between the ages of 18-25 years healthy of any hematological diseases.

The Figure 1 shows that 165 girls (80.9%) had changes in their menstruation during exams, whereas 39 girls (19.1%) stated no changes.

Table 1 shows that 112 girls (54.9%) had changes related to the timing of their monthly bleeding onset, whereas 103 girls (50.5%) had changes related to the menstruation blood flow, 122 girls (59.8%) had changes related to the level of their menstrual pain and 113 girls (55.4%) had more than one change in characteristics. This result clearly declares the menstrual pain as the most affected characteristic during exams.

The previously mentioned Table 2 explains how every menstrual characteristic is affected during exams. Out of the 204 girls, it showed that 67 girls (32.8%) had earlier monthly start, whereas 45 girls (22.1%) had later monthly start with 0.000 P value (<0.01). Also, the table shows that out of the 204 girls, 61 girls (29.9%) had their menstrual flow increased (hypermenorrhea), whereas 42 girls (20.6%) had their menstrual flow decreased (hypermenorrhea) with 0.000 P value (<0.01). It finally shows that 117 girls (57.4%) had an increased pain of their menstruation (dysmenorrhea), whereas 5 girls (2.5%) had a decreased pain of their menstruation with 0.000 P value (<0.01).

The chi-square test of independence results support that menstrual changes regarding the monthly start, bleeding intensity and menstrual pain do happen during exams.

The Figure 2 showing the percentage of each change arranged from the most common to the least common. It shows that (57.40%) has increased in pain (dysmenorrhea), whereas (32.80%) has an earlier

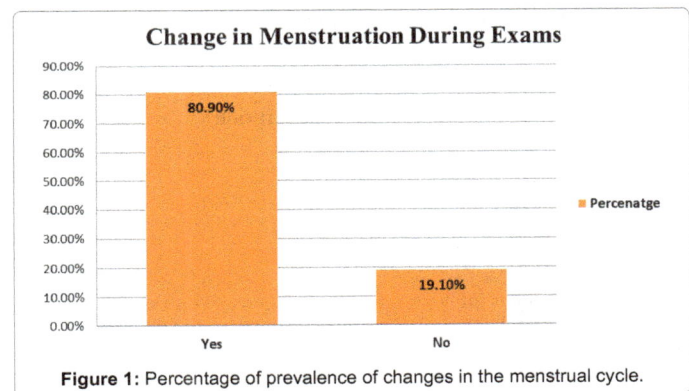

Figure 1: Percentage of prevalence of changes in the menstrual cycle.

Characteristics	Frequency	Percentage
Timing change	112	54.9%
Intensity of the flow change	103	50.5%
Change in the level of pain	122	59.8%
Change in several characteristics	113	55.4%

Table 1: Affected characteristics of the menstrual cycle during exams.

time start, also (29.90%) had an increase in the flow (hypermenorrhea), (22.10%) had a late time start, (20.60%) had a decrease in flow (hypermenorrhea) whereas (2.5%) had a low-grade pain.

Discussion

The first finding in this study is that 80.9% of our sample has menstrual changes during exams whereas 68% had more than one change. This finding has been supported by a study which demonstrated a significant association between academic stress and menstrual disorder among undergraduate females as for those who reported high level of academic stress were two times likely to suffer menstrual changes [11]. But it's conflicted with a study that investigated the impact of pre-examination stress in the second year medical students and reported changes in pre-examination menstruation in only 15.91% of the sample [3]. This difference could be partially due to the fact that the study was measuring different effects of stress and not focusing on the menstruation hence a part of the sample were males.

But why these changes happen is a question that needs to be answered. Some of the theories which might explain what's happening is the physiology of the stress which leads to an increase in cortisol in the body which leads, among others, to the disruption of normal ovulation and menstrual cycle [12] which might be the explanation of the timing change reported by 54% of the sample (earlier in 32.8% and later in 22.1%).

In addition to that, what's worth pointing out is dysmenorrhea, the most common reported dysfunction in 57.4% of the sample that might be explained by the suggestion that there's a possible neural mechanism through which stress could facilitate pain. This stress-induced hyperalgesia is due to the activation of stress-related circuitry in the hypothalamus to activate pain-facilitating neurons to increase the sensitivity towards pain [12].

Conclusion

The prevalence of menstrual changes is high among students during exams. The common dysfunctions are: increase in the level of pain (most common), earlier menstruation (2nd most common) and an increase in blood flow (3rd most common).

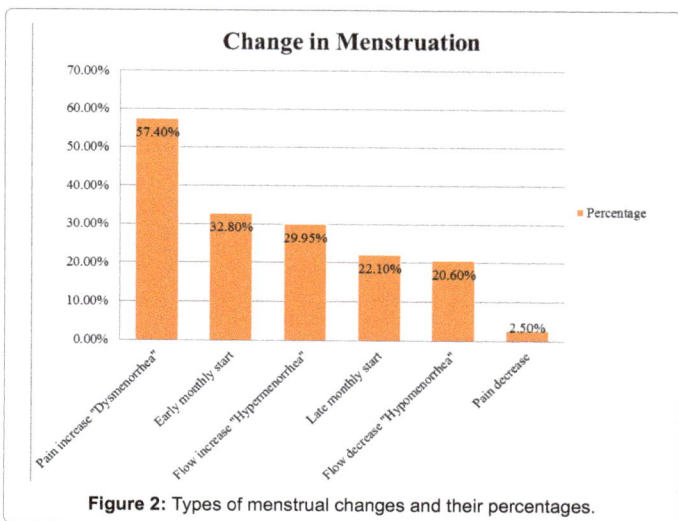

Figure 2: Types of menstrual changes and their percentages.

Characteristics	Changes	N (%)	P Value
Date	On date	92 (45.1%)	0.000**
	Early	67 (32.8%)	
	Late	45 (22.1%)	
	Total	204 (100%)	
Flow	No change	101 (49.5%)	0.000**
	Increase	61 (29.95%)	
	Decrease	42 (20.6%)	
	Total	204 (100%)	
Pain	No change	82 (40.2%)	0.000**
	Increase	117 (57.4%)	
	Decrease	5 (2.5%)	
	Total	204 (100%)	

Table 2: Prevalence of changes in menstrual cycle during exams. *P<0.05; **P<0.01.

Recommendations

Based on the results of the research, it's recommend that universities should provide their female students with short courses to teach deep breathing techniques, meditation and yoga as forms of relaxation methods previous to the exams. In addition to offer warm beverages in exam halls to reduce stress and boost students' mood and provide over-the-counter analgesics and warm packs to help with the pain. In addition, there should be a psychosocial specialist to help students succeed academically by providing counseling, instruction, and mentoring for those who are struggling in exams which will benefit students in reducing exams' stress. Lastly, it should be noted that exams are stressful times hence any healthy options for reducing stress should be considered.

References

1. Allsworth JE, Clarke J, Peipert JF, Hebert MR, Cooper A, et al. (2007) The influence of stress on the menstrual cycle among newly incarcerated women. Women's Health Issues 17: 202-209.

2. Harlow SD, Matanoski GM (1991) The association between weight, physical activity, and stress and variation in the length of the menstrual cycle. American journal of epidemiology 133: 38-49.

3. Rizvi AH, Awaiz M, Ghanghro Z, Jafferi MA, Aziz S (2010) Pre-examination stress in second year medical students in a government college. J Ayub Med Coll Abbottabad 22: 152-55.

4. Begum J, Hossain AM, Nazneen SA (2009) Menstrual pattern and common menstrual disorders among students in Dinajpur Medical College. Dinajpur Med Col J 2: 37-43.

5. Karout N, Hawai SM, Altuwaijri S (2012) Prevalence and pattern of menstrual disorders among Lebanese nursing students. Eastern Mediterranean Health Journal 18: 346-52.

6. Barsom SH, Mansfield PK, Koch PB, Gierach G, West SG (2004) Association between psychological stress and menstrual cycle characteristics in perimenopausal women. Women's Health Issues 14: 235-241.

7. Fenster L, Waller K, Chen J, Hubbard AE, Windham GC, et al. (1999) Psychological stress in the workplace and menstrual function. American Journal of Epidemiology 149: 127-134.

8. Sood M, Devi A, Azlinawati AMD, Razali S, Hapizah Nawawi S, et al. (2012) Poor correlation of stress levels and menstrual patterns among medical students. Journal of Asian Behavioural Studies 2: 59-66.

9. Matteo S (1987) The effect of job stress and job interdependency on menstrual cycle length, regularity and synchrony. Psychoneuroendocrinology 12: 467-476.

10. Ekpenyong CE, Davis KJ, Akpan UP, Daniel NE (2011) Academic stress and menstrual disorders among female undergraduates in Uyo, South Eastern Nigeria – the need for health education. Niger J Physiol Sci 26: 193-198.

11. Aronson D (2009) Cortisol-its role in stress, inflammation, and indications for diet therapy. Today's Dietitian 11: 38.

12. Martenson ME, Cetas JS, Heinricher MM (2009) A possible neural basis for stress-induced hyperalgesia. Pain 142: 236-244.

30

Women's Performance of Breast Cancer Screening (Breast Self-Examination, Clinical Breast Exam and Mammography)

Somaya Aljohani*, Israa Saib and Muatasim Noorelahi

Intern, College of Medicine, Taibah University, Medina, Saudi Arabia

Abstract

Background: Breast cancer is the most common malignancy among women in Saudi Arabia. Despite the availability of early detection methods to diagnose breast cancer, a huge number of women are still unaware about these methods. This study was conducted to identify the attitude of women in Medina toward breast cancer screening methods, including breast self-examination (BSE), clinical breast examination (CBE) and mammography.

Materials and methods: A cross sectional survey has been conducted on 124 women aged from 39 and older, who attended Taibah Medical Center for cancer screening either by doctor's recommendation, family or friends advice, or by herself. Face to face questionnaire was used to collect data. All data were analyzed by statistical analysis system software.

Results: The results showed only 35.5%, 27.4% and 37.8% of participants reported that they practiced BSE, CBE and annual mammography, respectively. Only 27.3% of women practiced BSE once per month, and 8.8% visited doctor annually for CBE. Both educational level and family history were significantly related to BSE. 57.7% of the participants who had positive family history practiced BSE, and 56.0% of the participants who practiced BSE were highly educated. Lacking awareness about BSE is the most important barrier in not practicing BSE, while not having a breast lump was the reason for not undergoing either clinical breast examination (38.7%) or periodic mammography (54.9%).

Conclusion: This study emphasized the need for massive health education program to increase awareness, and improve the attitude of women toward breast cancer screening methods.

Keywords: Breast cancer; Screening; Self-examination; Mammography

Introduction

Breast cancer is the most frequent malignancy among Saudi women and the ninth leading cause of death in Saudi Arabia in 2010 [1,2]. Breast cancer incidents have been escalating faster in the Kingdom and is currently ranked number one among cancerous diseases in women in the country of Saudi Arabia [3,4]. Breast cancer is the second leading cause of mortality and morbidity in women of western countries [5].

Breast cancer is preventable through early detection and healthy lifestyles that improve women's health and decrease the costs relating to cancer death [6]. Therefore, effective screening programs are the best way to detect cancer before experiencing any symptoms [7]. Breast cancer screening methods include breast self-examination (BSE), clinical breast examination (CBE) and mammograms [8]. These effective ways of screening are consistent with and show that there is relatively little current emphasize on the first published results of the New York randomized control trial in 1997 [9].

Ravichandran et al. conducted a study in the Riyadh region that revealed only 23.1% of studied subjects practiced BSE [10]. Hussein et al. carried out a study on 1000 participants in Hail city and its rural neighborhoods, and found that 50% of all female participants >16 years old did not practice BSE [11]. Some studies were based on selected groups, like students, and findings revealed an imbalance between the knowledge and practice of BSE, CBE and mammogram [12]. However, in the Gulf region, specifically in Saudi Arabia several previous studies conducted in different regions that assessed the awareness, knowledge, and attitude towards breast cancer among female Saudi teachers, female university students, and women respectively, indicated that many women are still lacking information about breast cancer screening [13,14].

Despite the spread of breast cancer screening centers in Saudi Arabia that offer free screening service, many women have no access to the screening program due to several factors like cultural, environmental, lack of education and awareness among females; and most importantly, lack of social support that incorporates lack of encouragement by a physician [15].

Health care should keep in mind that social support within hospitals and clinics are an essential component of a clinical encounter [16]. A study by Jensen et al. indicated that a low level of social support was strongly associated with non-participation in and non-adherence to breast cancer screening [17]. Thus, posing a major public health concern. The review of literature revealed that there are no published studies about this community issue in Medina, Saudi Arabia. We aimed to further evaluate such conditions for these women in this city and help them become more pragmatic in their own life.

Objective

To identify the prevalence and effectiveness in breast cancer screening methods among women.

---

*Corresponding author: Somaya Aljohani, Intern, College of Medicine, Taibah University, Alsalam Street, 41431, Medina, Saudi Arabia,
E-mail: somaya.aljohani@gmail.com

Subjects and Methods

This study carried out to investigate the attitude of women about breast cancer screening by using a cross-sectional survey of women aged from 39 years and older who were attending Taibah Medical Center for breast cancer screening for a period of four months (2015-2016). The sample comprised 124 Saudi and non-Saudi females who visited the center for a mammogram. A face-to-Face survey (10 minutes per each subject) was used to collect the data after obtaining written consent from each participant.

The study employed a predesigned structured, reliable and validated questionnaire to collect the data. Those who refused to participate or gave incomplete information were excluded from the study. Study approval was obtained from the Ethics Committee of Taibah College of Medicine, Medina, Saudi Arabia (TUCD-REC). A consent form was given at the beginning of the questionnaire explaining the purpose of the study, and requested their voluntary participation. The women's privacy and confidentiality were assured. The questionnaire was constructed based on the objective of the study, including questions on socio-demographic data (such as: age, marital status, nationality, education level, work status and income), a commitment to do a breast checkup including breast self-examination, breast clinical examination and mammogram as well as their reasons for not doing them.

All data was analyzed using the statistical analysis system (SAS) software package [18]. Data was presented using frequencies. The women's practice of breast cancer screening (breast self-examination, clinical breast examination and mammography) was assessed and compared by women's characteristics using appropriate statistical tests (Chi square and Fischer exact test). The criteria of significance were considered at a P-value of ≤ 0.05. Furthermore, the barrier items preventing women from the practice of the studied breast cancer screening methods were assessed by the frequency number and percent of each studied barrier item for each studied breast cancer screening.

Results

During the study period, 124 women were interviewed at Medina cancer screening center at Medina city, Saudi Arabia. Fifty women (40.3%) visited the center according to doctors' recommendation, 27 women according to their family and friends talks and 47 (38%) by women herself. Of the studied 124 women, there were 71 women (57.3%) reported that they practiced mammography for the first time during their life and the remaining 53 (42.7%) women had reported to practice mammography regularly. Of those 53 women, 20 (37.8%) had practiced mammography once every year, 7 (13.2%) every two years, 26 (49%) every three years. Of all the women studied, 63 women reported that they have been referred by doctors to do the mammography. Of the studied 124 women, there were 44 (35.5%) reported that they practice BSE and 34 (27.4%) reported that they practice clinical examination.

Among the studied women reporting breast self-examination (44 out of 124), there have been 13 women (27.3%) practicing BSE once monthly, only 5 women (11.3%) do it 2-3 days after their period ends, 26 women (59%) examine the breast while lying down, 34 (77.3%) raise their arms up and look for changes, 23 (52.3%) examine and press their nipples for any type of discharge, and 32 (73%) examine lymph nodes in their armpit. Of the studied women practicing clinical breast examination (34 out of 124), 3 women (8.8%) reported that they visited a doctor to examine their breasts every 2 months, 13 (38.3%) every 6 months, 3 (8.8%) every year and 15 (44.1%) every three years.

In Table 1 presented the characteristics of the studied 124 women.

Half of the studied women were aged ≥ 50 years, and 76.6% of the studied women were Saudis. About three-fourth of the studied women were married (72.6%), and didn't work (house wife) (76.6%), and less than university educated (79.8%). The majority of the studied women (96.8%) reported less than 20,000 SR as family's monthly income. The studied women reported that they have had a positive family history regarding breast cancer and having breast problems were 21.0% and 34.7%, respectively. The contraceptive pill use was 2.4% among all studied women while the ex-users were 56.7%.

In Table 2 showed the distribution of breast self-examination among the studied women by their characteristics. The higher significant proportion of women who practice breast self-examination are young women less than 40 years (100%) and those from 40 to less than 50 years (38.9%), highly educated women (56%), high monthly income women (75%) and those reported positive family history for breast cancer (57.7%). Although not significant, the proportion of breast self-examination was higher among non-Saudis, married and divorced, employed and retired, women having breast problems, and contraceptive pill users and ex-users.

In Table 3 presented practice of clinical breast examination among the studied women by their characteristics. Significant high proportions of women were found to do clinical breast examination among employed (41.1%), retired women (57.0%) and those with a monthly family income from 5000-20000 SR (38.5%) and those with monthly

Characteristics*	N=124
Age in years <40 40-<50 ≥ 50	3 (2.4) 59 (47.6) 62 (50.0)
Nationality Saudi Non Saudi	95 (76.6) 29 (23.4)
Marital status Single Married Widow and divorced	1 (0.8) 90 (72.6) 33 (26.6)
Occupation House wife Employed Retired	95 (76.6) 22 (17.7) 7 (5.7)
Educational level Illiterate Basic University and higher	25 (20.2) 74 (59.6) 25 (20.2)
Family monthly income in SR <5000 5000-20000 >20000	50 (40.3) 70 (56.5) 4 (3.2)
Family history of breast cancer Yes No	26 (21.0) 98 (79.0)
Having breast problem Yes No	43 (34.7) 81 (65.3)
Contraceptive use Users Ex-users No	3 (2.4) 70 (56.5) 51 (41.1)
Practice of breast cancer screening BSE** Clinical breast exam. Mammography for first time	44 (35.5) 34 (27.4) 71 (57.5)

*Data are presented by n (%).
**Breast self-examination.
Table 1: Characteristics of the studied women.

Socio-demographic characteristics	Breast self-examination		P value
	Yes (n=44)	No (n= 80)	
Age in years <40 40-<50 ≥ 50	3 (100.0) 23 (38.9) 18 (29.3)	0 (0.0) 36 (61.1) 44 (70.7)	0.03*
Nationality Saudi Non Saudi	31 (32.6) 13 (44.8)	64 (67.4) 16 (55.2)	0.23
Marital status Single Married Widow and divorced	0 (0.0) 35 (38.9) 9 (27.3)	0 (0.0) 35 (38.9) 9 (27.3)	0.43
Occupation House wife Employed Retired	24 (30.5) 11 (50.0) 4 (57.1)	66 (69.5) 11 (50.0) 3 (42.9)	0.1
Educational level Illiterate Basic University and higher	3 (12.0) 27 (36.5) 14 (56.0)	22 (88.0) 47 (63.5) 11 (44.0)	0.004*
Family monthly income in SR <5000 5000-20000 >20000	13 (26.0) 28 (40.0) 3 (75.0)	37 (74.0) 42 (60.0) 1 (25.0)	0.04*
Family history of breast cancer Yes No	15 (57.7) 29 (29.6)	11 (42.3) 69 (70.1)	0.01*
Having breast problem Yes No	17 (39.5) 27 (33.3)	26 (60.5) 54 (66.7)	0.49
Contraceptive use Users Ex-users No	2 (66.7) 29 (41.4) 13 (25.5)	1 (33.3) 41 (58.6) 38 (74.5)	0.09

*Significant.

Table 2: Breast self-examination among the studied women by their characteristics.

incomes of more than 20000 SR (25%). With no statistically significant differences, the proportion of clinical breast examination was also high among young aged women, Saudis, married women, basic and highly educated women, women with positive history for breast cancer, those with breast problems and users and ex-users of contraceptive pills

In Table 4 showed the distribution of the studied women by mammography practice and their characteristics. Of the studied women, there have been statistically significant differences between women who were practicing mammography for the first time and those reported frequent practice according to their educational level and monthly family income. The frequent mammography was more among the highly educated (56%) and higher family income (66.7%) women. on the other hand; however, the proportion of women practicing mammography for the first time was higher in relation to other studied variables, although not significant.

In Table 5 presented the barrier items preventing the studied women from contributing or conducting breast cancer screening. Among all the studied women, the most important barrier items preventing women from practice breast self-examination were lack of awareness about this method (41.0%) and not having breast lumps (21.8%). The barrier items preventing the studied women to seek clinical breast examination were not having a breast lump (38.7%) and lack of awareness (29.0%). Among women who practice mammography for the first time during their life, the most important barriers to contribute frequent mammography were not having a breast lump (54.9), a lack

of awareness (40.9%) and not being requested by a doctor to do so (16.9%).

Discussion

Globally, breast cancer is the second leading cause of death in women and ranked number one among cancerous diseases in women who live in Saudi Arabia [3-5]. The aim of this study was to investigate the attitude of women toward breast cancer screening. In the present study, breast self-examination, clinical breast examination and periodic mammography screenings were reported by 35.5%, 27.4%, 37.8% of women who participated in the study, respectively. The reported results of practicing breast cancer screening from other studies conducted in neighboring countries (Qatar and Jordan) showed BSE, CBE and periodic mammography screening were 13.9%, 31.3% and 26.9%, respectively in Qatar, [19] while 34.9%, 16.8% and 8.6%, respectively in Jordan [20]. Similarly, on regular performance of BSE, our data found 27.3% of participants have performed BSE once per month. However, previous study was conducted among Iranian women showed the regular performance of BSE was 10.1% [21]. Theses reported results reflect the differences of attitude toward BCS among different societies.

Regarding the performance of BSE, our findings in the present study emphasized the importance of social campaigns and mass media in teaching women the correct performance of practicing BSE. The data showed that the performance level of practicing BSE among the participants according to baseline technique of BSE was lacking, only 59% of participants examine breast in lying down position, 77.3% raise their arm up and look for changes, 52.3% examine and press their nipple for any type of discharge and 73% examine lymph nodes in their armpit. Our data indicated that young women (less than 40) have 100% practicing BSE while 38.9% and 29.3% among 40 to less 50 year old and more than 50 year old women, respectively. These reported results were not in line with Ravichandran et al. study, where he found that there is no significant association between the different age groups and practicing BSE [10].

In our study, positive family history was remarkable and a promoting factor to keep practicing BSE among the participants. More than one half (57.7%) of positive family history participants practiced BSE while only 29.6% of negative family history participants practiced BSE. As stated in study was conducted on 374 women in Riyadh, those women who perceives family history as a risk factor that increases her susceptibility of having breast cancer would be more likely to be committed to do breast examinations in regular manner [22]. These findings reflect a positive attitude among women who have family history of breast cancer.

According to the present study more than half (56.0%) of educated women (university and higher education) have a positive attitude about BSE. The data in this study showed practicing BSE were 30.5%, 50.0% and 57.1% for housewife, employed participants and retired respectively, this result was not in line with previous study that showed employment was the only significant socio-demographic predictor of BSE practice [22].

In terms of barrier for BSE, lacking awareness of this method (41.0%) was the most important factor in not practicing BSE among the participants in this study. This proportion is much lesser than a study in Jeddah reported that 47.5% of females participants knew how to perform BSE [4]. As well, based on the study conducted in King Abdulaziz Medical City, Riyadh, Saudi Arabia, had shown that

Socio-demographic Characteristics	Clinical breast examination		P value
	Yes (n=34)	No (n=90)	
Age in years			
<40	1 (33.3)	2 (66.7)	
40-<50	19 (32.2)	40 (67.8)	
≥ 50	14 (22.6)	48 (77.4)	0.4
Nationality			
Saudi	29 (30.5)	66 (69.5)	
Non Saudi	5 (17.2)	24 (82.8)	0.16
Marital status			
Single	0 (0.0)	1 (100.0)	
Married	29 (32.2)	61 (67.8)	
Widow and divorced	5 (15.2)	28 (84.8)	0.12
Occupation			
House wife	21 (22.1)	74 (77.9)	
Employed	9 (41.1)	13 (59.9)	
Retired	4 (57.0)	3 (43.0)	0.03*
Educational level			
Illiterate	5 (20.0)	20 (80.0)	
Basic	21 (28.9)	53 (71.1)	
University and higher	8 (32.0)	17 (68.0)	0.6
Family monthly income in SR			
<5000	6 (12.0)	44 (88.0)	
5000-20000	27 (38.5)	43 (61.5)	
>20000	1 (25.0)	3 (75.0)	0.003*
Family history of breast cancer			
Yes	8 (30.7)	18 (69.3)	
No	26 (26.5)	72 (73.5)	0.66
Having breast problem			
Yes	15 (34.9)	28 (65.1)	
No	19 (23.5)	62 (76.5)	0.17
Contraceptive use			
Users	1 (33.3)	2 (66.7)	
Ex-users	23 (32.9)	47 (67.1)	
No	10 (19.6)	41 (80.1)	0.18

*Significant

Table 3: Clinical breast examination among the studied women by their characteristics.

Barrier items	n (%)
Breast self examination (n=124)	
1. Lacking of awareness	51 (41.0)
2. Not having breast problem	27 (21.8)
3. Forgetting to do it	9 (7.3)
4. Unimportant test	4 (3.2)
5. Fearing of finding lump	2 (1.6)
Clinical breast examination (n=124)	
1. Not having breast problem	48 (38.7)
2. Lacking of awareness	36 (29.0)
3. Embarrasment	8 (6.4)
4. Fearing of finding lump	2 (1.6)
Mammography (n=71)*	
1. Not having breast problem	39 (54.9)
2. Lacking of awareness	29 (40.9)
3. Not requested by doctor	12 (16.9)
4. Fearing of results	2 (2.8)
5. Fearing of pain	1 (1.4)

*Significant

Table 4: Frequency distribution of mammography among the studied women by their characteristics.

Barrier items	n (%)
Breast self examination (n=124)	
1. Lacking of awareness	51 (41.0)
2. Not having breast problem	27 (21.8)
3. Forgetting to do it	9 (7.3)
4. Unimportant test	4 (3.2)
5. Fearing of finding lump	2 (1.6)
Clinical breast examination (n=124)	
1. Not having breast problem	48 (38.7)
2. Lacking of awareness	36 (29.0)
3. Embarrasment	8 (6.4)
4. Fearing of finding lump	2 (1.6)
Mammography (n=71)*	
1. Not having breast problem	39 (54.9)
2. Lacking of awareness	29 (40.9)
3. Not requested by doctor	12 (16.9)
4. Fearing of results	2 (2.8)
5. Fearing of pain	1 (1.4)

*Analyses including only those practice mammography for first time during their life time.

Table 5: Reasons of not performing breast cancer screening among the studied women.

the reasons for not doing BSE as reported by 235 women were: not knowing how to examine their breast [22].

Despite breast cancer screening is being offered for free in our city, the study revealed that only 12% of the families with low monthly income (<5000 SR) came for CBE and 30.0% of them came to do frequent mammography screening in comparable with 25% of high monthly income (>20,000 SR) came for CBC and 66% of them came to do frequent mammography screening. While in a another study, found that the cost of screening had a crucial effect on women not seeking breast cancer screening [23].

Barriers preventing women from seeking clinical breast examination were: not having breast lumps (38.7%) and lacking awareness (29.0%). Similarly, a recent study reported that not having symptoms (92%) and not knowing that screening was needed (40%) were the main reasons for not undergoing either clinical breast examination or mammography [24].

In reference to another study, Women were not obtaining access to the screening program due to several factors, and most importantly, lack of education and awareness [15]. Data in this study were in concordance with the previous study which indicated that education level has a strong impact on women performance toward breast cancer screening. Out of 124 studied women, 56% of highly educated females do mammogram frequently, while only 16% of illiterate females do mammogram frequently. According to women who practiced mammography for first time, the data revealed not having a breast lump (54.9%) is the most significant barrier that contribute doing frequent mammography. This contrasts with another study, where lack of knowledge and awareness of breast screening were found to be the most important barrier [25].

The strengths of this study include that the study questionnaire was comprehensive and addressed almost all items as well as wide range of personal and belief barrier factors discussed in previously published Saudi and non-Saudi studies. The study questionnaire has also been validated by specialist in this filed; including radiologist, oncologist and an epidemiologist. To the best of our knowledge, this study is the first to study practice and barriers of different breast cancer screening methods in Medina region in Saudi Arabia. Dissemination of these findings to Medina Cancer Breast Screening Center (MCBSC) will help to know the current situation and to plan different breast awareness and health education programs to correct some incorrect beliefs preventing women in Medina and to encourage them attending the center.

The limitations of this study should not be overlooked. Self-selection bias may have been a limitation factor in this study because all women were selected from single center, which should not attract women from different educational and family income sectors to attend. However, because of socio-demographic distributions observed in this study, the sample appeared representative and this factor appeared to have no role in the study findings.

Conclusions

Our results support the need for new emphasis in health educational program throughout promotion campaigns, mass media or even encouragement by health professionals. Moreover, increase the nationwide breast cancer screening awareness to engage them in breast cancer preventive practice. Further research is needed to shed more light on this occurrence, particularly on Medina's population, and suggests future barriers and solution direction.

Acknowledgements

We are grateful to the healthcare providers at Taibah Breast Cancer Screening Center in Medina for their contributions to reach the goals of the study. The authors would like to thank all patients participated in this study.

References

1. Mokdad AH, Jaber S, Aziz MIA, AlBuhairan F, AlGhaithi A, et al. (2014) The state of health in the Arab world, 1990-2010: an analysis of the burden of diseases, injuries, and risk factors. Lancet 383: 309-320.

2. El Bcheraoui C, Basulaiman M, Wilson S, Daoud F, Tuffaha M, et al. (2015) Breast cancer screening in saudi arabia: free but almost no takers. PLoS One 10: e0119051.

3. Desouky DE, Taha AA (2015) Effects of a training program about breast cancer and breast self-examination among female students at Taif University. J Egypt Public Health Assoc 90: 8-13.

4. Radi SM (2013) Breast Cancer awareness among Saudi females in Jeddah. Asian Pac J Cancer Prev 14: 4307-4312.

5. American Cancer Society (2012) Breast Cancer Facts and Figures.

6. Noroozi A, Tahmasebi R (2011) Factors influencing breast cancer screening behavior among Iranian women. Asian Pac J Cancer Prev 12: 1239-1244.

7. Bleyer A, Welch HG (2012) Effect of three decades of screening mammography on breast-cancer incidence. N Engl J Med 367: 1998-2005.

8. Rafi Baig M, Subramaniam V, Chandrasegar AA, Mehmood Khan T (2011) A population based survey on knowledge and awareness of breast cancer in the suburban females of Sungai Petani, Kedah, Malaysia. Int J Collab Res Intern Med Public Heal 3: 671-679.

9. Shapiro S (1977) Evidence on screening for breast cancer from a randomized trial. Cancer 39: 2772-2782.

10. Ravichandran K, Al-Hamdan NA, Mohamed G (2011) Knowledge, attitude, and behavior among Saudis toward cancer preventive practice. J Family Community Med. Medknow Publications and Media Pvt. Ltd. 18: 135-142.

11. Hussein DM, Alorf SH, Al-Sogaih YS, Alorf SH, Alaskar RS, et al. (2015) Breast cancer awareness and breast self-examination in Northern Saudi Arabia. A preliminary survey. Saudi Med J 34: 681-688.

12. Latif R (2015) Knowledge and attitude of Saudi female students towards breast cancer: A cross-sectional study. J Taibah Univ Med Sci 9: 328-334.

13. Habib F, Salman S, Safwat M, Shalaby S (2010) Awareness and Knowledge of Breast Cancer Among University Students in Al Madina Al Munawara Region. Middle East Journal of Cancer, pp: 159-166.

14. Dandash KF, Al-Mohaimeed A (2007) Knowledge, attitudes, and practices surrounding breast cancer and screening in female teachers of Buraidah, Saudi Arabia. Int J Health Sci (Qassim) 1: 61-71.

15. Abulkhair OA, Al Tahan FM, Young SE, Musaad SM, Jazieh ARM (2015) The first national public breast cancer screening program in Saudi Arabia. Ann Saudi Med 30: 350-357.

16. Usta YY (2012) Importance of Social Support in Cancer Patients. Asian Pacific J Cancer Prev 13: 3569-3572.

17. Jensen LF, Pedersen AF, Andersen B, Vedsted P (2015) Social support and non-participation in breast cancer screening: a Danish cohort study. J Public Health 38: 335-342.

18. SAS Institute Inc. (1999) Proprietary Software Release 8.2. Cary, NC, SAS Institute Inc.

19. Donnelly TT, Khater AH, Al-Bader SB, Al Kuwari MG, Malik M, et al. (2015) Factors that influence awareness of breast cancer screening among Arab women in Qatar: results from a cross sectional survey. Asian Pac J Cancer Prev 15: 10157-10164.

20. Abu-Helalah MA, Alshraideh HA, Al-Serhan AA, Kawaleet M, Nesheiwat AI (2015) Knowledge, barriers and attitudes towards breast cancer mammography screening in jordan. Asian Pac J Cancer Prev 16: 3981-3990.

21. Hajian Tilaki K, Auladi S (2015) Awareness, Attitude, and Practice of Breast Cancer Screening Women, and the Associated Socio-Demographic Characteristics, in Northern Iran. Iran J cancer Prev 8: e3429.

22. Abolfotouh MA, Bani Mustafa AA, Mahfouz AA, Al-Assiri MH, Al-Juhani AF, et al. (2015) Using the health belief model to predict breast self-examination among Saudi women. BMC Public Health 15: 1163.

23. Wagner M, Anderson KH, Broxton L (2016) Assessment of Barriers to Screening Mammograms for Rural, Poor, Uninsured Women and a Community Plan of Action. J Community Health Nurs. Routledge 33: 42-53.

24. Islam RM, Bell RJ, Billah B, Hossain MB, Davis SR (2016) Awareness of breast cancer and barriers to breast screening uptake in Bangladesh: A population based survey. Maturitas 84: 68-74.

25. Mukem S, Sriplung H, McNeil E, Tangcharoensathien V (2014) Breast cancer screening among women in Thailand: analyses of population-based household surveys. J Med Assoc Thai 97: 1106-1118.

31

Association Studies of *DRD2* and *COMT* Gene Polymorphisms with Risperidone-induced Amenorrhea in Female Schizophrenia Patients

Chengye Hou[1,4], Jintian Xu[2,3], Jing Yan[1], Zhenguo Zhao[1], Yan Sun[2,3], Zhiyong Li[1], Yang Shen[1], Yichen Huang[1], Songnian Hu[2]* and Ying Liang[1]*

[1]National Clinical Research Center for Mental Disorders, Peking University Sixth Hospital, Institute of Mental Health, Key Laboratory of Mental Health, Ministry of Health, Peking University, Beijing, China
[2]CAS Key Laboratory of Genome Sciences and Information, Beijing Institute of Genomics, Chinese Academy of Sciences, Beijing, China
[3]University of Chinese Academy of Sciences, Beijing, China
[4]Liaoning Province Demobilize Soldiers Hospital, Huludao, China

Abstract

Object: To study the association between *dopamine D2 receptor* (*DRD2*) and *catechol-O-methyltransferase* (*COMT*) gene polymorphisms and the risperidone-induced amenorrhea resulted from hyperprolactinemia in female schizophrenia patients.

Patients and methods: According to International Diagnostic and Classification of Diseases tenth edition (ICD-10) criteria, 45 Chinese female schizophrenic patients (25 patients with amenorrhea, and 20 patients with eumenorrhea) were recruited by trained psychiatrists in this study. Sanger sequencing was utilized to determine the *DRD2* and *COMT* genotypes from peripheral venous blood samples.

Results: There were no significant differences between amenorrhea patients and eumenorrhea patients in age, disease courses and risperidone dosages (P>0.05). Also, no significant differences were observed in rs6277, rs1079598 and rs4680 polymorphisms between the two groups.

Conclusion: These results suggest that *DRD2* rs6277, rs1079598 and *COMT* rs4680 gene polymorphisms show no significant correlation with risperidone-induced amenorrhea in Chinese female schizophrenia patients.

Keywords: Schizophrenia; Amenorrhea; *DRD2*; *COMT*

Introduction

Schizophrenia is a serious mental disorder that affects social function of patients. Clinical characteristics of schizophrenia are early onset age and prolonged disease course. With the extensive application of antipsychotics, there are significant improvements in the remission rate of psychotic symptoms such as impaired social function in schizophrenic patients. However, in recent years, disruption of endocrine system was observed in the patients especially for women with long-term use of antipsychotic drugs. It has been reported that antipsychotic drugs could lead to delayed and reduced menstruation or even life-long amenorrhea by blocking the dopamine receptors [1]. This adverse drug reaction has a broad impact on medication compliance and life quality in women with schizophrenia. Thus, this concern has become one of the main problems in the treatment of female psychiatric patients for many years. Therefore, more correlation studies should focus on the disrupted endocrine system and antipsychotic drugs.

Risperidone is a new atypical antipsychotic drug which has good effects on both positive and negative symptoms of schizophrenia. And fewer side effects such as extrapyramidal motor symptoms (EPS) and excessive sedation were observed after usage of risperidone. Therefore, the risperidone is one of the most widely used antipsychotic drugs in the treatment of schizophrenia [2]. Side effects of risperidone such as hyperprolactinemia which leads to amenorrhea, decreased libido, weight gain and infertility have also been reported [3-5]. However Not all risperidone-induced hyperprolactinemia would result in amenorrhea in female. The agnogenic adverse reaction of risperidone varies in patients, which indicates that genetic differences are a key factor. The mechanism of risperidone-induced amenorrhea needs to be further studied.

Dopamine dysfunction has been considered to be an important reason for the pathogenesis of schizophrenia, and the treatment of schizophrenia with risperidone mainly by antagonizing dopamine receptors [6,7]. Recent studies have shown that the gene polymorphisms in *dopamine D2 receptor gene* (*DRD2*) and *catechol-O-methyltransferase gene* (*COMT*) are associated with schizophrenia, antipsychotic treatment efficacy, and adverse reactions. For instance, polymorphism of *DRD2* rs6277 was found to be a susceptible factor of schizophrenia, and patients with *DRD2* rs6277 and rs1079598 variants have high risk for antipsychotic-induced weight gain [8,9]. Besides, *COMT* rs4680(Val>Met) polymorphism showed associated with schizophrenia, and the Met allele was also associated with the improvement of negative symptoms after risperidone treatment [10,11]. Furthermore, the *DRD2* rs6277 variants have been associated with clozapine-induced hyperprolactinemia [12]. It has been reported that the prolactin level in patients carrying *COMT* rs4280 Met allele is higher than that in patients without this allele after treated with risperidone [13]. However, the relationship between genetic factors and amenorrhea caused by risperidone-induced hyperprolactinemia has not been reported. In this study, in order to explore the genetic mechanism of risperidone-induced amenorrhea in female schizophrenia patients,

*Corresponding authors: Ying Liang, National Clinical Research Center for Mental Disorders, Peking University Sixth Hospital, Institute of Mental Health, Ministry of Health, Peking University, Beijing, Haidian District, Huayuanbeilu 51, 100191, China, E-mail: liangying1980@bjmu.edu.cn

Songnian Hu, Beijing Institute of Genomics, Chinese Academy of Sciences, No.1 Beichen West Road, Chaoyang District, Beijing 100101, China, E-mail: husn@big.ac.cn

we studied the schizophrenia susceptible *DRD2* rs6277, rs1079598 gene polymorphism and risperidone-induced hyperprolactinemia related *COMT* rs4680 gene polymorphism.

Materials and Methods

Clinical data

Clinical data of hospitalized patients with schizophrenia was collected at the Demobilized Soldiers Corning Hospital in Liaoning Province in February 2015.

Inclusion criteria were 1) meeting the diagnostic criteria for schizophrenia in ICD-10; 2) female patients; 3) age 18-40 years old; 4) treatment for at least 6 months with single medication of risperidone; 5) hyperprolactinemia (hyperprolactinemia defined as: prolactin>566 uIU/ml) occurred after the use of risperidone.

Exclusion criteria were 1) associated with metabolic diseases, endocrine diseases or connective tissue diseases; 2) taking medicine which may affect women menstrual; 3) history of ovarian resection; 4) suffering from other mental or neurological diseases; 5) eating disorders, alcohol abuse or dependence; 6) pregnant or lactating women. Women with schizophrenia whose menstrual interrupted after taking risperidone for at least 6 months were classified as amenorrhea group. Women with schizophrenia who have normal menstruation after taking risperidone for at least 6 months were classified as menstrual normal group. A total of 45 patients were included, 25 patients with amenorrhea and 20 patients with eumenorrhea.

The protocol and informed consent were approved by the Ethics Committee of the Peking University Institute of Mental Health in accordance with the guiding principles of the Guideline for Good Clinical Practice of the International Conference on Harmonization (ICH-GCP). Prior to the enrolment, written informed consent was obtained from the subjects or their legal guardians.

Clinical evaluation

Questionnaires about patient's general information and disease related situation including age, sex, date of birth, education level, ethnicity, marital status, age of onset, course of disease, past medical history and medication history, as well as the current medication list were conducted by all patients.

Laboratory evaluation

Blood collection: The venous blood was collected from the subjects at 6-7 AM after 8-12 hours fasting by nurses. The blood samples were kept in 5 mL coagulation tubes produced by a domestic mountain medical company.

Blood sample testing: (1) Prolactin: UniCel DxI800 Access automatic micro particle chemiluminescence instrument manufactured by Beckman Coulter Inc. was used for detection, and chemiluminescence immunoassay was used for determination. PRL detection range is 5.3~4240 μIU/mL, the normal range is 58-566 μIU/mL.

(2) *DRD2*, *COMT* genotype determination: The PCR primers were designed by Primers 3.0 software online according to the gene sequence of *DRD2* rs6277, rs1079598 and *COMT* rs4680 gene locus, upstream primer of rs4677: AGTCTTCAGAGGGGGAAAGG, downstream primer of rs4677: GGAATGGGACCTTTCACAGA, upstream primer of rs1079598: AGGCTAAGTCCTCCTTCTAC, downstream primer of rs1079598: TCAGGGAAGGCTTTCTAGAGG, upstream primer of rs4680: ACCAGGGAGGTGAAATACCC, downstream primer of rs4680: GATGACAAGGCCCCACTCT. PCR reacted in a 20 μL system, which include 1.0 μL of template DNA, 2.0 μL of $10 \times NH_4^+$ buffer, 0.5 μL of dNTP, 0.2 μL of EXTaq enzyme and 0.8 μL of each pair of primers. The PCR conditions were as follows: pre-denaturation at 95°C for 3 min; denaturation at 95°C for 30 s, annealing at 58°C for 45 s, extension at 72°C for 1 min, a total of 35 cycles; extension at 72°C for 10 min. Finally, sequencing of the PCR products was carried out using the ABI 3730XL automatic sequencer.

Statistical methods

The independent samples t-test was used to compare the general demographic data, and the $\chi 2$ test was used to determine whether the genotype distribution accorded with Hardy-Weinberg equilibrium. The difference of genotype and allele distribution was analyzed by $\chi 2$ test and Fisher's exact test. All data were analysed using SPSS 19.0, $P<0.05$ for the difference was statistically significant.

Results and Discussion

The basic characteristics of the two groups of subjects

The mean age of the amenorrhea patients was (32.6 ± 6.0) years, the course of disease (10.7 ± 3.4) years, the risperidone dosage (5.4 ± 2.2) mg; the mean age of the normal menstrual patients was (35.6 ± 4.7) years, the course of disease (9.4 ± 3.9) years, risperidone dosage (4.9 ± 2.5) mg. There were no significant differences in age, course of disease and dose of risperidone between the two groups ($P>0.05$), showed in Table 1.

There was no significant difference between the two groups in the prolactin level ($P>0.05$), and the prolactin level is (1741.7 ± 1073.1) uIU/mL in menorrhea patients and (1485.2 ± 772.8) μIU/mL in normal menstrual patients.

Hardy-Weinberg equilibrium test

There was no significant difference in frequency distribution of *DRD2* rs6277, rs1079598 and *COMT* rs4680 gene polymorphism genotype ($P>0.05$), which accorded with Hardy-Weinberg equilibrium law.

Association analysis of *DRD2* rs6277, rs1079598 and *COMT* rs4680 polymorphisms with risperidone-induced hyperprolactinemia resulted in amenorrhea

In the amenorrhea group and normal menstruation group, results of *DRD2* rs6277, rs1079598 and *COMT* rs4680 gene polymorphism

Variable	Amenorrhoea	Normal menstruation	P
Age (years old)	32.6 ± 6.0	35.6 ± 4.7	>0.05
Course of disease (years)	10.7 ± 3.4	9.4 ± 3.9	>0.05
Risperidone dosage (mg)	5.4 ± 2.2	4.9 ± 2.5	>0.05
Prolactin level (uIU/mL)	1741.7	1485.2 ± 772.8	>0.05

Table 1: Demographics and clinical data for the studied subjects.

SNP	Group	Number	Allele frequency		P	Genotype frequency			P
			C	T		CC	CT	TT	
rs6277	Amenorrhoea	25	49	1	>0.05	24	1	0	>0.05
	Normal menstruation	20	36	4		17	12	1	

Table 2: Allele and genotype distribution of rs6277.

SNP	Group	Number	Allele frequency		P	Genotype frequency			P
			G	A		GG	GA	AA	
rs4680	Amenorrhoea	25	39	11	>0.05	15	9	1	>0.05
	Normal menstruation	20	27	13		10	7	3	

Table 3: Allele and genotype distribution of rs4680.

SNP	Group	Number	Allele frequency		P	Genotype frequency			P
			T	C		CC	CT	TT	
rs1079598	Amenorrhoea	25	29	21	>0.05	9	11	5	>0.05
	Normal menstruation	20	24	16		8	8	4	

Table 4: Allele and genotype distribution of rs1079598.

were showed in Tables 2-4. The results showed that there were no significant differences in genotype frequency and allele frequency between the two groups (P>0.05).

Discussion

Dopamine is the one of the most important regulator of Prolactin (PRL), and in vivo and in vitro studies showed that dopamine is a potent inhibitor for prolactin. In the hypothalamic arcuate nucleus, dopamine is released from tuberoinfundibular dopamine (TIDA) neurons to the anterior pituitary, which inhibits the secretion of prolactin continuously. Risperidone is a strong antagonist of DRD2, which increases the level of prolactin by antagonizing DRD2 on the anterior pituitary prolactin cells to influence the prolactin level significantly. The incidence of hyperprolactinemia caused by risperidone is reaching to as high as 72-100%. Hyperprolactinemia could lead to reduction of estrogen by inhibiting the secretion of gonadotropin (GnRH), resulting in amenorrhea in female [14].

Risperidone is widely used in the treatment of schizophrenia, and the main adverse reaction of this drug is hyperprolactinemia, but not all risperidone-induced hyperprolactinemia in female patients will cause amenorrhea. In this study, the patients with hyperprolactinemia caused by taking risperidone were recruited, and we found that a part of the patients had amenorrhea, while others were normal, and the levels of prolactin were not significantly different between the two groups. This result indicates that this individual difference may be due to genetic differences among patients. In previous studies, individual differences of adverse effects such as efficacy and weight gain in risperidone therapy have been reported, but the genetic mechanism of amenorrhea caused by risperidone-induced hyperprolactinemia in female schizophrenia patients has not been reported [9,15].

Catechol-O-methyltransferase (COMT) is a widely existed enzyme in the human body, which can catalyze the degradation of catecholamine's including dopamine, norepinephrine, and epinephrine [16]. rs4680 is a well-studied SNP in the COMT gene. The 158th codon of COMT is mutated from valine (Val) to methionine (Met). This reduced the activity of COMT enzyme, and leading to slow down the degradation of dopamine, which may be responsible for central nervous disease [17]. Gao et al. studied 83 cases of Chinese patients with schizophrenia, and found that the prolactin levels of schizophrenia patients with Met allele were significantly higher than

Val/Val patients after 8 weeks immunotherapy with risperidone [13]. Another study has shown that the cognitive function of schizophrenia patients with homozygous Met allele was significantly better than that with other alleles after receiving risperidone therapy [18].

Risperidone functions as a blocking agent for D2 receptors, and the side effects such as risperidone-induced hyperprolactinemia and risperidone efficacy has been confirmed to have association with the polymorphism of the gene. It has been reported that female schizophrenia patients with TaqIA gene polymorphism had a higher level of prolactin secretion after taking risperidone [19]. The rs6277 locus changes the stability and translation level of DRD2 mRNA and alters the expression of DRD2 in dopamine channel [20]. Rs6277 had association with plasma prolactin increasing and schizophrenia in the study of different populations, which is also one of susceptible locus in Chinese Han population schizophrenia patients [21-23]. A DRD2 haplotype (-141delC and TaqIA) tended to correlate with better clinical performance of risperidone in Japanese schizophrenia patients [24]. Moreover, patients with DRD2-141C Ins/Del polymorphism had a better treatment with risperidone. Prolactin secretion of patients with A-241G polymorphism was significantly higher than that of non-carriers [19].

In this study, a total of 45 Chinese female schizophrenic patients were recruited, which were divided into amenorrhea group and normal menstrual group. It has shown that there was no significant association between DRD2 rs6277, rs1079598 and COMT rs4680 gene polymorphism and amenorrhea caused by risperidone-induced hyperprolactinemia. This may suggest that amenorrhea caused by risperidone-induced hyperprolactinemia in female schizophrenia patients is due to multiple gene interaction or cumulative effect [25]. In addition, this adverse event may also be associated with more complex metabolic pathways.

Conclusion

An important limitation of this study is the number of patients; therefore, the result can't explain the whole situation of this region, China and Asian people. However, the present findings generate important hypotheses in a sample of Chinese schizophrenia patients that may lay the foundation for future study in other populations. In the follow-up research, we will further increase the number of cases. Furthermore, we will also expand the relevant gene list by searching for possible regulatory pathways through metabolic pathways and regulatory network analysis between risperidone target gene set and the amenorrhea-related gene set, and re-sequencing the target genes using high-throughput sequencing. To carry out a stratified study on schizophrenia patients with high prolactin caused by risperidone treatment, study the relevance between gene polymorphism and normal menstruation and amenorrhea phenotype and hormone levels and other indicators by association analysis. We hope to improve the safety and tolerance of risperidone in the treatment of schizophrenia, and to achieve the precise medical treatment of schizophrenia by studying the genetic polymorphism of patients with amenorrhea induced by risperidone.

Acknowledgements

We thank Ms Qianhui Zhu participate in data analysis and paper revise.

Disclosure

The authors report no conflicts of interest in this work.

References

1. Haddad PM, Wieck A (2004) Antipsychotic-induced hyperprolactinaemia. Drugs 64: 2291-2314.

2. Bhana N, Spencer CM (2000) Risperidone: a review of its use in the management of the behavioural and psychological symptoms of dementia. Drugs & aging 16: 451-471.

3. David SR, Taylor CC, Kinon BJ, Breier A (2000) The effects of olanzapine, risperidone, and haloperidol on plasma prolactin levels in patients with schizophrenia. Clinical therapeutics 22: 1085-1096.

4. Dickson RA, Dalby JT, Williams R, Edwards AL (1995) Risperidone-induced prolactin elevations in premenopausal women with schizophrenia. The American journal of psychiatry 152: 1102-1103.

5. Kim YK, Kim L, Lee MS (1999) Risperidone and associated amenorrhea: a report of 5 cases. Journal of Clinical Psychiatry 60: 315-317.

6. Leysen JE, Gommeren W, Eens A, De Courcelles DDC, Stoof JC, et al. (1988) Biochemical profile of risperidone, a new antipsychotic. Journal of Pharmacology and Experimental Therapeutics 247: 661-670.

7. Hänninen K, Katila H, Kampman O, Anttila S, Illi A, et al. (2006) Association between the C957T polymorphism of the dopamine D2 receptor gene and schizophrenia. Neuroscience letters 407: 195-198.

8. Hoenicka J, Aragüés M, Rodriguez-Jimenez R, Ponce G, Martinez I, et al. (2006) C957T DRD2 polymorphism is associated with schizophrenia in Spanish patients. Acta Psychiatrica Scandinavica, 114: 435-438.

9. Müller DJ, Zai CC, Sicard M, Remington E, Souza RP, et al. (2012) Systematic analysis of dopamine receptor genes (DRD1–DRD5) in antipsychotic-induced weight gain. The pharmacogenomics journal, 12: 156-164.

10. González-Castro TB, Hernández-Díaz Y, Juárez-Rojop IE, López-Narváez ML, Tovilla-Zárate CA, et al. (2016) The role of a Catechol-O-Methyltransferase (COMT) Val158Met genetic polymorphism in schizophrenia: a systematic review and updated meta-analysis on 32,816 subjects. Neuromolecular medicine 18: 216-231.

11. Kang CY, Xu XF, Shi ZY, Yang JZ, Liu H, et al. (2010) Interaction of catechol-O-methyltransferase (COMT) Val108/158 Met genotype and risperidone treatment in Chinese Han patients with schizophrenia. Psychiatry research 176: 94-95.

12. Young RM, Lawford BR, Barnes M, Burton SC, Ritchie T, et al. (2004) Prolactin levels in antipsychotic treatment of patients with schizophrenia carrying the DRD2* A1 allele. The British Journal of Psychiatry 185: 147-151.

13. Gao S, Hu Z, Cheng J, Zhou W, Xu Y, et al. (2012) Impact of catechol-o-methyltransferase polymorphisms on risperidone treatment for schizophrenia and its potential clinical significance. Clinical biochemistry 45: 787-792.

14. Melkersson K (2005) Differences in prolactin elevation and related symptoms of atypical antipsychotics in schizophrenic patients. The Journal of clinical psychiatry 66: 761-767.

15. Zhao QZ, Liu BC, Zhang J, Wang L, Li XW, et al. (2012) Association between a COMT polymorphism and clinical response to risperidone treatment: a pharmacogenetic study. Psychiatric genetics 22: 298-299.

16. Lachman HM, Papolos DF, Saito T, Yu YM, Szumlanski CL, et al. (1996) Human catechol-O-methyltransferase pharmacogenetics: description of a functional polymorphism and its potential application to neuropsychiatric disorders. Pharmacogenetics and Genomics 6: 243-250.

17. Maria K, Charalampos T, Vassilakopoulou D, Stavroula S, Vasiliki K, et al. (2012) Frequency distribution of COMT polymorphisms in greek patients with schizophrenia and controls: A study of SNPs rs737865, rs4680, and rs165599. ISRN psychiatry.

18. Weickert TW, Goldberg TE, Mishara A, Apud JA, Kolachana BS, et al. (2004) Catechol-O-methyltransferase val108/158met genotype predicts working memory response to antipsychotic medications. Biological psychiatry 56: 677-682.

19. Calarge CA, Ellingrod VL, Acion L, Miller DD, Moline J, et al. (2009) Variants of the dopamine D2 receptor and risperidone-induced hyperprolactinemia in children and adolescents. Pharmacogenetics and genomics 19: 373.

20. Duan J, Wainwright MS, Comeron JM, Saitou N, Sanders AR, et al. (2003) Synonymous mutations in the human dopamine receptor D2 (DRD2) affect mRNA stability and synthesis of the receptor. Human molecular genetics 12: 205-216.

21. Bilibio JP, Matte Ú, de Conto E, Cunha-Filho JS (2015) Recurrent miscarriage is associated with the dopamine receptor (DRD2) genotype. Gynecological Endocrinology 31: 866-869.

22. Lawford BR, Young RM, Swagell CD, Barnes M, Burton SC, et al. (2005) The C/C genotype of the C957T polymorphism of the dopamine D2 receptor is associated with schizophrenia. Schizophrenia research 73: 31-37.

23. Fan H, Zhang F, Xu Y, Huang X, Sun G, et al. (2010) An association study of DRD2 gene polymorphisms with schizophrenia in a Chinese Han population. Neuroscience letters 477: 53-56.

24. Yamanouchi Y, Iwata N, Suzuki T, Kitajima T, Ikeda M, et al. (2003) Effect of DRD2, 5-HT2A, and COMT genes on antipsychotic response to risperidone. The pharmacogenomics journal 3: 356-361.

25. Zhang JP, Malhotra AK (2011) Pharmacogenetics and antipsychotics: therapeutic efficacy and side effects prediction. Expert opinion on drug metabolism & toxicology 7: 9-37.

32

A Pilot Study Evaluating the Effect of Daily Education by a Pharmacist on Medication Related HCAHPS Scores and Medication Reconciliation Satisfaction

Megan Huebner*, Mary E Temple-Cooper, Melissa Lagzdins, Jun-Yen Yeh
Hillcrest Hospital, Cleveland Clinic, USA

Abstract

Purpose: The purpose of this study is to determine if daily pharmacist counseling improves Hospital Consumer Assessment of Healthcare Providers and Systems (HCAHPS) medication scores in a 25 bed medical surgical unit. Secondary objectives included determination of Full-time equivalent (FTE) hours required to complete the task of a pharmacist completing daily counseling and medication reconciliation for each patient on a 25 bed hospital unit, as well as determining if medication reconciliation performed on each patient improved satisfaction survey scores among staff.

Methods: This was a single center, controlled, parallel study in two medical surgical units. Patients included were those admitted to the control or intervention unit, and the primary investigator (PI) completed daily counseling in the intervention unit and counseling once during admission on the control unit. Medication reconciliation was also completed by the PI on the intervention unit, and satisfaction was assessed through a survey provided to caregivers before and after the study. An FTE analysis was completed to determine the FTE and cost burden to implement this practice model.

Results: A total of 128 patients were included in the study over 27 days. Overall medication communication scores increased by 11.4% and decreased by 0.9% in the intervention and the control unit, respectively. Communication about side effects increased by 43% (p = 0.007) and 13.3% (p = 0.013) in the intervention and control units, respectively. A number of medication reconciliation satisfaction endpoints trended towards significance including decreased number of medication misadventures (p = 0.107), increased efficiency of patient admission (p = 0.157) and decreased interference with patient discharge (p = 0.157), and decreased total time to complete the discharge process (p=0.058). The FTE cost analysis indicated that on average, an additional 16 minutes of counseling is required per 3 day admission. Therefore, an additional four to seven FTEs will be required to incorporate this model into our institution.

Conclusion: Daily counseling by a pharmacist resulted in a statistically significant increase in communication about side effect HCAHPS survey scores and an overall increase in medication communication compared counseling once during admission.

Background

Pharmacists provide pharmaceutical care with other healthcare workers to improve medical outcomes for patients. Pharmacists have a responsibility to take an active role in patient care and ensuring patients understand their drug regimens. Medication non-adherence costs the United States of America $100 billion and noncompliance has caused 2 million hospital admissions per year [1]. Pharmacists can increase adherence and decrease readmission rates by counseling patients about the purpose, appropriate use, most common side effects and management of side effects for their medications [1]. Pharmacists also improve pharmaceutical care by preventing medication errors [2].

The Center for Medicare and Medicaid (CMS) established reimbursement criteria based on a number of endpoints, including pharmaceutical care and medication communication. Medication communication criteria are measured through a Hospital Consumer Assessment of Healthcare Providers and Systems (HCAHPS) Survey. Institutions seeking CMS reimbursement are required to distribute these surveys to their patients discharged from their hospital.2 The HCAHPS Survey measures medication communication and assesses patient satisfaction with caregiver communication about their medications and potential side effects [2]. Survey scores are based on the percentage of patients that answer "always" to the survey questions. These percentages are then ranked into percentiles. CMS utilizes the HCAHPS survey to standardize measuring patients' perspectives on hospital care. This is a method that allows collection and public reporting of patients' perspectives of care information that will allow comparisons to be made across all hospitals [3].

Thorough and complete admission medication histories are also critical in preventing medication errors. Medication reconciliation (MR) is a tool to aid in admission and discharge of patients. MR ensures all appropriate medications are being discontinued or held upon admission and appropriately restarted at discharge. Medication history discrepancies may increase medication misadventures, increase patient harm and costs and reduce caregiver time with patients while discrepancies are resolved [4]. An accurate and efficient MR process is required to assure success in the process, prevent patient harm and to prevent delays in admission and discharge. Assessment of healthcare team satisfaction with the MR process is essential to assure the best practice is utilized in admitting and discharging patients [2].

Increasing the frequency of medication counseling to patients by pharmacists may contribute to improved HCAHPS scores [5].

*Corresponding author: Megan Huebner, PGY2 Ambulatory Care Resident, Cleveland Clinic Health Systems, USA, E-mail: HUEBNEM@ccf.org

Pharmacists may require additional time to counsel patients when increasing the frequency of patient counseling. The feasibility of increased counseling time added to other pharmacists' duties requires an assessment before such a practice is incorporated into daily work flow. Currently, there is no data available to describe the feasibility and time requirement for a pharmacist to complete daily counseling and MR on an adult medical surgical unit. Our primary hypothesis was that pharmacists can be utilized to improve HCAHPS medication communication scores by counseling patients daily versus once during admission. Our secondary hypothesis was that a MR intervention completed by pharmacists would improve healthcare worker satisfaction. This study was conducted at Hillcrest Hospital, a 500-bed Cleveland Clinic community hospital. Researchers conducted the study in two similar, 25-bed, medical surgical units. The Cleveland Clinic Foundation Institutional Review Board reviewed the study protocol and approval was received prior to study initiation.

Methods

Study Design

This was a 27 day prospective, pilot-study performed on two similar medical/surgical units within a 500-bed community hospital. The study was composed of three main parts as shown in Figure 1, a patient counseling intervention, MR intervention and satisfaction survey, and a full-time equivalent analysis. The primary objectives of this study were to determine if the initiation of a daily pharmacist-based counseling service improved HCAHPS medication scores compared to HCAHPS medication scores in a second group of patients counseled only once during admission. Secondary objectives included assessment of the number of full time equivalent hours required to complete admission medication counseling, daily and discharge counseling, and MR for each patient on a 25 bed hospital unit. Other secondary outcomes were analyzed, including the number of orders a pharmacist was able to process while doing MR and patient counseling versus how many orders were verified by the pharmacist staff verifying the control unit orders. Finally, we sought to determine if MR performed on each patient in the intervention unit improved satisfaction survey scores among nursing, physician and ancillary staff.

Pharmacy Counseling Intervention

Patients were included for the pharmacy counseling intervention if they were admitted to either the control or intervention unit and did not have dementia unless a family member was present to receive medication counseling from the pharmacist. Patients were excluded if they were scheduled to be discharged to a skilled nursing facility, rehabilitation facility, long-term acute care facility, or nursing home. The pharmacy counseling intervention was performed on two similar

medical/surgical units. The control unit was a 25 bed unit where the Primary Investigator (PI) counseled each patient once upon admission. The intervention unit was a 25 bed unit where the PI counseled each patient on a daily basis and performed MR for each patient on admission and at discharge. Patient counseling was completed on these two units by one primary evaluator (pharmacist) for 27 consecutive days from the hours of 10 am to 6 pm. Each patient on the control unit was counseled about their medications within 24-48 hours after admission. Medication counseling included the indication for each medication and potential side effects. If the patient was incapable of interpreting or understanding the counseling as assessed by the diagnosis of dementia, a family member received the counseling. Patients on the intervention unit received daily counseling. Counseling occurred within 24 hours of admission, on each day of hospital stay, and prior to discharge. Each day the pharmacist addressed any ongoing medication issues with the patient in addition to providing counseling on new medications. The pharmacist also reviewed discharge medications ordered for the patient and any changes made to the patients' drug regimen as compared to prior to admission. An inpatient note was recorded after each counseling session in the patient's chart documenting the patient counseling for that specific intervention. Patient counseling was not performed by any other pharmacist on either the control unit or intervention unit during the 28 day study to control for bias and variability.

The HCAHP survey was distributed at random to a group of individuals on both the control and intervention units. The Cleveland Clinic hires an independent group to disperse their HCAHP surveys to patients after they are discharged from the hospital. The researchers were blinded regarding which patients received the survey. Selected patients received a phone call after discharge asking them to evaluate their stay at Hillcrest Hospital. The patients could have taken the survey or refused at will. The researchers did not know how many declined the survey, just how many took the survey. The portion of HCAHP survey of interest in this study were the two medication related questions (Appendix 1 and 2). The HCAHP percentage for each question only included the "always" answers or the top-box choice. The percentages of patients who answered "always" to the medication question were given to an independent reporter and were reported to the researchers. The total percentage of participants who answered "always" to one or both of the medication questions of the HCAHP survey were recorded and reported by the quality office and this data was used to determine the difference in HCAHP scores before and after the interventions.

Prescription order verification was completed by the PI for the intervention unit. Stat or immediate orders were required to be verified within fifteen minutes of order entry by the ordering provider. If stat orders were not verified by the PI within fifteen minutes, another pharmacist in the hospital verified the order. Non-stat orders remained in the order verification screen for thirty minutes before a pharmacist outside the intervention unit verified the order [6]. A report was run identifying how many orders were verified by the PI and how many were verified by the other pharmacists.

Medication Reconciliation Intervention and Satisfaction Survey

MR was performed by a pharmacist for each patient in the intervention unit. MR was performed for each patient in one of two ways. The first method occurred in the emergency room (ER). The ER pharmacist spoke with the patient, patient representatives, the patient's pharmacy or primary physician office to clarify current medications. The emergency room pharmacist completed the MR when they were

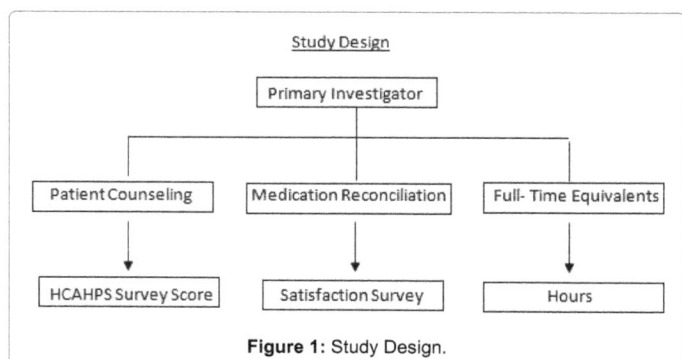

Figure 1: Study Design.

A Pilot Study Evaluating the Effect of Daily Education by a Pharmacist on Medication Related HCAHPS...

173

available. The emergency room pharmacist works seven days on and seven days off. The PI completed MR for all other patients admitted to the intervention unit. A note was added to each patient's chart indicating the MR had been completed. A MR template was used by both the PI and the pharmacist in the emergency room.

MR satisfaction was assessed before and after the MR intervention on the intervention unit. A ten question survey was designed using a likert scale and approved by the IRB as a quality tool. The survey was distributed as part of a quality initiative and was phase one of this study. The survey was distributed to nurses, physicians, and social workers during this phase. Phase two of the MR study involved a reassessment of nurses, physicians, and social workers satisfaction with the MR process after the PI finished the 27 day pilot program. The survey in phase 1 was used to assess the overall evaluation of the current MR process in the hospital during the time prior to the study initiation. The phase 2 survey was distributed within one week of completion of the pharmacist intervention month to reevaluate the overall satisfaction of the caregivers for the MR process in the hospital. The same ten questions were distributed to the same individuals and the differences in answers pre and post intervention were analyzed.

Full-time Equivalent Analysis

A full-time equivalent analysis was performed in order to assess the feasibility of incorporating the tasks of daily pharmacist counseling and MR into a pharmacy practice model. FTEs were calculated based on the time allotted for the task of the primary evaluator in addition to order entry. The minutes spent on each task were recorded after each patient counseling session (admission, interim, and discharge), each record of the patient note, and each MR during admission and at discharge for the intervention unit. The researchers also recorded the minutes spent counseling on the control unit. Average minutes spent counseling was compared between the control and intervention unit. A cost analysis was completed to determine the financial requirement of implementing a pharmacy practice model similar the one demonstrated in this study. The following assumptions were made to complete our cost-analysis: 500-bed hospital, average of 47 non-ICU adult admissions per day, average length of stay three days.

Statistical Analysis

The sample size calculation was based on the primary endpoint; change in HCAHPS survey scores before and after the intervention. This calculation was based on 95% confidence interval, a power set at 80%, and an effect size of 5% which required a sample size of 64 patients pre-intervention and 64 patients post-intervention. The 64 pre-intervention patients included the patients completing the HCAHPS survey 1 month prior to the study month. The 64 patients post-intervention included the patients completing the HCAHPS survey during the study. The primary endpoint was the change in percentage of daily counseled patients rating the medication counseling portion of the HCAHP survey as "always" from baseline versus change in percentage from baseline in a second group of patients counseled only on admission. This was analyzed using a Fisher's exact test. The Wilcoxon signed rank matched pairs test was used to analysis the change in HCAHP survey scores within each group compared to their historical HCAHP survey data.

The secondary endpoints included FTE hour calculation required by a pharmacist performing daily counseling in a 25 bed unit versus counseling only on admission on the control unit, MR for each new admission on a 25 bed unit, and the number of orders entered by the PI on the unit during a 10 hour shift. The difference in full-time equivalent

requirements was analyzed using a t-test. We hypothesized that an additional four hours or 0.5 FTEs might be required to counsel each patient daily and perform MR on admission and discharge. Also, the change in MR satisfaction in assigned unit from baseline was assessed. The MR satisfaction survey data was analyzed by determining the mode for each question as well as evaluating the change in the percentage of answers for each individual question after the MR intervention. This change was analyzed using the Wilcoxon signed ranks matched pairs test. All data was analyzed using SigmaPlot 10.0 [7].

Results

One-hundred and twenty-eight patients were included in the study population with 71 on the intervention unit and 58 on the control unit (Table 1). The average age of the patients was 61 years and 62% were female. The primary admitting diagnoses on the intervention unit were orthopedically related, including patients who were post-hip and knee arthroplasty. Orthopedic admission accounted for 24% of the admissions included from this unit. The primary admitting diagnoses on the control unit were gastrointestinal related, accounting for 47% of the patients included from this unit. Approximately 80 patients were excluded secondary to skilled nursing, long-term care, or acute rehabilitation placement at discharge. An additional 10 patients were excluded for communication barriers such as language and hearing.

HCAHPS Counseling

Two days into the study, the time allotted per day for patient counseling and MR was changed from 10 hours per day (10am to 8pm) to 8 hours per day (10am to 6pm). This change was based on the determination the completion of study tasks was feasible in an 8 hour period. A total of 10 and 14 surveys were completed on the intervention and control units, respectively, by patients discharged during the study month (February 2013). The overall change in medication communication scores, as compared to one month prior to the study intervention (January 2013), increased by 11.4% and decreased by 0.9% in the intervention and control units, respectively (Figure 2 and 3). The percentage of patients answering always to question 1 (Communication about what the medication is for) decreased on both units compared to January 2013: 26% (p = 0.186) and 15.2% (p = 0.179) percent decrease in the intervention and control units, respectively. A statistically significant increase in the percentage of patients who answered "always"

Demographic	Intervention Unit	Control Unit	Total
Average Age (years)	63 (20-93)	59 (25-88)	61
Males	36 (51%)	14 (24%)	50 (39%)
Females	35 (49%)	44 (76%)	79 (61%)
Total Patients	71	58	129

Table 1: Baseline Characteristics.

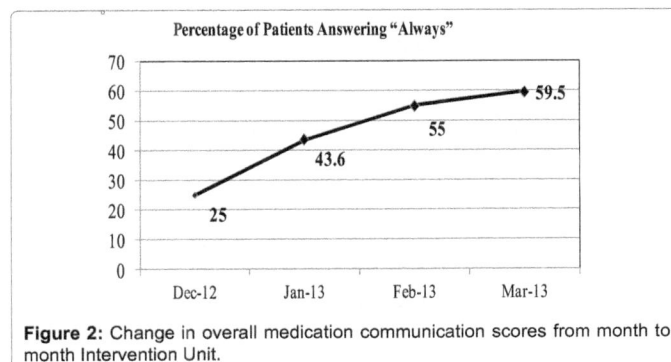

Figure 2: Change in overall medication communication scores from month to month Intervention Unit.

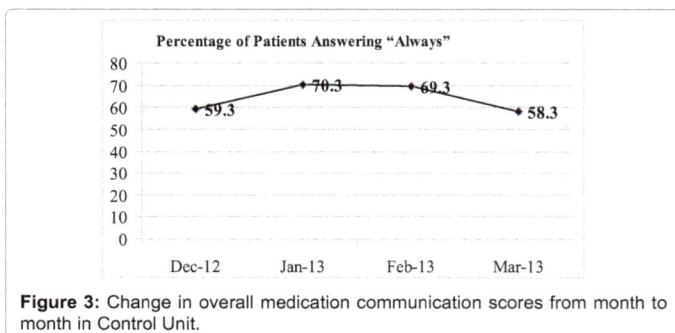

Figure 3: Change in overall medication communication scores from month to month in Control Unit.

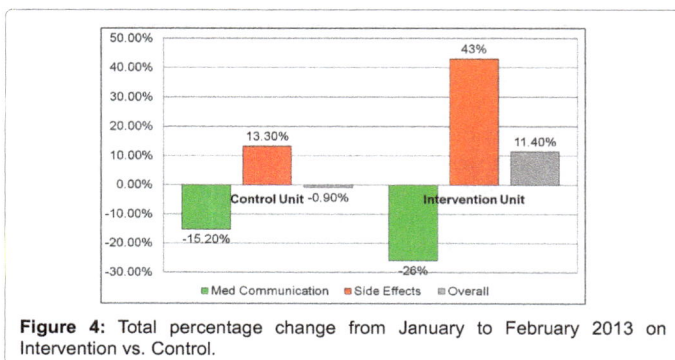

Figure 4: Total percentage change from January to February 2013 on Intervention vs. Control.

to question 2 (Communication about side effects) compared to January 2013, occurred on both units: 43% (p = 0.007) and 13.3% (p = 0.013) increase in the intervention and control units, respectively (Figure 4).

Scores from 2013 were compared to the average scores in 2012 from both units. Increased patient counseling resulted in a non-significant change in the scores for both questions when comparing average scores from 2012 versus 2013. A total of 144 surveys were completed in 2012 and 25 surveys completed in 2013 on the intervention unit. The percentage of patients answering "always" to question 1 was 66% vs. 72% in 2013 (p = 0.374). The percentage of patients answering "always" to question 2 was 29.2% in 2012 vs. 25% in 2013 (p = 0.889). A total of 177 surveys were completed for the control unit in 2012 and 30 surveys were completed in 2013. The total percentage of patients answering "always" to question 1 was 79.2% in 2012 vs. 86.7% in 2013 (p = 0.87). The total percentage of patients answering "always" to question 2 was 39.8% in 2012 vs. 53.3% in 2013 (p = 0.9). No significant differences in patient satisfaction with respect to either question one (p = 0.326) or two (p = 0.527) were noted between the units from 2013 (25 surveys from the intervention unit and 30 from the control unit) (Figure 4).

Medication Reconciliation Intervention

MR was successfully completed for each patient admitted on the intervention unit and documented in the patients' chart. The first phase of the MR survey was administered to staff working on the intervention unit approximately 6 months prior to the study month. A total of 28 individuals (71% nurses) completed the first phase of the MR survey. The second phase of the MR survey was completed within approximately 2 weeks of the completion of the MR intervention. Only 13 (46%) of the individuals completed the second phase of the survey. We were unable to contact certain nurses who had left the health-system, or were relocated to a different floor within the hospital, and therefore they would not be able to adequately assess MR on the intervention unit. Four of the ten questions that assessed various aspects of the MR process trended

towards a significant change of improvement when compared before and after the study. These included decreased number of medication misadventures (p = 0.107), increased efficiency of patient admission (p = 0.157), decreased interference with patient discharge (p = 0.157), and decreased total time to complete the discharge process (p = 0.058).

FTE Analysis

A total of 256 counseling sessions were completed during the 27 day study. The pharmacist spent an average of 10 minutes per counseling session on the intervention unit and an average of 13 minutes per session on the control unit. Each patient on the intervention unit received an average of 2.7 counseling sessions versus one counseling session on the control unit. A total of 16 extra minutes were required to counsel patients daily throughout their three day admission if they were on the intervention unit versus the control unit.

A total of 1613 orders were verified on the intervention unit by the PI during the hours of 10 am and 6 pm. Seventy-four percent (1194) orders were verified successfully by the PI. Approximately 15 orders were not verified by the PI daily. The investigators discovered this was likely caused by pharmacists who were working "as needed" within our institution and were unaware of the research project. Education was provided to those individuals throughout the month to reinforce the need to defer the orders to the primary investigator.

An FTE cost-analysis was completed to determine the potential financial requirement to incorporate the type of pharmacy practice model conducted in this study throughout our 500-bed hospital. We utilized an additional 16 minutes of counseling would be required per each patient's three day admission on the intervention unit versus the control unit. Based on the assumptions stated in our methods, we calculated our required FTEs based on these assumptions as well as the total number of pharmacists we would need to be placed in each adult medicine unit throughout the hospital. Therefore, we would require an additional 4 to7 FTEs (approximately $400,000-$700,000) to implement this practice model throughout our institution. We could utilize a minimum of 4 additional FTEs if we allowed cross-coverage between units where our volume was lower.

Discussion

We found that counseling by a pharmacist statistically significantly improved side effect communication when provided to a patient multiple times versus once throughout their admission. Additionally, a trend was seen towards improvement in overall medication communication scores. Communication about the purpose of medications decreased after the study intervention on both units. This may be explained by the fact that the actual questions on the HCAHPS survey identify "hospital staff" in general as being responsible for the medication communication. Patients likely considered the communication by nursing and physician staff instead of pharmacists alone. Patients consider this question to pertain to the direct administration of medications, and how often a nurse explains to them the use of a medication when it is administered. Therefore, pharmacists can make an impact on these endpoints, but ultimately, multiple healthcare providers contribute to the medication communication HCAHPS survey results. Our institution can rework our patient counseling processes and continue to work with our nursing team to improve medication communication and remind each other as colleagues to touch on these points when administering or discussing medications.

The impact of increased counseling by pharmacists was assessed in a study including 125 patients with low literacy [8]. Patients were randomized 1:1 to have medication counseling completed by either a pharmacist or a nurse or physician taking care of the patient. The patients randomized to the pharmacist group received counseling upon admission, discharge, and follow-up after discharge. A survey was provided to patients to assess the utility of the different components of the intervention after the intervention was completed. Seventy-two percent of the patients reported it was "very helpful" to talk to the pharmacist about their medications. Sixty-three percent and 72% of patients said the intervention was "very helpful" in preventing and managing side effects and understanding how to take their medications, respectively [8]. Our study had similar results, although the number of patients that completed the HCAHPS survey was much lower. The survey provided to patients in the aforementioned survey identified the pharmacist as the healthcare provider in the question [8].

A MR intervention was included in this study to improve our current processes within the hospital. The key difference with our study was that a pharmacist completed the process as opposed to nursing staff. Authors conducted a study to evaluate the effect of pharmacist driven medication reconciliation on preventable medication errors post-discharge in low-literacy patients.9 Patients were randomized 1:1 to have medications reconciled by a pharmacist or a nurse or physician taking care of them. Authors included 851 patients, in which 432 (51%) experienced one or more clinically important medication errors during 30 days after hospital discharge. Mean number of medication errors were similar per patient in the intervention and control groups, 0.87 per patient versus 0.95, respectively (p=0.92). Authors concluded that no statistical difference existed between the prevention of medication errors when a pharmacist completed medication reconciliation versus a physician or nurse [9]. Our survey results showed a trend towards reduction in medication errors post intervention by a pharmacist. This data is based on opinion, and actual incidence of medication errors is important to study in the future similar to the aforementioned study [9].

Our FTE analysis was completed to accurately reflect the financial burden that may be required to implement a pharmacy practice model within our hospital similar to the one utilized in our study: a pharmacist providing daily counseling, completing MR, and verifying all medication orders for a patients on a 25 bed unit. The major difference between the practice model utilized in our study and the one that would be implemented within our hospital, is that patients being discharged to skilled nursing facilities and long-term care facilities would not be excluded from MR and patient counseling. This likely will increase the amount of time spent completing MR and patient counseling by the pharmacist and may limit the time a pharmacist could spend with each patient, thus affecting the quality of the counseling sessions.

Several limitations existed within our study including differences between the patient populations on the intervention and control units, low return on completed HCAHP and medication reconciliation satisfaction surveys, barriers to complete medication reconciliation interventions, and limited ability to apply our FTE cost analysis elsewhere within our institution. We attempted to include the most similar units within the hospital when choosing our intervention and control units, although there were inherit differences that could have affected our results. The primary differences included admitting indications. On the control unit, most patients were admitted post-orthopedic surgery. Medication communication often included pain management topics as well as bowel regimen control. These patients require a considerably larger amount of pain medications compared to the control unit, where the primary indication was gastrointestinal

related surgeries. Patients were discharged post-operatively sooner on the control unit (within 24-48 hours) than the intervention unit (within 72 hour average or longer), indicating the need for a longer duration of pain management post-operatively on the intervention unit. Increased pain levels as well as pain medication use, could have affected the patients' overall experience within the hospital, and in turn contributed to their survey results. Additionally, we did not meet our required number of completed patient surveys to accurately measure the impact of daily counseling on this patient population.

Although, MR was reviewed upon admission for each patient included on the intervention unit, a number of barriers may have limited the success of this process. The medication orders for most MR interventions were already approved by the physician by the time the patient arrived on the intervention unit. This required the PI to make MR changes only after speaking to the physician. If the patient's MR was completed overnight, the PI had to make the changes the next day, and the patient may have received medications in error in the mean time. The greatest disadvantages to MR conducted in this manner, included increased time requirement to contact the physician and inability to catch the errors before administration to the patient (i.e. if patient was admitted overnight). Ideally, the MR could be completed either in the emergency room by a pharmacist or by a pharmacist on the floor prior to physician orders being placed. We hope to conduct MR in this manner in the future. Additionally, the second phase of our MR survey was not completed by over half of the staff members who completed phase I of the survey. This limited our ability to fully evaluate the effect of MR completed by a pharmacist versus the nursing staff.

Lastly, our cost analysis was based on the average length of stay on one of our adult medical-surgical units which was 3 days. This does not reflect the varying length of stays throughout our other adult medicine units; therefore the additional time requirement per patient admission for daily counseling may be greater in other hospital units.

Conclusion

Our data indicated that daily counseling by a pharmacist can improve medication communication related HCAHPS scores, and thus improve patient care. Although our results were limited by low numbers of completed HCAHPS and MR satisfaction surveys, our trends towards significance indicates the positive impact this practice model could have on patient care if implemented into practice. Our study provides data for a larger study to completely validate the effectiveness of pharmacists in improving medication communication and the medication reconciliation process. In the future, when medication reconciliation is completed, pharmacists should document the number of changes made to the medication regimen and the incidence of medication errors should be evaluated. Our FTE analysis indicated that additional time will be required to counsel daily throughout admission on the intervention unit. The counseling requirements and lengths of stay vary from unit to unit within our hospital and therefore this practice model should be tested on other adult medicine units within our facility. Further study is needed to assess the impact of a pharmacist on patient readmission rates and improved medication communication when a program similar to ours is instituted.

References

1. Griffith NL, Schommer JC, Wirsching RG (1998) Survey of inpatient counseling by hospital pharmacists. Am J Health Syst Pharm 55: 1127-1133.

2. Federal Register, Daily Journal of the United States Government. Medicare Program; Hospital Inpatient Value-Based Purchasing Program. A Rule by the Centers for Medicare & Medicaid Services.

3. Centers for Medicare & Medicaid Services, Baltimore, MD.

4. Kramer JS, Hopkins PJ, Rosendale JC, Garrelts JC, Hale LS, et al. (2007) Implementation of an electronic system for medication reconciliation. Am J Health Syst Pharm 64: 404-422.

5. Temple ME, Jakubecz MA, Link NA (2013) Implementation of a training program to improve pharmacy services for high-risk neonatal and maternal populations. Am J Health Syst Pharm 70: 144-149.

6. Physician's orders: accepting, writing, transcribing (2012) Euclid, Hillcrest, and South Pointe Hospitals Hospital Policy Manual Clinical Services.

7. Systat Software. Cranes Software International, Ltd.

8. Cawthon C, Walia S, Osborn CY, Niesner KJ, Schnipper JL, et al. (2012) Improving care transitions: the patient perspective. J Health Commun 17 Suppl 3: 312-324.

9. Kripalani S, Roumie CL, Dalal AK, Cawthon C, Businger A, et al. (2012) Effect of a pharmacist intervention on clinically important medication errors after hospital discharge: a randomized trial. Ann Intern Med 157: 1-10.

33

Assessment of Community Health and Health Related Problems in Debre Markos Town, East Gojjam, Ethiopia, 2013

Belayneh Kefale Gelaw[1]*, Gobezie Temesgen Tegegne[1] and Yeshanew Asinake Bizuye[2]

[1]Department of Pharmacy, College of medicine and Health Sciences, Ambo University, Ambo, Ethiopia
[2]Debire Markose Hospital, North East Ethiopia, Ethiopia

Abstract

Community Based Training is an on-site training program tailored to an employer's specific hiring needs. The training takes place in the actual work area in the workplace, and a professionally trained job coach is located on-site to provide additional support in training. The study was conducted in Keble 05 Debre markos town found in Amhara region, East Gojjam Zone, which is located 299 km for away from Addis Ababa and 265 km away from Bihar Dar town. The Administration has 8 sefer the keble has 8551 population of these 4447 were female and 4104 male, its climate condition, woynadega and had 45 government and private health institution. The aim of the study was to assess the community health status and health related condition in Keble 05 Debre Markos town, East Gojjam Zone, Ethiopia, 2013.

Method: Community based cross sectional survey conducted from 25/08/2013-24/09/2013 by using interviewer administrative questioner and observation. The study conducted in urban population Keble 05 Debire markos town.

Result: The cross sectional descriptive study, 94% of house hold in the keble had latrine facility Among this 50% of house don't have hand washing facility connected with latrine among women who were pregnant 100% were attained at least 1st ANC and 90 of them deliver in the health facility from breast feeding 18% of children stop breast feeding before the age of 6 month and early and late feeding also present in 9% of children.

Conclusion: Most of the house hold in the kebel had latrine constructed but most of them had no hand washing facility connected with latrine and low coverage of solid and liquid waste disposal system. There were also different problems like low immunization coverage's, low family planning, utilization poor wining and exclusive breast feeding.

Keywords: Debre Markos; Kebele; Latrine; Sanitation; Community health; ANC; PNC

Acronyms and Abbreviations: ANC: Antenatal Care; CBE: Community Based Education; CBTP: Community Based Training Program; CDI: Community Directed Intervention; EDHS: Ethiopia Demographic Health Survey; EPI: Expanded Program of Immunization; HEP: Health Extension Program; HC: Health Center; HP: Health Post; IUCD: Intrauterine Contraceptive Device; MCH: Maternal and Child Health; MDG: Millennium Development Goal; ORS: Oral Rehydration Salt; PAB: Prevention at Birth; PMTCT: Prevention of Mother to Child Transmission; PNC: Postnatal Care

Introduction

Community based training program

Community Based Training is an on-site training program tailored to an employer's specific hiring needs. The training takes place in the actual work area in the workplace, and a professionally trained job coach is located on-site to provide additional support in training [1]. CBTP (community based training program) is one parts of community based education (CBE) which is designed to train health science students, about community diagnosis to identify the problems related to health in the community, it provide health science students to apply the theoretical knowledge in to practical application.

Sustaining a healthy community is the goal of every part of the world. However, achieving this goal requires careful planning and organized community members, health organizations, academic institutions, and various government agencies. Although, in terms of education, technology, health resources, and per capita purchasing power are higher in United States, it fails to deliver the best health care at a reasonable cost. About 45 million (15.6%) US population is not covered by health insurance [2]. The United States, which spends 16% of its GDP on health care, spends more on health care per capita than any other industrialized country. For example, Switzerland and Germany (which also spend a relatively high percentage of their GDP on health care) each spend 11% of their GDP on health care [1].

Neglected populations living under poverty throughout the developing world are often heavily burdened by communicable and non-communicable diseases, and are highly marginalized by the health sector due to their limited access to health and social support services [3]. The population density and diversity of urban communities offers formidable challenges for healthcare delivery. The constant mobility (within urban areas, rural–urban–rural cycles) further complicates the delivery of appropriate health interventions. The current approaches and systems in urban areas are unable to reach agreed-upon goals and targets (e.g., the MDGs, RBM, national targets) [4]. Without improved delivery of health services, the present obstacles – accessibility, affordability and utilization of the health systems-will perpetuate disparities and likely increase the risk factors, incidence and

*Corresponding author: Belayneh Kefale Gelaw, Department of Pharmacy, College of medicine and health science, Ambo University, P.O.Box 19, Ambo, Ethiopia, E-mail: belayneh.kefale@yahoo.com

prevalence of treatable and manageable health conditions as the size of vulnerable and marginalized urban populations grows. Reduction in disease burden would enable these communities and groups to become more economically active and, thereby, further reduce the socio-economic factors contributing to disease occurrence.

Achieving reduction in disease burden lies in ensuring available health interventions reach at risk. Many simple, affordable and effective disease control measures have had limited impact due to poor access especially by the poorer populations (urban and rural) and inadequate community participation [5]. 'Community Directed Interventions (CDI) for major health problems in Africa' was found to be effective and efficient thus providing overwhelming evidence for its use as a strategy in delivering multiple interventions at the community level in rural Africa should be mandatory [6]. There is thus a need to test the feasibility, acceptability and effectiveness of the CDI strategy.

During 2011-12, the World Health Organization's Special Programme for Research and Training in Tropical Diseases (TDR) sponsored a multi-country situation analysis in four large and medium-sized urban settings throughout Africa-including Ghana (Bolgatanga, Wa), Liberia (Monrovia), Nigeria (Ibadan) and the Democratic Republic of Congo (Kinshasa) - to explore the feasibility of the CDI approach in addressing multiple disease intervention in urban communities [7].

Statement of the problem

Ethiopia is one of the developing country in which most of its population (85%) mainly depends on agricultures [8]. Different factors like lack of professional committeemen, population awareness about the problems of waste disposal, adequate and necessary medical equipment, in accessible health facility and low health seek behavior leads to the community to have low health status.

Communicable dieses, nutritional problems, maternal and child health problems are the major challenging health care related problems in Ethiopia.

Even though the sanitary coverage of this zonal town was relatively higher, there is still lack of proper utilization of latrine [9]. The town municipality has attempted to manage the solid and liquid waste by converting in to compost for agricultural activities. Although the above measure has been taken, there is a problem in collection, transportation, and disposal of wastes on time as a result this the community is exposed to different communicable disease.

Justification of the study

As most of health related problems in Ethiopia are preventable, community health assessment is an important tool to identify health status, health related problems, and factors that could affect the society's health. The result of this survey can be used by governmental and non-governmental institutions to solve the community health related problems. This study can also be used as a base line data for further study (Figure 1).

Objective of study

General objective: To assess community health and health related problems in Keble 05 Debre markos town, East Gojjam Zone, Amhara, Ethiopia, 2013.

Specific objective

- To assess socioeconomic status of the community

- To assess environmental health and sanitation condition of community

- To assess MCH status of community

- To assess major morbidity statues of communicable disease

Methodology

Study area and period

Debre Markos is a capital city of East Gojjam Zone. It was established around 1852. Its name was menkorer. It is 299 km away from Addis Ababa, capital city of Ethiopia. Debre Markos town consists of 7 Keble's. It has 86,786 populations, of which 41,618 are male. It has an altitude of 2420 m above sea level with annual rainfall of 1380 mm and average temperature is 16°C. The weather condition of Debre Markos town is Woynadega. In Debre markos town, there are 17 KG, 23 primary school, 2 high school, 1 preparatory, 15 adult

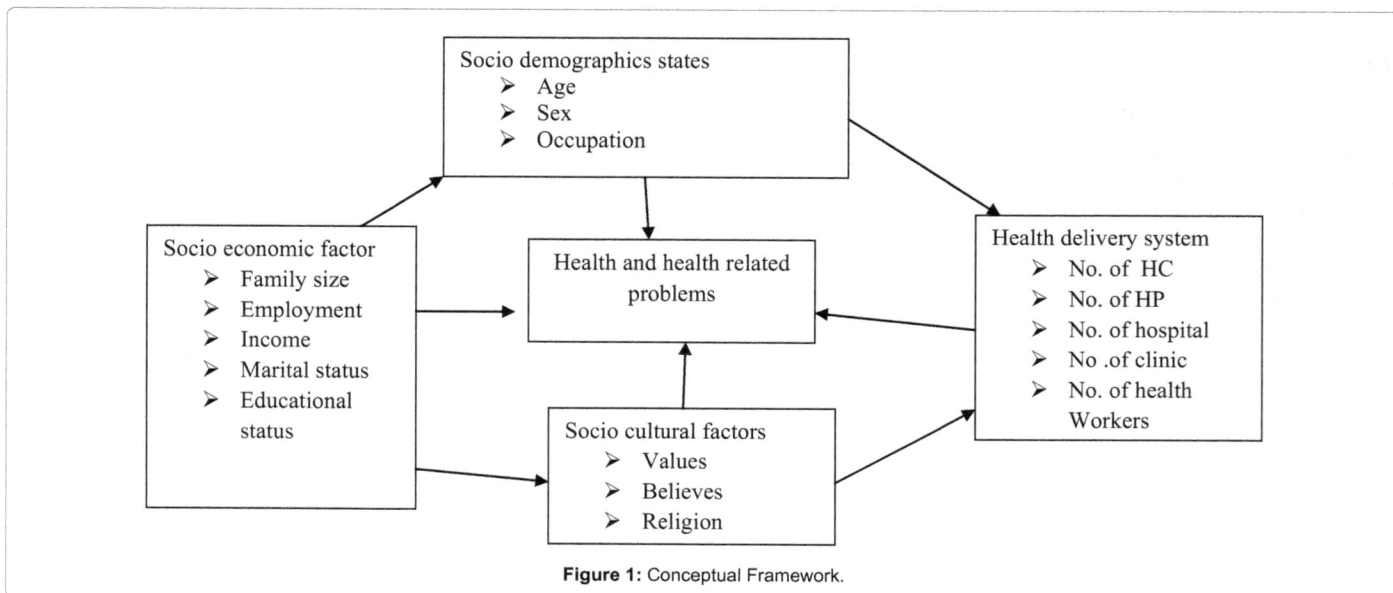

Figure 1: Conceptual Framework.

education schools, 11 different colleges and one University. It has also 1 Hospital, 3 health center, 7 health post, 21 private pharmacy, 11 private clinic, 2 diagnostic laboratory, and 13 traditional healers, which are from different professional expertise. The study was conducted in Debre Markos town Keble 05. The study was done from 25/08/2013-24/09/2013.

Study design

A community based descriptive cross sectional survey was conducted.

Population

- Source population- our source of population was all people who live in Debre Markos town,

- Study population- all population who live in Keble 05.

- Study unit- The representative of household

- Sampling unit- house holds

Inclusion and exclusion criteria

- Inclusion criteria: The house hold of the study in keble 05 Debre Markos town

- Exclusion criteria:

- Individual who were seriously ill

- A house hold members who lived for less than 6 month in town

- Absence of household's members during visit.

Sample size determination and sampling techniques

Among the 7 Kebles of Debre Markos town administration, kebele 05 was selected by lottery method (probability sampling techniques).

Systematic sampling technique, which was taken in 8 house hold intervals, was used.

Variables of the study

- Dependent variables

- Hygiene and sanitation problems

- Maternal and neonatal, child health problems

- Major communicable disease and morbidity and mortality problems.

- Independent variables

- Health care delivery system

- Socio economic states of the population

- Educational status

- Socio cultural factors

- Demographic factors sex, age, religion.

Data collection tool

The data was collected by using structured questionnaire and an interview. The questionnaire consists of socio demographic situation, environmental sanitation, mother and child health and diseases condition in the house hold. The interview was undertaken among nine households for one hour in environmental sanitation, mother and child health and diseases condition in the house hold.

Data quality management

To ensure quality, data were cheeked for completeness, accuracy, clarity, and consistency by the principal investigator. The structured questionnaire was translated to their local language (Amharic).

Data processing and analysis

Tally sheet was used to analyze the data. The results were presented in tables and graphs.

Ethical considerations

Approval and permission was sought from Ethical Review Board of College of medicine and health Sciences of Debre Markose University. An official letter of cooperation was written from the Department of Pharmacy to Debre markos woreda Keble 05 administration office to obtain their consent the necessary explanation about purpose of the study and its procedures was done informed consent was also avils from each respondents. Unwilling participants in the study ware not encountered more over any omission was not present to ensure confidentiality anonymous interviewer was conducted.

Operational definition

- Traditional birth attendant -birth attendants who attends birth out of health institution.

- Skilled birth attendant: Birth attendants who attend birth in the health institution with scientific skill and knowledge.

- Community diagnosis: It is quantitative and qualitative description of health status of citizen and the factor which influence the health. It identifies problem, proposes area for improvement and stimulate action.

- Health status: The health condition of the community, assessed on morbidity, mortality, disability and utilization of health services.

- Head of house hold: is a person with either sex, who is considered to be the head by other member of that house hold, for polygamous wife living in separate house hold, the house hold is considered to be head only.

- Maternal and Child Health: Include those who are aged 15-49 year women and those under five years' old children.

- Live birth: Number of infants born alive during the last 12 months including anyone who were born alive.

Result

Scio demographic data

The study consisted of 201 individuals found in 50 households. Of which 94 (46.77%) of them were males, while 31.28% of them were under 14 years of old. Individual that couldn't read and write consisted of 19.9% on the other hand 1.6% of them were farmers (Table 1).

Environmental sanitation

All the studied houses had a roof that was made of sheet. 94.6% of the houses had smooth wall which is not cracked and scratched while the remaining 5.4% were scratched. 83.3% of studied houses had floor made of soil, and the rest 17.4% is made from cement.

During visiting, 30 (60.6%) houses' window was opened. Half of them have been opened daily and the other 40.6% windows have

	Year	M	F	Total	%
Age	0-4	6	4	10	4.98
	5-14	25	28	53	26.3
	15-24	16	23	39	19.41
	25-64	44	46	90	44.78
	>65	3	6	9	4.48
Religion	Orthodox	94	107	201	100
	Muslim	-	-	-	-
	Catholic	-	-	-	-
	Protestant	-	-	-	-
	Other	-	-	-	-
Ethnicity	Amhara	94	107	201	100
	Others	-	-	-	-
Educational status	Can't read & write	16	24	40	19.9
	Can read write	9	9	18	8.96
	1-8 grade	24	31	55	27.37
	9-12 grade	14	19	33	16.4
	Higher education	19	26	45	22.39
Occupation	Civil servants	3	6	9	4.48
	Private worker	9	5	14	6.97
	Merchants	3	5	8	3.98
	Daily labor	4	9	13	8.47
	Farmer	2	1	3	1.6
	Others	81	73	154	76.62
Marital status	Single	24	42	66	32.8
	Married	25	26	51	25.38
	Divorce	0	10	10	4.98
	Widow	0	10	10	4.98
	Live separate	0	1	1	0.5
	Not reach to marriage	31	32	63	31.35
Monthly income	<500 birr	9	15	24	48.00
	501-1000 birr	7	5	12	24
	1001-2500 birr	5	1	6	12
	>2500 birr	3	5	8	16

Table 1: Socio-demographic status of Debre Markose 05 kebele individuals in 2013.

opened occasionally. From the total selected houses, 57.78% of them have an additional door to escape during emergency cases. Most of the houses (91%) have enough light, from which 30.12% obtain morning light. 17.39% of the selected houses gain light afternoon and the rest 52.49% obtain both morning and afternoon light. Out of the studied houses 70.4% of them are separated from the neighboring house and the other 29.6% of them are joined with the nearby houses. Regarding the owner ship of the houses, 65.6% of them are private while the

remaining is rented. Most of the family members sleep on bed and the rest sleep on floor (`medeb`).

89.22% of the selected households have kitchen of which 86.58% of them are separated from the main houses, and 12.8% are joined with the main houses. From 29 households only 2 (6.87%) of them have kitchen with windows.

Regarding stove utilization, 30 houses holds (60%) have traditional stove. From these 17 stoves (35.55%) have chummy. From the selected houses only one house hold use electrical stove. 49 (98%) households use wood, charcoal, can dung & fuel gas for cooking. All households have electric supply.

Regarding latrine condition, 47(94%) households have latrine while all have common latrine. 35(70.32%) households do not have cover for their latrine. 22(44.5%) households have good sanitation condition.

Regarding water supply, all households are suspired with the current water supply. Most households have (47) domestic animals. Household fly, flea, mosquito, rodent (rat) and bed bug are common rodents (Figure 2). These problems that need special attention on the health of the community of the selected households.

Maternal and child health result

In the study population, 50 of them were in the reproductive age group (15-49 years). Among 47 couples, 13 (6.47%) and 30 (14.41%) of them married in the age less than 18 and greater than 18 years respectively.

Among couples, 12(25.54%) number of women gave birth in the age of less than 18 years old while 23 (48.94%) of them gave birth between the age of 18-35 years old. No abortion case (legal and illegal) was found in the last 12 month.

Among the reproductive age group individual, 5(10%) and 4(8%) were pregnant and gave birth in past 12 months respectively. All of them gave birth in health institution. All pregnant mothers attained ANC services at least one times. When we see post natal care services at health facility, two of them within 2 days, one in first 7 days and one in the 42 days of delivery. 18 numbers of women used contraceptive, of which 12(85.4%) of them used Depo-Provera (Tables 2 and 3).

Child health status

In our community assessment there was 11(5.48%) under five children from the total 201 sample population (Table 4). Harmful traditional practice like Tonsillectomy, FGM and Tooth Extraction

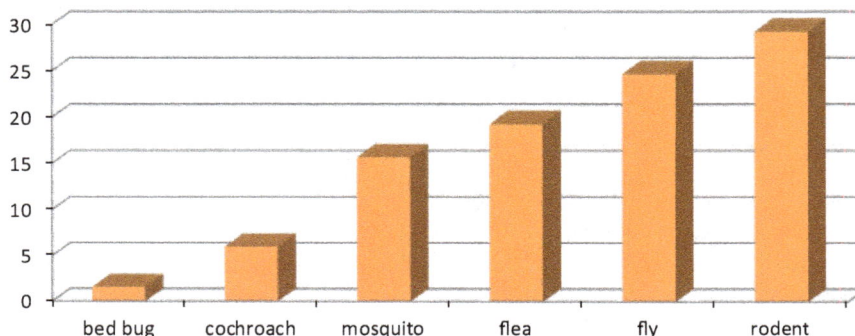

Figure 2: The magnitude of rodents and insects in Debre Markos town in 05 Keble in 2013.

No	Types of contraceptive methods	Frequency	Percentage
1	Depo-Provera	12	66.6
2	Oral contraceptive	2	11.1
3	Nor plant	2	11.1
4	IUCD	1	5.5
5	Rhythmic periodic	1	5.5
	Total	18	100%

Table 2: The type of contraceptive use and frequency of these contraceptive in Debremarkose kebele 05 in 2013.

S. No	TT Vaccination	Frequency
1	TT1	20
2	TT2	16
3	TT3	14
4	TT4	13
5	TT5	7

Table 3: Immunization status of reproductive age (15-49) women for tetanus in Debre Markose kebele 05 in 2013.

S. No	Criteria	Age	No.	%
1	Breast feeding	< 6 months	2	18.18
		6-24 months	8	72.73
		>24 months	1	9.09
2	Complementary feeding	< 6 months	1	9.09
		at 6 months	9	81.82
		>6 months	1	9.09

Table 4: The length of breast feeding in less than 5 year children in Debre Markose kebele 05 in 2013.

weren't practiced in selected households (Table 5). Dropout rate of penta and meseales was 33.34%.

Morbidity status

There were two individual who were physically disable due to injection error and fracture. AS we interviewed the selected house hold in Debre Markos town 05 kebele almost all the houses respond that if one of the members of household is sick, they tried to go to health institutions (Table 6).

Discussion

According to our study 94% of households had latrine, while EDHS 2011data showed relatively lower number of households (62% of house hold) [8,10,11]. This may be due to adequate health education about latrine construction and utilization by co- coordinating health extension worker, health development army, health center, also health office. In our study 52% and 36% of house hold had no solid and liquid waste disposal pit respectively, but according to Amhara regional state health be roué 2012 annual reported slow performance in inspection of solid and liquid waste disposal pit was 84%and 88% respectively [9,12,13].

According to our study there is no maternal death related to pregnancy and delivery but the maternal mortality rate of Ethiopia is 676 deaths from 100,000 live births according to EDHS 2011[8,14]. The result may indicate that health extension worker, woreda health office, hospital and other supporters of community create awareness on maternal health.

In our finding, measles fully immunization coverage was low (60%). This may be due to urban health extension workers didn't give immunization service, and low community awareness about immunization default. There was poor practice about exclusive breast

feeding and complementary feeding which showed, 9% of infant start complementary feeding before six months while 9% of not started complementary feeding at the age of >6 month. This indicates the awareness of the community about exclusive breast feeding & complementary feeding is low.

ANC follow-up was good (100%), on the contrary EDHS 2011report showed, it was 34% [8,15]. This may be due to increase awareness of the pregnant women.

In our study show, skill birth attendant is high/100%/ but in EDHS/2011/ it was 10% [8,16]. This may be due to the cooperative work of health care professionals by giving information regarding to mother and child health.

This study found, marriage before the age of 18 yrs was 6.47%, but EDHS 2011 report found 63% [17,18]. This result may be due to strong legal issue that prohibits marriage before age 18 years and most females spent their time on school.

From the interview, harm full traditional practice was not exercised. This indicates there was community awareness in the negative health impact of harmful traditional practice.

Conclusion

Most health extension packages were not properly utilized. Although all deliveries were under taken in health institution, vaccination and complementary feeding of the child were not taken properly and in appropriate time. Asthma and gastritis were most

S. No	Types of vaccination	No infant <1 yrs	Vaccination infant	%
1.	Polio 0		1	20
	Polio 1		3	60
	Polio 2		3	60
	Polio 3		2	40
2.	Penta 1		3	60
	Penta 2		3	60
	Penta 3		2	40
3.	BCG		3	60
4.	Measles	5	2	40
5.	PCV 1		2	40
	PCV 2		2	40
	PCV 3		2	40
6	PAB		2	40
7	Fully immunized		2	40

Table 5: Vaccination of infants and frequency of each vaccination in Debre Markos 05 kebele in 2013.

S. No	Types of disease	Frequency	Percent
1	Headache	1	8.33
2	Common cold	1	8.33
3	Hypertension	1	8.33
4	Heart failure	1	8.33
5	HIV	1	8.33
6	Asthma	2	25
7	Diabetes mellitus	1	8.33
8	Gastritis	2	25
9	Idiopathic	1	8.33
10	Pneumonia	1	8.33
	Total	12	

Table 6: List of disease other than diarrheal diseases that occur in the last two weeks in Debre Markos Town administration, kebele 05 in 2013.

frequently encountered disease. Harmful traditional practice was exercised, especially early married. There is High dropout rate of penta and measles and also low TT vaccine coverage.

Recommendation

The following recommendations were forwarded.

1. The town administration and woreda health office with concerned stakeholders should work to improve the awareness of the community about proper placement and utilization of liquid and solid waste burning materials, kitchen and latrine utilization, and alternate energy source for cooking.

2. The health office stake holder should work to create awareness about immunization.

3. Health care providers:- to teach hand washing.

4. for those working in Family planning:-to teach the different forms of family planning.

Acknowledgements

We are very grateful to our college staff members for unreserved guidance and constructive suggestions and comments from the stage of proposal development to this end.

We would like to thank Debire Markos University for supporting the budget which required for this research.

Finally our deepest gratitude goes to Debire Markos kebele 05 administration offices that help and allow us in collecting and gathering data from the households.

References

1. National Center for Health Statistics (2006) Health, United States, with chart book on trends on the health of Americans. Hyattsville, MD.

2. US (2005) Bureau of the Census. Statistical Abstract of the United States: 2006. Washington, DC.

3. Holveck JC, Ehrenberg JP, Ault SK (2007) Prevention, control, and elimination of neglected diseases in the Americas: pathways to integrated, inter-programmatic, inter-sectoral action for health and development. BMC Public Health 7: 6.

4. Measure DHS: DHS surveys and national reports on health situations in different African countries.

5. Odeyemi AO, Nixon J (2013) Assessing equity in health care through the national health insurance schemes of Nigeria and Ghana: a review-based comparative analysis. Int J Equity Health 12: 9.

6. Ssengooba F, Rahman S, Hongoro C, Rutebemberwa E, Mustafa A, et al (2007) Health sector reforms and human resources for health in Uganda and Bangladesh: mechanisms of effect. Human Resource Health 5: 3.

7. WHO (2008) Community-directed interventions for major health problems in Africa: a multi-country study, Geneva, Switzerland: Special Programme for Research & Training in Tropical Diseases (TDR) World Health Organization.

8. Ethiopia health demography survey 2011.

9. Debre Markose (2013) Debre markos ketma health office, health extension program annual report, 23-25.

10. Department of Community Health (1988) Team Training Programme Manual, Part II. Jimma: Jimma Institute of Health Sciences 1-26.

11. Department of Community Health (1996) Manual for Student Research Project. Jimma: Jimma Institute of Health Sciences 1-71.

12. Woodward C (1992) Some reflections of evaluations of outcomes of innovative medical education Programme during the practice period Annals of Community-Oriented Education 5: 181-191.

13. WHO study groups (1993) Increasing the relevance of education for health professionals. WHO Technical Report Serves No 838.

14. Kamien M, Boelen C, Heck J (1999) Measuring social responsiveness of medical schools. Education for Health, 12: 9-19.

15. Moja EA, Ghetti V (1995) Assessing performance of medical schools. Annals of Community-Oriented Education, 8:247-253.

16. Department of Community Health (1987) Community Based Training Program Manual, Part I. Jimma: Jimma Institute of Health Sciences 1-63.

17. Seefeldt M (2000) Evaluating community-based health programmes. In: Schmidt M et al., (ed). Handbook of community-based education: theory and practices. Maastricht: Network Publications 345-360.

18. Sims P (1997) Community-based education-the Zambian experience. Education for Health 10: 301-310.

34

Anthropometric Measures and Insulin Resistance in Rural Indian Adolescents

Bhattacharya S[1,2]*, Smith GD[3], Shah SH[1,4], Ben-Shlomo Y[5] and Kinra S[6]

[1]Duke Global Health Institute, Duke University Medical Center, Durham, NC, USA
[2]Duke Translational Research Institute, Duke University, Durham, NC, USA
[3]MRC, Translational Centre, Bristol, UK
[4]Division of Cardiovascular Medicine, Duke University Medical Center, Durham, NC, USA
[5]School of Social and Community Medicine, University of Bristol, Bristol, UK
[6]Department of Epidemiology and Population Health, London School of Hygiene and Tropical Medicine, London, UK

Abstract

Aims: To evaluate the relationship of anthropometric measures with insulin resistance (IR) in 1162 Indian adolescents from the follow-up survey of the Hyderabad Nutrition trial.

Methods: Analysis was done on data collected from 1162 adolescent participants of the Hyderabad Nutrition trial follow up survey. Participation included an interview, physical examinations and blood draws. Associations of body mass index (BMI), fat mass index (FMI), fat free mass index (FFMI), central to peripheral skinfold ratio (CPR), percent of body fat, waist circumference (WC) and waist-hip ratio (WHR) with IR were studied using linear regression models accounting for village clustering and adjusting for age and pubertal stage. Anthropometric indices were calculated from height, weight, skinfold thickness, waist and hip circumferences and IR was calculated by the homoeostasis model assessment (HOMA).

Results: We observed strong associations of BMI, FMI and FFMI with HOMA. Interestingly, FFMI (β (95% confidence interval) -0.03 (0.01, 0.06); $P=0.007$ (girls) and 0.06 (0.03, 0.09); $P<0.0001$ (boys)) was as strongly associated with IR as BMI (0.03 (0.01, 0.06); $P=0.006$ (girls) and 0.06 (0.03, 0.09); $P<0.0001$(boys)) and FMI (0.03 (0.01, 0.05); $P=0.02$ (girls) and 0.05 (0.02, 0.07); $P=0.001$ (boys)) We explored the relationship of lean mass with IR relative to fat mass and the associations remained strong.

Conclusions: We conclude that lean mass is as strongly associated with IR as fat mass in rural Indian adolescents. These findings appear contrary to the belief that higher rates of IR in South Asians reflect greater central adiposity. Future research needs to increase our understanding of the underlying mechanisms that lead to these associations in both obese and lean populations.

Keywords: Adolescents, Anthropometry, Body Composition, Body Mass Index, IR

Introduction

The rates of diabetes in India are rising dramatically, with the number of people with diabetes projected to rise to 57.2 million by 2025 [1]. The diabetes epidemic, in part, can be explained by the rapid globalization leading to westernizations of diets, more sedentary lifestyles, and transitions from rural to urban living. As observed in adults, South Asian children and adolescents have high rates of IR compared to children and adolescents of other ethnicities [2]. IR predicts the future risk of cardiovascular disease (CVD) [3]. Additionally Indian adolescents have an increased sensitivity to adiposity, high percent of body fat, abdominal obesity and high subcutaneous fat levels [4,5]. Studies in adolescents have shown that obesity, particularly visceral obesity, is associated with the development of IR in this age group, with evidence of a 50% increase in IR in overweight adolescents with every half unit increase in body mass index (BMI) [6-8].

There has been a growing interest in studying different anthropometric measures as indicators of IR and diabetes; especially to understand the increased susceptibility of leaner Indian populations to diabetes. Measurement of WC is a useful measure of obesity-related diabetes risk in Indians, who are more prone to abdominal obesity at normal BMI [9,10]. Additionally, Indians have greater amounts of visceral adipose tissue and a higher percentage of body fat than individuals of European ancestry [11,12]. Percent of body fat and central obesity (measured by WHR) as compared to generalized obesity (measured by BMI) have been evaluated as risk factors for diabetes with conflicting reports in Indian populations. In the INTERHEART study, waist hip ratio was the strongest marker of myocardial infarction in South Asians, followed by waist circumference and then BMI [13].

There is lack of consensus on a single anthropometric measure as the best indicator of IR in adolescents. WHR, WC and BMI showed similar correlations with fasting insulin and IR in Chinese children [14]. In Greek schoolchildren BMI, WC and waist-to-height ratio were highly associated with IR [15]. Subscapular skinfold thickness better identified fasting hyper insulinemia than BMI and WC in urban Indian adolescents, however this study did not have data on sexual maturity, which may play an important role on insulin sensitivity in adolescents [16].

Our objective was to evaluate the associations of anthropometric measures with IR in a cohort of rural Indian adolescents who are leaner than their urban counterparts and represent a different socio-economic

*Corresponding author: Sayanti Bhattacharya, Duke Global Health Institute, Duke Translational Medicine Institute, MURDOCK Study 310 Trent Drive, Room #330 Durham, NC 27707, USA, E-mail: sayanti.bhattacharya@duke.edu

stratum of Indian society. A better understanding of this relationship in adolescents will shed more light on the mechanisms and risks involved with development of early IR, a predictor of adverse health outcomes later in life.

Materials and Methods

Design of the follow up survey of the Hyderabad Nutrition Trial

Details of design of the Hyderabad Nutrition trial and the follow up survey have been previously published [17]. All adolescents born to participants of the Hyderabad Nutrition trial during the years 1987-1990 were eligible to participate in the follow up study and were included in the current analysis. Participants were recruited from 29 Indian villages. Participation included completion of an interview administered via a questionnaire, clinical examinations and collection of fasting blood samples by a venous blood draw and a brief interview of the mothers. Height, weight, skinfold thickness at four sites, waist and hip circumference, blood pressure and temperature were measured [17]. Data collection was done from 2003 through 2005. The Ethics committee of the National Institute of Nutrition of India, Hyderabad approved the study. Village heads and their committees in each of the 29 villages approved the study as well. In our study we have 1162 adolescents between 12-18 years of age, including 535 girls and 627 boys.

Physical examination

All measurements were conducted in light, minimal clothing and no shoes. Weight was measured by a digital weighing machine (Model HD 305; Tanita, Japan) to the nearest 100 gm and height was measured to the nearest mm by a portable plastic stadiometer (Leicester height measure; Chasmors Ltd, London, UK). WC was measured on the bare skin with a non-stretch metallic tape, at the midpoint between the iliac crest below and the costal margin above. Hip circumference was measured in a single layer of light clothing at the widest part, between the greater trochanter and the lower buttock level, with the legs together. The arm measurements were made on the non-dominant side of the participant, with the arm flexed at 90 degrees. A Holtain skinfold caliper calibrated to 0.2 mm was used to measure the thickness of the skinfolds. Triceps skinfold thickness, biceps skinfold thickness, subscapular skinfold thickness and upper supraihiac skinfold thickness were measured. Blood pressure was assessed in the supine position using a validated oscillometric device with appropriate cuff sizes (OMRON HEM 705 CP; Omron, Matsusaka Co, Japan) and the mean of two measurements was used.

Pubertal status was classified into early, middle, late puberty and post pubertal stages based on time since the onset of menstruation (girls) and testicular volume (boys) [18]. The data on menstruation was collected through interview with the participant. Self-assessed testicular volume was determined by participants with the help of a Prader's orchidometer and recorded by study staff.

Interview

Trained social workers administered the questionnaire, developed from questions already tested and used in other studies. Data collection included demographic information, education and employment, household circumstances, socio-economic status, smoking and alcohol consumption and general health. A short questionnaire was used to interview the mothers.

Blood sample collection and processing

Fasting blood samples (at least 8 hours) were collected in vacutainers and transferred to an icebox (4-8°C) to be processed within four hours. Glucose, total cholesterol, HDL cholesterol, triglycerides were assayed on the same day using an autoanalyser (ACE Clinical System; Schiapparelli Biosystems, NJ, USA) and the recommended kits for it (Alfa Wasserman, NJ, USA). Fasting serum insulin concentrations were estimated by radioimmunoassay in batches within four to six weeks [19].

Statistical analysis

We calculated IR from the homoeostasis model assessment (HOMA) by dividing the product of fasting glucose (mmol/L) and insulin (mU/mL) by the constant 22.5 in participants with fasting glucose <7 mmol/l [20]. Body density was calculated as the log of the sum of four skinfolds by using the equation of Durnin and Wormsley [21]; and then converted into percent body fat by Siri's equation (body fat%= (4.95/body density-4.50) X 100) [22]. Body fat percent was converted to fat mass and fat-free mass by using body weight (total body fat (kg) = body fat% x weight (kg) x 0.01) and (total body fat free mass (kg)=weight (kg)-body fat (kg)). Fat and fat-free mass were converted into corresponding indices after dividing them by the square of height in meters [23]. Central to peripheral skin fold ratio was estimated as a ratio of central (subscapular plus suprailiac) to peripheral (biceps plus triceps) skinfolds. Low density lipoprotein cholesterol was measured from triglycerides, total cholesterol, and high density lipoprotein cholesterol by using the Friedewald-Fredrickson equation [24].

Distribution of the anthropometric indices and metabolic risk factors in the whole study cohort, and specifically in girls and boys are presented as means and standard deviations. We used t-tests to compare the means of the variables between boys and girls. Insulin and HOMA scores were positively skewed and we applied log transformations to these variables. To ensure comparability of the models including different anthropometric measures (which have unique measurement units and some are ratios without units) we converted the anthropometric measures to standardized z-scores. These z-scores are standardized scores generated for every observation by using the standard deviations of the individual observations from the observed mean. All models were run using these standardized z-scores.

Associations between anthropometric measures and HOMA, fasting glucose and insulin were tested by using univariable and multivariable linear regression models with generalized estimating equations accounting for clustering by villages. We used models adjusting for age and pubertal development and used separate models for each of the anthropometric measures as the degree of correlation among these indices is very high. Associations of the ratio of FMI to FFMI with HOMA, fasting glucose and insulin was evaluated by using uni variable and multivariable linear regression models accounting for clustering by villages. Multivariable models were additionally adjusted for age and pubertal stage.

Sub group analyses were done within categories of pubertal development separately in boys and girls, to study whether the correlations of these indices with HOMA differed by sexual maturity. Earlier studies have indicated that levels of IR are higher with increasing age and pubertal maturity in adolescent boys and girls [25]. In addition to adjusting for age and pubertal status in our models, we explored the relationship between anthropometric measures and HOMA within categories of pubertal development.

	Total (N=1162)	Girls (N=535)	Boys (N=627)	T test p value
Age	15.9, 0.9	15.8, 0.9	15.9, 0.9	0.001
Anthropometric measures				
Height (cm)	155.4, 8.2	151.5, 5.7	158.8, 8.5	<0.0001
Weight (kgs)	41.8, 7.2	41.0, 6.1	42.4, 8.0	<0.0001
WC (cm)	61.3, 5.5	60.6, 5.8	62.0, 5.2	<0.0001
BMI (kg/m²)	17.2, 2.2	17.8, 2.2	16.7, 2.1	<0.0001
WHR	0.8, 0.1	0.8, 0.1	0.8, 0.1	<0.0001
Percent body fat (%)	18.1, 4.6	21.2, 3.6	15.4, 3.5	<0.0001
FMI (kg/m²)	2.6, 1.4	3.8, 1.1	1.6, 0.7	<0.0001
Lean mass index (kg/m²)	14.6, 1.5	14.1, 1.3	15.1, 1.5	<0.0001
Central to peripheral skin ratio	1.5, 0.3	1.4, 0.2	1.5, 0.2	<0.0001
Puberty stages				
Early	171	0	171	
Middle	365	43	322	
Late	316	205	111	
Post-pubertal	272	272	0	
CVD risk factors				
Total cholesterol (mmol/l)	3.5, 0.7	3.7, 0.7	3.3, 0.6	<0.0001
LDL cholesterol (mmol/l)	2.0, 0.6	2.2, 0.6	1.9, 0.6	<0.0001
HDL cholesterol (mmol/l)	1.0, 0.2	1.0, 0.2	1.0, 0.2	0.07
Triglycerides (mmol/l)	0.9, 0.4	1.0, 0.4	0.8, 0.3	<0.0001
Glucose (mmol/l)	4.7, 0.7	4.7, 0.7	4.7, 0.6	0.43
Insulin (mU/l)	19.4, 11.2	20.1, 11.5	18.8, 10.8	<0.0001
Systolic blood pressure (mmHg)	109.1, 10.2	107.4, 9.1	110.6, 10.9	<0.0001
Diastolic blood pressure (mmHg)	62.4, 6.5	62.7, 6.5	62.1, 6.6	0.04
HOMA	4.1, 2.6	4.2, 2.7	4.0, 2.5	<0.0001

Values are presented as means, standard deviations

Table 1: Characteristics of the study population.

	Girls				Boys			
	Unadjusted model* (n=468)		Minimally adjusted model** (n=468)		Unadjusted model*(n=366)		Minimally adjusted model**(n=364)	
	β (95% CI)	P	β (95% CI)	P	β (95% CI)	P	β (95% CI)	P
BMI	0.03 (0.01, 0.05)	0.01	0.03 (0.01, 0.06)	0.006	0.06(0.03, 0.08)	<0.0001	0.06 (0.03, 0.09)	<0.0001
FMI	0.03 (0.00, 0.05)	0.02	0.03 (0.01, 0.05)	0.02	0.05 (0.02, 0.07)	0.0008	0.05 (0.02, 0.07)	0.001
FFMI	0.03 (0.01, 0.05)	0.02	0.03 (0.01, 0.06)	0.007	0.06 (0.03, 0.08)	<0.0001	0.06 (0.03, 0.09)	<0.0001
CPR	0.05 (0.02, 0.07)	<0.0001	0.05 (0.03, 0.07)	<0.0001	0.02 (-0.01, 0.05)	0.14	0.02 (-0.02, 0.05)	0.25
Percent of body fat	0.02 (0.00, 0.05)	0.04	0.03 (0.00,0.05)	0.03	0.04(0.01, 0.06)	0.004	0.03(0.01, 0.06)	0.008
WC	0.03 (0.01, 0.05)	0.01	0.03 (0.01, 0.05)	0.009	0.03(0.01, 0.06)	0.01	0.03 (0.01, 0.06)	0.02
WHR	0.01 (-0.01, 0.04)	0.24	0.01 (-0.01, 0.04)	0.27	-0.03 (-0.06, -0.01)	0.01	-0.03 (-0.06, -0.01)	0.02

* Adjusted for village clustering only
**Adjusted for age, pubertal stage and village clustering

Table 2: Association of anthropometric measures with insulin resistance (HOMA) in girls and boys from linear regression models.

All statistical analyses were performed using SAS version 9.2 (Cary NC). No adjustments were made for multiple comparisons.

Results

Distribution of anthropometric indices and metabolic risk factors

The characteristics of the study population are represented in Table 1. Of the 1162 adolescents in our study, 535 were female and 627 were male. Participants with missing data on important variables like pubertal status (n=38), body composition (n=95), incomplete questionnaires (n=31), and unavailable blood samples (n=63) were excluded. Children who were fasting for less than eight hours prior to blood sample collection were also excluded from the analyses (n=8). Participants with HOMA scores above 7 mmol/L were excluded

from analyses (n=5). Glucose and insulin data were available on 1008 adolescents, mainly as insulin assay reagents could not be obtained for the last batch of samples (n=48) [17].

The mean age was 15.9 years, with boys being older (p=0.001), taller and weighing more than the girls. Our study population was very lean, with a mean BMI of 17.2 kg/m². Only 3.6% of the population was overweight or obese, using age and sex specific BMI cutoffs determined for Indian adolescents, corresponding to the WHO recommended BMI cutoff for overweight (23 kg/m²) and obese (28 kg/m²) in South Asians [26]. Girls had an overall higher mean BMI than boys (p<0.0001) and a higher percentage of body fat. The girls were further along in the pubertal development than boys; with none of the girls in early stages of development, 39.4% in late stages and 52.3% in post pubertal stage of development. In comparison, most boys were in middle stages

| | Early* | Middle* | | Late* | | Post pubertal* |
| | Total, all boys (N=97) | Girls (N=40) | Boys (N=200) | Girls (N=184) | Boys (N=67) | Total, all girls (N=245) |
	β (95% CI); P	β (95% CI); P	β (95% CI); P	β (95% CI); P	β (95% CI); P	β (95% CI); P
BMI	0.07 (0.01, 0.13); 0.02	0.14 (0.04, 0.24); 0.006	0.06 (0.03, 0.10); 0.0008	0.02 (-0.02, 0.06); 0.40	0.04 (-0.02, 0.11); 0.17	0.03 (-0.00, 0.06); 0.05
FMI	0.08 (0.01, 0.15); 0.03	0.10 (-0.00, 0.20); 0.06	0.05 (0.01, 0.08); 0.01	0.03 (-0.01, 0.07); 0.22	0.03 (-0.02, 0.08); 0.26	0.02 (-0.01, 0.05); 0.18
FFMI	0.06 (0.00, 0.11); 0.04	0.13 (0.04, 0.22); 0.004	0.06 (0.03, 0.10); 0.0009	0.01 (-0.03, 0.05); 0.67	0.05 (-0.02, 0.12); 0.17	0.03 (0.00, 0.07); 0.03
CPR	-0.01 (-0.06, 0.05); 0.95	0.07 (-0.00, 0.15); 0.07	0.04 (0.00, 0.08); 0.03	0.04 (0.00, 0.09); 0.04	-0.01 (-0.06, 0.04); 0.73	0.05 (0.02, 0.08); 0.002
Percent Body Fat	0.06 (-0.00, 0.11); 0.06	0.05 (-0.02, 0.13); 0.18	0.04 (0.00,0.07); 0.05	0.03 (-0.01, 0.07); 0.15	0.03 (-0.03, 0.08); 0.32	0.01 (-0.02, 0.04); 0.44
WC	0.04 (-0.02,0.11); 0.19	0.06 (-0.04, 0.16); 0.22	0.05 (0.01, 0.08); 0.02	0.04 (-0.01, 0.08); 0.10	0.01 (-0.04, 0.07); 0.65	0.02 (-0.00, 0.05); 0.10
WHR	-0.05 (-0.10, -0.01); 0.03	-0.01 (-0.10, 0.07); 0.70	-0.02 (-0.06, 0.01); 0.21	0.04 (-0.00, 0.08); 0.05	-0.03 (-0.09, 0.03); 0.31	0.01 (-0.02, 0.04); 0.64

* Adjusted for village clustering only

Table 3: Associations of anthropometric measures with insulin resistance (HOMA) in different pubertal stages in girls and boys.

of pubertal development (53.3%) followed by early (28.3%) and late (18.3%) and none were in the post pubertal stage. Mean fasting insulin levels (p=0.006) and mean HOMA scores (p=0.03) were also higher in girls than the boys.

Associations of anthropometric indices with HOMA

Correlation of the anthropometric measures with HOMA, fasting insulin and fasting glucose are shown in Appendix 1. Associations between anthropometric indices and HOMA in girls and boys are represented in Table 2. Excluding those with missing data on outcome and other variables, 468 girls were included in the analyses and 366 and 364 boys were included in the unadjusted and the adjusted models respectively. BMI, FMI and interestingly FFMI showed consistently strong associations with IR in both boys and girls. FFMI showed associations with IR (β=0.06) that were as strong as associations with BMI and FMI (β=0.05) in boys even after adjusting for age and pubertal stage. In girls as well, associations of FFMI with IR (β=0.03) were as strong as associations with FMI (β=0.03). CPR showed strong associations with HOMA in girls but not in boys.

To further evaluate the relationship of FFMI with IR relative to FMI, we explored the associations of the ratio of FMI to FFMI with HOMA (Appendix 3). We found similar associations of FMI/FFMI with HOMA in boys (β=1.01; unadjusted and β=0.95; adjusted models) and in girls (β=0.29; unadjusted and β=0.46; adjusted models).

Associations of anthropometric indices with HOMA within pubertal development stages

It has been observed in earlier studies that IR (HOMA) in adolescents was higher with increasing age in both boys and girls [25]. We explored the associations by stages of pubertal development in each sex in sub-group analyses (Table 3). FFMI along with BMI and FMI showed consistent strong associations with IR and associations tended to be stronger in earlier stages of pubertal development, contrary to findings from earlier studies. All analyses were done using generalized estimating equations to account for clustering by villages and using standardized z-scores. Since there were no girls in early stage of development, and no boys in post pubertal stage comparisons within these groups by sex were not possible. In middle stages of pubertal development anthropometric indices were relatively more strongly associated with HOMA in girls than in boys, however there were very few girls (n=40) in this stage of pubertal development compared to boys (n=200).

Associations of anthropometric indices with fasting glucose and fasting insulin

All analyses evaluating the association of fasting insulin and fasting

glucose with anthropometric indices were done using standardized z-scores for the anthropometric measures and adjusted for age and stage of pubertal development in addition to accounting for village clustering. Similar to HOMA, fasting insulin levels showed strong associations with FFMI, BMI and FMI (Appendix 1). Fasting glucose levels did not show any associations with anthropometric measures with the exception of WHR in boys (p=0.02). We found similar associations of FMI/FFMI with fasting insulin in both boys and girls (Appendix 3).

Discussion

In this study we evaluated the relationship of anthropometric measures with IR, fasting glucose and fasting insulin in rural Indian adolescents. This is a cohort of rural Indian adolescents, which sets it apart in terms of ethnicity, socioeconomic conditions and geographic region from other studies done on adolescents. We found that FFMI was as strongly associated with IR as FMI and BMI in this study. These observations were consistent in both sexes and within different stages of pubertal development. This is an interesting finding in the light of multiple studies indicating adiposity as a risk for IR [6-8,27].

BMI has proved to be a strong indicator of IR in the adolescents in multiple studies [16,27,28] similar to the findings in our study. By breaking BMI into FMI and FFMI, we can look at the effect of sarcopenic obesity and study the effects of muscle mass and fat mass independently [29]. Our findings indicate that lean mass is as strongly related to IR as fat mass. Hence the observed associations of IR with obesity (and BMI) could be attributed to a larger body mass mainly comprised of fat free/lean mass instead of body fat/adiposity. To further explore this relationship we looked at the association of the ratio of FMI/FFMI with IR, fasting glucose and fasting insulin levels. Strong associations were observed with HOMA and with fasting insulin in both boys and girls. The relationship of lean mass with IR appears to be independent of fat mass. This finding challenges the known relationship between adiposity and IR and emphasizes the need for a better understanding of the mechanisms mediating these associations.

Our observations are contrary to earlier studies that showed an increase in lean muscle mass improves insulin sensitivity [30]. A study in lean Indian men showed that a loss of muscle mass contributes to IR [31] and that a low lean mass compared to fat mass contributes to IR in lean South Asian populations with a high burden of IR and diabetes [30]. Another study emphasized that maintaining a higher muscle mass is instrumental in preventing obesity, IR and diabetes [32]. In view of these associations, there has been an interest on studying skeletal muscle metabolism and its contribution to the development of IR [33].

Interestingly, early studies in women showed that higher lean mass and higher truncal fat content were associated with insulin resistance

[34] and higher lean mass along with higher visceral fat content was associated with metabolic syndrome [35]. It has been established that adiposity contributes to the development of IR, but interestingly in this cohort of older women a larger lean mass also contributed to metabolic syndrome. The findings of these studies were validated in more recent studies in obese post-menopausal women using dual-energy X-ray absorptiometry to measure body composition and computed tomography (CT) to measure body fat distribution [36,37]. Lean mass was independently associated with insulin levels and glucose homeostasis, and the association of visceral fat with IR was enhanced by an increase in lean mass in post-menopausal women [37]. All these studies were done in obese post-menopausal women. We found similar associations in lean Indian adolescents. Further research on the metabolism of skeletal muscle and its role in the development of IR is required to better understand these associations.

CPR, a measure of central adiposity, was strongly associated with HOMA in girls but not in boys; even within categories of pubertal development. The observed difference between the sexes can be partly explained by the difference in fat distribution in the two sexes and due to the difference in metabolic actions of insulin in men and women, including deposition of adipose tissue [38]. Girls had a higher fasting insulin levels and HOMA scores than boys, and higher BMI and body fat, a difference expected due to hormonal effects [5]. Excess truncal subcutaneous adipose tissue independently predicts IR in post pubertal Indian adolescents [5] and there is evidence to indicate that subcutaneous adipose tissue is more closely correlated to IR than intra-abdominal fat [39]. In Indians an excess of visceral adipose tissue is usually accompanied by central subcutaneous adiposity (measured by subscapular/triceps skin fold thickness) [11], the effects of which need to be studied in greater detail.

Though all observed associations were slightly stronger in boys than in girls, but we cannot comment on these gender differences due to the small magnitude of the difference and the possibility of it being a chance occurrence. As pubertal development is known to play a considerable role in these associations [25], we studied the gender differences after adjusting for pubertal maturity. Within the same stage of pubertal development the strength of association in boys was not consistently stronger than in girls. The strength of the associations weakened as the girls and boys moved forward along stages of puberty. This finding was contrary to earlier studies that indicated IR increases with an increase in age and pubertal maturity in adolescents.

Other studies in European adolescents found BMI, WC, weight height ratio, skinfold sum and total fat mass were more strongly associated with IR than with WHR [27]. BMI and subscapular skinfold thickness were most useful in predicting hyperinsulinemia in urban Indian adolescents; and BMI, WC and subscapular skinfold thickness were better at identifying boys with metabolic syndrome than girls [16]. In India, urban populations are typically more overweight, have a different diet and more sedentary lifestyles than rural populations. Moreover, both these studies [16,27], did not look within levels of pubertal maturity to explore differential pubertal development in the two sexes as an explanation for the gender differences they observed.

Strengths and limitations

We used pubertal development data to stratify the associations of anthropometric measures with HOMA in each sex, which sets our study apart from most other studies that were limited by absence of data on pubertal development. Sexual maturation has considerable influence on insulin sensitivity, and we were able to look within stages

of development and compare correlations in both the sexes. As our study population included adolescents from ages 12 years through 18 years, we could explore the relationships of the indices with HOMA in the complete age range of adolescence and study the differences of these associations at different ages and stages of pubertal development.

A limitation of our study is that more accurate measures of body composition such as dual-energy X-ray absorptiometry (DEXA) scan for measurement of total and regional body fat and computerized tomography for measurement of abdominal fat were not used though these have now been obtained as part of a new follow-up so in future work we will be able to examine these more direct measures of adiposity. This analysis from a follow up survey of the Hyderabad Nutrition Trial was cross sectional in nature; hence we could not study progression of IR or other risk factors of diabetes with age but a new follow-up has been recently completed so future work will enable us to examine risk factors for age-related changes. We used a more crude method of pubertal stage classification than full Tanner staging. However a full Tanner staging can be difficult to conduct for a large epidemiological study and the methods we used for determination of pubertal development have been shown to be quite adequate for a broad classification of children into the main stages of maturation and in distinguishing children undergoing peak growth spurt from those before and after [40]. Our cohort is lean and very young; hence the findings are not generalizable to adults and populations burdened with more overweight and obesity.

Conclusion

In conclusion, we observed a strong association of IR with FFMI similar to associations of BMI and FMI with IR. These associations were consistent across stages of pubertal development in both boys and girls. The association of FFMI with IR as independent of fat mass and hence indicates that lean mass may play an important role in IR contrary to the well-established relationship between adiposity and IR. Further research is needed to better understand the epidemiology of early IR, a predictor of adverse health outcomes later in life and to elucidate the underlying mechanisms of the association of lean mass with IR especially in high risk populations.

Acknowledgement

Institutional support was provided by the National Institution of Nutrition, Hyderabad. We are extremely thankful to our study participants without whom this study would not have been possible.

Contributors

The study was conceived and designed by Sayanti Bhattacharya, Svati H. Shah, and Sanjay Kinra. Sanjay Kinra was instrumental for implementation of the fieldwork and trained and supervised the field teams. Sayanti Bhattacharya did the statistical analyses and wrote the first draft of the paper. All authors contributed to writing the manuscript and saw and approved the final version. Sanjay Kinra is the guarantor.

References

1. King H, Aubert RE, Herman WH (1998) Global burden of diabetes, 1995-2025: prevalence, numerical estimates, and projections. Diabetes Care. 21: 1414-1431.

2. Whincup PH, Gilg JA, Papacosta O, Seymour C, Miller GJ, et al. (2002) Early evidence of ethnic differences in cardiovascular risk: cross sectional comparison of British South Asian and white children. BMJ. 324.

3. Ginsberg HN (2000) Insulin resistance and cardiovascular disease. The Journal of clinical investigation 106: 453-458.

4. Misra A, Vikram NK (2004) Insulin resistance syndrome (metabolic syndrome) and obesity in Asian Indians: evidence and implications. Nutrition 20: 482-491.

5. Misra A, Vikram NK, Arya S, Pandey RM, Dhingra V, et al. (2004) High prevalence of insulin resistance in postpubertal Asian Indian children is associated with adverse truncal body fat patterning, abdominal adiposity and excess body fat. Int J Obes Relat Metab Disord. 28:1217-1226.

6. Bacha F, Saad R, Gungor N, Janosky J, Arslanian SA (2003) Obesity, regional fat distribution, and syndrome X in obese black versus white adolescents: race differential in diabetogenic and atherogenic risk factors. J Clin Endocrinol Metab. 88: 2534-2540.

7. Krekoukia M, Nassis GP, Psarra G, Skenderi K, Chrousos GP, et al. (2007) Elevated total and central adiposity and low physical activity are associated with insulin resistance in children. Metabolism 56: 206-213.

8. Keskin M, Kurtoglu S, Kendirci M, Atabek ME, Yazici C (2005) Homeostasis model assessment is more reliable than the fasting glucose/insulin ratio and quantitative insulin sensitivity check index for assessing insulin resistance among obese children and adolescents. Pediatrics 115: e500-3.

9. Balkau B, Deanfield JE, Despres JP, Bassand JP, Fox KA, et al. (2007) International Day for the Evaluation of Abdominal Obesity (IDEA): a study of waist circumference, cardiovascular disease, and diabetes mellitus in 168,000 primary care patients in 63 countries. Circulation. 116:1942-1951.

10. Ramachandran A, Snehalatha C, Dharmaraj D, Viswanathan M (1992) Prevalence of glucose intolerance in Asian Indians. Urban-rural difference and significance of upper body adiposity. Diabetes Care 15: 1348-1355.

11. Chandalia M, Abate N, Garg A, Stray-Gundersen J, Grundy SM (1999) Relationship between generalized and upper body obesity to insulin resistance in Asian Indian men. J Clin Endocrinol Metab. 84: 2329-2335.

12. Shelgikar KM, Hockaday TD, Yajnik CS (1991) Central rather than generalized obesity is related to hyperglycaemia in Asian Indian subjects. Diabet Med. 8: 712-717.

13. Yusuf S, Hawken S, Ounpuu S, Bautista L, Franzosi MG, et al. (2005) Obesity and the risk of myocardial infarction in 27,000 participants from 52 countries: a case-control study. Lancet. 366: 1640-1649.

14. Yan W, Wang X, Yao H, Dai J, Zheng Y, et al. (2006) Waist-to-height ratio and BMI predict different cardiovascular risk factors in Chinese children. Diabetes Care 29: 2760-2761.

15. Manios Y, Kourlaba G, Kafatos A, Cook TL, Spyridaki A, et al. (2008) Associations of several anthropometric indices with insulin resistance in children: The Children Study. Acta Paediatr. 97: 494-499.

16. Misra A, Madhavan M, Vikram NK, Pandey RM, Dhingra V, et al. (2006) Simple anthropometric measures identify fasting hyperinsulinemia and clustering of cardiovascular risk factors in Asian Indian adolescents. Metabolism 55: 1569-1573.

17. Kinra S, Rameshwar Sarma KV, Ghafoorunissa, Mendu VV, Ravikumar R, et al. (2008) Effect of integration of supplemental nutrition with public health programmes in pregnancy and early childhood on cardiovascular risk in rural Indian adolescents: long term follow-up of Hyderabad nutrition trial. BMJ 337.

18. Tanner JM (1962) Growth at adolescence; with a general consideration of the effects of hereditary and environmental factors upon growth and maturation from birth to maturity. 325.

19. Clark PM, Hales CN (1994) How to measure plasma insulin. Diabetes/Metabolism Reviews 10: 79-90.

20. Matthews DR, Hosker JP, Rudenski AS, Naylor BA, Treacher DF, et al. (1985) Homeostasis model assessment: insulin resistance and beta-cell function from fasting plasma glucose and insulin concentrations in man. Diabetologia. 28: 412-419.

21. Durnin JV, Womersley J (1974) Body fat assessed from total body density and its estimation from skinfold thickness: measurements on 481 men and women aged from 16 to 72 years. British Journal of Nutrition 32: 77-97.

22. Siri WE (1993) Body composition from fluid spaces and density: analysis of methods. 1961. Nutrition 9: 480-491.

23. Wells JC (2001) A critique of the expression of paediatric body composition data. Arch Dis Child. 85: 67-72.

24. Friedewald WT, Levy RI, Fredrickson DS (1972) Estimation of the concentration of low-density lipoprotein cholesterol in plasma, without use of the preparative ultracentrifuge. Clin Chem. 18: 499-502.

25. Pinhas-Hamiel O, Lerner-Geva L, Copperman NM, Jacobson MS (2007) Lipid and insulin levels in obese children: changes with age and puberty. Obesity (Silver Spring) 15: 2825-2831.

26. Khadilkar VV, Khadilkar AV, Borade AB, Chiplonkar SA (2012) Body mass index cut-offs for screening for childhood overweight and obesity in Indian children. Indian Pediatr. 49: 29-34.

27. Kondaki K, Grammatikaki E, Pavon DJ, Manios Y, Gonzalez-Gross M, et al. (2011) Comparison of several anthropometric indices with insulin resistance proxy measures among European adolescents: The Helena Study. Eur J Pediatr. 170: 731-739.

28. Hirschler V, Ruiz A, Romero T, Dalamon R, Molinari C (2009) Comparison of different anthropometric indices for identifying insulin resistance in schoolchildren. Diabetes Technol Ther. 11: 615-621.

29. Dulloo AG, Jacquet J, Solinas G, Montani JP, Schutz Y (2010) Body composition phenotypes in pathways to obesity and the metabolic syndrome. Int J Obes (Lond). 34 Suppl 2:S4-17.

30. Lear SA, Kohli S, Bondy GP, Tchernof A, Sniderman AD (2009) Ethnic variation in fat and lean body mass and the association with insulin resistance. J Clin Endocrinol Metab. 94: 4696-4702.

31. Unni US, Ramakrishnan G, Raj T, Kishore RP, Thomas T, Vaz M, et al. (2009) Muscle mass and functional correlates of insulin sensitivity in lean young Indian men. European journal of clinical nutrition. 63: 1206-1212.

32. Wolfe RR (2006) Skeletal muscle protein metabolism and resistance exercise. The Journal of nutrition 136: 525S-528S.

33. Krotkiewski M (1994) Role of muscle morphology in the development of insulin resistance and metabolic syndrome. Presse Med. 23:1393-1399.

34. Krotkiewski M, Bjorntorp P (1986) Muscle tissue in obesity with different distribution of adipose tissue. Effects of physical training. International journal of obesity 10: 331-341.

35. You T, Ryan AS, Nicklas BJ (2004) The metabolic syndrome in obese postmenopausal women: relationship to body composition, visceral fat, and inflammation. J Clin Endocrinol Metab. 89: 5517-5522.

36. Karelis AD, Faraj M, Bastard JP, St-Pierre DH, Brochu M, et al. (2005) The metabolically healthy but obese individual presents a favorable inflammation profile. J Clin Endocrinol Metab. 90: 4145-4150.

37. Brochu M, Mathieu ME, Karelis AD, Doucet E, Lavoie ME, et al. (2008) Contribution of the lean body mass to insulin resistance in postmenopausal women with visceral obesity: a Monet study. Obesity (Silver Spring). 16: 1085-1093.

38. Magkos F, Wang X, Mittendorfer B (2010) Metabolic actions of insulin in men and women. Nutrition 26: 686-693.

39. Misra A, Garg A, Abate N, Peshock RM, Stray-Gundersen J, et al. (1997) Relationship of anterior and posterior subcutaneous abdominal fat to insulin sensitivity in nondiabetic men. Obes Res. 5: 93-99.

40. Cameron N (1993) Assessment of growth and maturation during adolescence. Horm Res. 3: 9-17.

Permissions

List of Contributors

Kathy Sexton-Radek
A Reporting of College Student Health Knowledge, Elmhurst College, USA

Mohammed J Alramadan, Afsana Afroz and Baki Billah
Department of Epidemiology and Preventive Medicine, Monash University, Melbourne, Australia

Mohammed Ali Batais and Turky H Almigba
College of Medicine, King Saud University, Riyadh, Saudi Arabia

Hassan Ahmad Alhamrani and Fatimah A Alramadan
Diabetes Centre, Directorate of Health Affair, Hofuf, Saudi Arabia

Ahmed Albaloshi
Diabetes Centre, Directorate of Health Affair, Jeddah, Saudi Arabia

Dianna J Magliano
Baker Heart and Diabetes Institute, Melbourne, Victoria, Australia

Ghaida Jabri, Alaa Sandokji, Nourah Alzughaibi, Ibrahim Alsehli, Hanan Neyaz, Khadijah Alhusaini, Mohammed Jabri and Mohammed Kareems
Faculty of Medicine, Taibah University, Kingdom of Saudi Arabia

Eric Worlanyo Deffor
University of Ghana Business School, Department of Organization and Human Resource Management Legon, Accra-Ghana West Africa

Nne Pepple
Salem University, Lokoja, Kogi State, Nigeria

Flávio Rocha da Silva and Alexandre de Oliveira Saísse
Instituto Oswaldo Cruz, Fundação Oswaldo Cruz, Rio de Janeiro, RJ, Brazil

Flávio Rocha da Silva and Bernardo Elias
Associação Nacional de Biossegurança, Rio de Janeiro, RJ, Brazil

Marli Brito M. de Albuquerque Navarro and Correa Soares
Núcleo de Biossegurança-Escola Nacional de Saúde Pública, Rio de Janeiro, Brazil

Salvatore Giovanni De Simone
Instituto Nacional de Ciência e Tecnologia de Inovação em Doenças Negligenciadas (INCT-IDN)/Centro de Desenvolvimento Tecnológico em Saúde (CDTS), Fundação Oswaldo Cruz, Rio de Janeiro, RJ, Brazil Departamento de Biologia Celulare Molecular, Instituto de Biologia Universidade Federal Fluminense Niterói, RJ, Brazil

Naoko Takayama
Department of Education, Asahi University, Japan

Hiromi Ariyoshi
Department of Medicine, Saga University, Japan

Osuala Eunice O
Department of Nursing Science, Nnamdi Azikiwe University, Nnewi Campus, South East, Nigeria

Adina Dreier-Wolfgramm, Sabine Homeyer, Angelika Beyer, Stefanie Kirschner and Wolfgang Hoffmann
Department of Epidemiology of Healthcare and Community Health, University Medicine Greifswald, Greifswald, Germany

Roman F. Oppermann
Department of Health, Nursing and Management, University of Applied Science Neubrandenburg, Germany

Shimizu Y, Iida H, Nenoi M and Akashi M
National Institute of Radiological Sciences, National Institutes for Quantum and Radiological Science and Technology, 4-9-1 Anagawa, Inage-ku, Chiba 263-8555, Japan

Hung-Hsiang Chiu and Bing-Jun Wang
Department of Electrophysics, National Chiao Tung University, Hsinchu 30010, Taiwan

Kumera Negash Amente
School of Music, College of Social Sciences and Humanity, Jimma University, Ethiopia

Teresa Iglesias M
Universidad Francisco de Vitoria, Spain

Wajiha Iffat and Sadia Shakeel
Dow College of Pharmacy, Dow University of Health Sciences, Karachi-Sind, Pakistan

Fatima Fasih
Dow International Medical College, Dow University of Health Sciences, Karachi-Sind, Pakistan

Yossef Alnasser, Habeeb AlSaeed and Hadeel Al-Sarraj
Department of Pediatrics, King Saud University, Riyadh, Saudi Arabia

Nourah Z Al-Beeshi, Haya Alotaibi, Kholoud AlAmari and Ayshah Jaber
Depatment of Medicine, King Saud University, Riyadh, Saudi Arabia

Patricia A Carney
Department of Family Medicine and Public Health and Preventive Medicine, Oregon Health and Science University, Portland, Oregon, USA

Elizabeth Jacob-Files
BJF Research, Seattle, Washington, USA

Susan J Rosenkranz
School of Nursing, Oregon Health and Science University, Portland, Oregon, USA

Deborah J Cohen
Department of Family Medicine, Oregon Health and Science University, Portland, Oregon, USA

Larry Green
Department of Family Medicine, Epperson-Zorn Chair for Innovation in Family Medicine and Primary Care, University of Colorado, Denver, Colombia, USA

Samuel Jones
Fairfax Family Medicine Residency Program, Fairfax, Virginia, USA

Colleen T Fogarty
Department of Family Medicine, University of Rochester, Rochester, New York, USA

Terri Rebmann, Amy M Strawn, Zachary Swick
Institute for Biosecurity, Saint Louis University, College for Public Health and Social Justice, St Louis, MO, USA

David Reddick
Bio-Defense Network, 116 Embassy Lane, Kirkwood, USA

Muaid H Ithman, Ganesh Gopalakrishna, Niels C Beck, Jairam Das and Gregory Petroski
University of Missouri-Columbia, Columbia, Missouri, USA

Ricardo Rodrigo Rech and Ricardo Halpe
Federal University of Health Sciences of Porto Alegre, Brazil. University of Caxias do Sul, Brazil

Sanchia S Goonewardene
Guys Hospital, Kings College London, UK

Persad R
Bristol Southmead, UK

Nanton V and Young A
University of Warwick, UK

Makar A
Worcestershire Acute Hospitals, Worcestershire, UK

Joaquim JF Soares and Eija Viitasara
Department of Public Health Sciences, Mid Sweden University, Sundsvall, Sweden

Örjan Sundin
Department of Psychology, Mid Sweden University, Östersund, Sweden

Maria Gabriella Melchiorre
Italian National Institute of Health and Science on Aging, INRCA, Ancona, Italy

Mindaugas Stankunas
Department of Health Management, Lithuanian University of Health Sciences, Kaunas, Lithuania School of Public Health, Griffith University, Gold Coast Campus, Queensland, Australia

Jutta Lindert
Department of Public Health Science, Protestant University of Applied Sciences, Ludwigsburg, Germany

Francisco Torres-Gonzales
Network of Biomedical Research on Mental Health Centers, University of Granada, Spain

Henrique Barros
Department of Hygiene and Epidemiology, University of Porto, Medical School, Porto, Portugal

Elisabeth Ioannidi-Kapolou
Department of Sociology, National School of Public Health, Athens, Greece

Broz Frajtag Jasenka
Department for Otolaryngology, University Clinical Hospital Center, Croatia

Babita Singh and Pratima Ghimire
National Medical College Nursing Campus, Birgunj, Nepal

Ying Ge and Jinfu Zhang
Faculty of Psychology, Key Laboratory of Personality and Cognition, Ministry of Education, Southwest University, Beibei, Chongqing, China

Yuanyan Hu
Laboratory of Cognition and Mental Health, Chongqing University of Arts and Sciences, Yongchuan, Chongqing, China

Mehrnosh Rabbani Zadeh
Department of Psychology, Science and Research Branch, Islamic Azad University, Fars, Iran

Sareh Behzadi Pour
Department of Psychology, Shiraz Branch, Islamic Azad University, Shiraz, Iran

Atilla Yaprak
Sabuncuoğlu Şerefeddin Training and Research Hospital, Amasya University, Turkey

Ayala Gonen
Nursing Department, School of Social and Community Science, Ruppin Academic Center, Israel

Lilac Lev-Ari
Behavioral Department, School of Social and Community Science, Ruppin Academic Center, Israel

Knox Van Dyke
Department of Biochemistry and Molecular Pharmacology, West Virginia University Medical School, Morgantown, WV 26506, USA

Muneerah Khalid AlJadidi, Ohoud Oadah AlMutrafi, Rawan Othman Bamousa, Sarah Safar AlShehri, Anwar Sattam AlRashidi, Huda Abdullah AlNijadi, Arwa Abdulrhman AMousa, Alanoud Saleh AlNami, Norah Mohammad AlSubaie, Norah Abdulaziz AlMulhim and Lamees Abdulla AlAbdulgader
College of Medicine, King Faisal University, Saudi Arabia

Somaya Aljohani, Israa Saib and Muatasim Noorelahi
Intern, College of Medicine, Taibah University, Medina, Saudi Arabia

Chengye Hou, Jing Yan, Zhiyong Li, Yang Shen, Yichen Huang and Ying Liang
National Clinical Research Center for Mental Disorders, Peking University Sixth Hospital,
Institute of Mental Health, Key Laboratory of Mental Health, Ministry of Health

Megan Huebner, Mary E Temple-Cooper, Melissa Lagzdinsm and Jun-Yen Yeh
Hillcrest Hospital, Cleveland Clinic, USA

Belayneh Kefale Gelaw and Gobezie Temesgen Tegegne
Department of Pharmacy, College of medicine and Health Sciences, Ambo University, Ambo, Ethiopia

Yeshanew Asinake Bizuye
Debire Markose Hospital, North East Ethiopia, Ethiopia

Bhattacharya S
Duke Global Health Institute, Duke University Medical Center, Durham, NC, USA
Duke Translational Research Institute, Duke University, Durham, NC, USA

Shah SH
Duke Global Health Institute, Duke University Medical Center, Durham, NC, USA
Division of Cardiovascular Medicine, Duke University Medical Center, Durham, NC, USA

Ben-Shlomo
School of Social and Community Medicine, University of Bristol, Bristol, UK

Kinra S
Department of Epidemiology and Population Health, London School of Hygiene and Tropical Medicine, London, UK

Index